Bone Tumors

Jim S. Wu · Mary G. Hochman

Bone Tumors

A Practical Guide to Imaging

Springer

Jim S. Wu, MD
Department of Radiology
Beth Israel Deaconess Medical Center
Harvard Medical School
Boston, MA, USA

Mary G. Hochman, MD
Department of Radiology
Beth Israel Deaconess Medical Center
Harvard Medical School
Boston, MA, USA

ISBN 978-1-4419-0807-0 e-ISBN 978-1-4419-0808-7
DOI 10.1007/978-1-4419-0808-7
Springer New York Dordrecht Heidelberg London

Library of Congress Control Number: 2012932312

Printed on acid-free paper

Springer is part of Springer Science+Business Media (www.springer.com)

To Ann, Alex, and Sonie, thanks for everything.

–JSW

With love and appreciation to my wonderful family and friends and with special thanks to Dr. R.E. Langevin for starting me on my radiology journey.

–MGH

Preface

The major goals of this book are to provide the reader with a practical way to analyze bone tumors and to highlight the most common tumors that one would expect to see in everyday clinical practice. We include high-yield facts and representative images for each tumor, focusing on their classic appearance and location, in order to provide a solid foundation for evaluating these tumors and to avoid the confusion that comes from including their uncommon presentations. In medicine, there are exceptions for almost everything; however, it is difficult to appreciate the extreme rarity of a chordoma in the tibia, if one does not first know that they occur almost exclusively in the axial skeleton.

The intended audience for this book is anyone interested in bone tumors, including radiologists, orthopedic surgeons, pathologists, and primary care physicians. However, we hope that the format of the book will make it particularly useful for the radiology resident who is preparing for rotations and for board exams. We imagine that this book is short enough to be read in a few days and we anticipate it being used as a quick reference during daily readouts.

We have divided the book into two sections: a didactic section and a section comprised of unknown cases. In the didactic section, we present key "bread and butter" facts and include a list of differential diagnoses with distinguishing features. We have tried to select images that illustrate the classic appearance and typical location for each tumor. Moreover, we also devote a chapter to lesions that can mimic bone tumors. In real life, physicians encounter many bone lesions that are not true tumors, but could be mistaken for a bone tumor. It would be impossible to adequately discuss the differential diagnosis for many bone tumors, without this section. In the unknown cases section, we have included a variety of cases, including: (1) tumors discussed in the didactic section but with a particular teaching point highlighted by the case; (2) examples of some unusual bone tumors; and (3) commonly-encountered "mimickers" that could be mistaken for true bone tumors. The cases are meant to be taken as if the reader were discussing them during an unknown case conference. We provide a short (usually relevant) clinical history, description of the imaging findings, a "best 3" differential diagnosis list, a short discussion that reveals the most likely diagnosis, and some relevant key facts.

It is our hope that after reading this book and working through the cases, you will find yourself with a solid foundation for evaluating bone tumors.

Jim S. Wu
Mary G. Hochman

Acknowledgments

This effort could not have been possible without the help and support of many people and we wish to express our sincere thanks and appreciation to all of them.

- The residents and fellows whom we have had the privilege of training, who have asked the hard questions and who have inspired us to delve deeper into this field.
- Our colleagues from across Beth Israel Deaconess Medical Center—and their patients—who have taught us so much about the field of orthopedic oncology and who have provided many of the insights that have been incorporated into this book: Drs. Mark Gebhardt, Megan Anderson, Jeff Goldsmith, Ferris Hall, Diane Savarese, Dimitrios Spentzos, Mary Ann Stevenson, and Nick Tawa.
- Our colleagues and mentors from across the field of Musculoskeletal Imaging, whose research and teaching has been instrumental to our own understanding of this field.
- Friends and colleagues who generously shared their case material and who kindly reviewed and commented on draft versions of this book. This effort has been incalculably enriched by contributions from Drs. Manjiri Didolkar, Jean-Marc Gauguet, Andy Haims, Mai-Lan Ho, Adam Jeffers, James Kang, Lee Katz, Justin Kung, Phil Kuo, Suzanne Long, Colm McMahon, Gul Moonis, Mark Murphey, Tony Parker, Johannes Roedl, Mark Schweitzer, Sanjay Shetty, Dan Siegal, Jennifer Son, and Corrie Yablon. Special thanks to Children's Hospital of Boston and our colleagues there, Drs. Susan Connolly and Paul Kleinman.
- Dr. Ron Eisenberg for his insightful comments and editing guidance.
- Donna Wolfe and Michael Larson for their invaluable expertise, in thinking about formatting and presenting text and images for this book and in creating illustrations for it.
- Clotell Forde for her expert assistance in preparing text and images for publication.
- Andrew Moyer from Springer and Abiramasundari Mahalingam from SPi Global for their support in bringing this project to fruition.
- Our families, for their on-going encouragement, understanding, and support.
- You, our readers, who have been our constant virtual companions as we have worked on this project. We hope you find this a useful resource and we very much welcome your feedback.

Jim S. Wu
Mary G. Hochman

Contents

Abbreviations

ABC	Aneurysmal bone cyst
ADC	Apparent diffusion coefficient
AIDS	Acquired immune deficiency syndrome
AJCC	American Joint Committee on Cancer Staging
ALL	Acute lymphoblastic leukemia
AML	Acute myelogenous leukemia
AP	Anteroposterior
AS	Angiosarcoma
AVN	Avascular necrosis
BPOP	Bizarre parosteal osteochondromatous proliferation of bone
CBC	Complete blood count
CLL	Chronic lymphocytic leukemia
CML	Chronic myelogenous leukemia
CMF	Chondromyxoid fibroma
CT	Computed tomography
CXR	Chest X-ray
DF	Desmoplastic fibroma
DDx	Differential diagnosis
EIC	Epidermoid inclusion cyst
EG	Eosinophilic granuloma
ESR	Erythrocyte sedimentation rate
ES	Ewing sarcoma
FCD	Fibrous cortical dysplasia
FD	Fibrous dysplasia
FDG	Fluoro-deoxy-glucose
FLAIR	Fluid attenuated inversion recovery
FNA	Fine needle aspiration
FOV	Field of view
FS	Fat-saturated
GCT	Giant cell tumor
G-CSF	Granulocyte colony-stimulating factor
GI	Gastrointestinal
GY	Gray
HME	Hereditary multiple exostoses
HU	Hounsfield unit
IV	Intravenous
JC	Jaffe–Campanacci syndrome
LCH	Langerhan cell histiocytosis
LSMFT	Liposclerosing myxofibrous tumor
MCL	Medial collateral ligament
MFH	Malignant fibrous histiocytoma
MGUS	Monoclonal gammopathy of undetermined significance
MRA	MR angiography
MRI	Magnetic resonance imaging
NHL	Non-Hodgkin lymphoma
NF1	Neurofibromatosis type 1
NOF	Non-ossifying fibroma
NOS	Not otherwise specified
NSAIDS	Nonsteroidal anti-inflammatory drug
NSF	Nephrogenic systemic fibrosis
OFD	Osteofibrous dysplasia
PCNB	Percutaneous core needle biopsy
PET	Positron emission tomography
POEMS	Polyneuropathy, organomegaly, endocrinopathy, monoclonal gammopathy
PNET	Primitive neuroectodermal tumor
PSA	Prostate specific antigen
PTH	Parathyroid hormone
PVNS	Pigmented villonodular synovitis
RCC	Renal cell carcinoma
RPMI	Roswell Park Memorial Institute (medium for flow cytometry of lymphoma)

SBC	Simple bone cyst
SBP	Solitary plasmacytoma of bone
SPECT	Single photon emission computed tomography
SPEP	Serum protein electrophoresis
STIR	Short tau inversion recovery
SUV	Standardized uptake value
T1W	T1-weighted
T2W	T2-weighted
TGFβ	Transforming growth factor beta
UPEP	Urine protein electrophoresis
US	Ultrasound
VEGF	Vascular endothelial growth factor
WBC	White blood cells
WHO	World Health Organization

Introduction to Bone Tumors

1

Focal lesions in bone are encountered frequently during everyday clinical practice. While some lesions are true neoplasms, many represent benign entities. Determining which lesions require evaluation and which should be left alone can be a daunting process. On occasion the imaging appearance is pathognomonic or highly suggestive of a specific entity; thus, imaging can play a determinative role in clinical management. Although the ultimate goal is always to arrive at a definitive correct diagnosis, this is often not possible based on the available clinical and imaging data. In practice, it is important to provide a short, reasonable list of relevant diagnoses, making sure that malignant tumors are not inappropriately omitted and that benign lesions are not overtreated. In order to do this effectively, it is important to understand some basic principles regarding the evaluation of bone tumors and their characteristic imaging features.

Classification of Bone Tumors

The World Health Organization (WHO) classification system of bone tumors provides uniformity for the reporting and treatment of bone tumors and is in common use (Table 1.1). The WHO classifies bone tumors based on their pattern of differentiation, meaning that they are grouped by the histologic tissue that they resemble. For instance, tumors that contain cartilaginous components are grouped under cartilage tumors and tumors that contain osseous matrix are grouped under osteogenic tumors. Many of these histologic subcategories contain both benign and malignant entities. Furthermore, there are several bone lesions that are not true neoplasms and therefore are not included in the WHO classification. These include bone islands, osteomas, and non-ossifying fibromas (NOF), among others. Bone islands and osteomas are hamartomas, in which normal cortical bone is seen in an atypical location. NOFs are considered developmental defects that resolve over time. Lastly, it is important to consider nonneoplastic lesions that can mimic a bone tumor on imaging, such as congenital anomalies, osteomyelitis, or posttraumatic changes. These are also not included in the WHO classification system.

J.S. Wu and M.G. Hochman, *Bone Tumors: A Practical Guide to Imaging*,
DOI 10.1007/978-1-4419-0808-7_1,

Incidence of Bone Tumors

The true incidence of each bone tumor is difficult to accurately assess and the reported numbers in the literature can be confusing, if not misleading. This is because many lesions are discovered incidentally on imaging and histologic diagnosis is not pursued in all cases. This is especially true for benign lesions, such as small asymptomatic enchondromas, osteochondromas, or intraosseous lipomas. Conversely, malignant lesions behave more aggressively and lead to symptoms if left untreated. It is therefore not surprising that three-fourths of all bone lesions that undergo biopsy are malignant. Moreover, there is more data on the epidemiology and features of malignant tumors than benign bone tumors, since malignant tumors are more likely to be evaluated.

Metastases are by far the most common tumor seen in bone. However, metastases are considered secondary tumors of bone because the primary tumor does not originate in bone. Primary tumors of bone, such as an osteosarcoma or chondrosarcoma, are actually quite rare. Prostate, breast, and lung cancers are the three most common primary sources of bone metastases. The ratio between primary and secondary (metastatic) bone lesions is believed to be around 20-to-1; however, this ratio is likely skewed in favor of metastases, since they are biopsied more commonly than benign lesions (Fig. 1.1).

Of the primary malignant tumors that occur in bone, plasma cell myeloma is most common; however, for practical purposes, it should only be considered in patients older than 40 years of age (Fig. 1.2). The various sarcomas of bone account for the next most common primary malignancies in bone. Of the primary bone sarcomas, the most common are: osteosarcoma—35%, chondrosarcoma—25%, Ewing sarcoma—16%, chordoma—8%, and malignant fibrous histiocytoma—5% (Fig. 1.3). Primary sarcomas of bone comprise only 0.2% of all neoplasms in the body and occur at one-tenth the rate of soft tissue sarcomas.

The incidence of primary benign tumors of bone is more difficult to determine since not every newly discovered lesion is biopsied or even completely evaluated. Biopsy or resection would be impractical and inappropriate in many instances if the lesion can be fully characterized as benign based on radiographic and clinical features. The most common benign neoplasms of bone are the following: osteochondroma—35%, enchondroma—20%, giant cell tumor of bone—15%, osteoid osteoma—10%, and fibrous dysplasia—5% (Fig. 1.4). Moreover, it is important to realize that even if a lesion is clearly benign based on radiographic and clinical data, the lesion nonetheless may require workup and treatment. For example, a giant cell tumor with extension to the tibial articular surface would be at risk for pathologic fracture and a fibular osteochondroma causing peroneal nerve compression would need to be resected to minimize nerve symptoms.

Table 1.1 World Health Organization (WHO) classification of bone tumors

Cartilage tumors
- Osteochondroma
- Chondroma
  - Enchondroma
  - Periosteal chondroma
  - Multiple chondromatosis
- Chondroblastoma
- Chondromyxoid fibroma
- Chondrosarcoma
  - Central, primary, secondary
  - Peripheral
  - Dedifferentiated
  - Mesenchymal
  - Clear cell

Osteogenic tumors
- Osteoid osteoma
- Osteoblastoma
- Osteosarcoma
  - Conventional
    - Chondroblastic
    - Fibroblastic
    - Osteoblastic
  - Telangiectatic
  - Small cell
  - Low grade central
  - Secondary
  - Parosteal
  - Periosteal
  - High grade surface

Fibrogenic tumors
- Desmoplastic fibroma
- Fibrosarcoma

Fibrohistiocytic tumors
- Benign fibrous histiocytoma
- Malignant fibrous histiocytoma

Ewing sarcoma/primitive neuroectodermal tumor
- Ewing sarcoma

Hematopoietic tumors
- Plasma cell myeloma
- Malignant lymphoma, NOS

Giant cell tumor
- Giant cell tumor
- Malignancy in giant cell tumor

Notochordal tumors
- Chordoma

Vascular tumors
- Hemangioma
- Angiosarcoma

Smooth muscle tumors
- Leiomyoma
- Leiomyosarcoma

Lipogenic tumors
- Lipoma
- Liposarcoma

Neural tumors
- Neurilemmoma

Miscellaneous tumors
- Adamantinoma
- Metastatic malignancy

Miscellaneous lesions
- Aneurysmal bone cyst
- Simple cyst
- Fibrous dysplasia
- Osteofibrous dysplasia
- Langerhans cell histiocytosis
- Erdheim–Chester disease
- Chest wall hamartoma

Joint lesions
- Synovial chondromatosis

Reproduced with permission from: Fletcher CD, Unni KK, Mertens F, eds. WHO classification of tumours: pathology and genetics of tumours of soft tissue and bone. Lyon, France: IARC, 2002

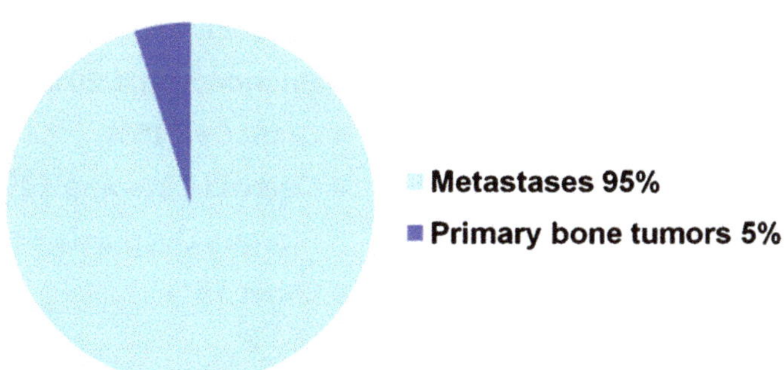

(adapted with permission from: Murphey MD. Musculoskeletal Neoplasms: Fundamental Concepts. Radiologic Pathology. 2nd Ed. 2006)

Fig. 1.1 Bone tumors

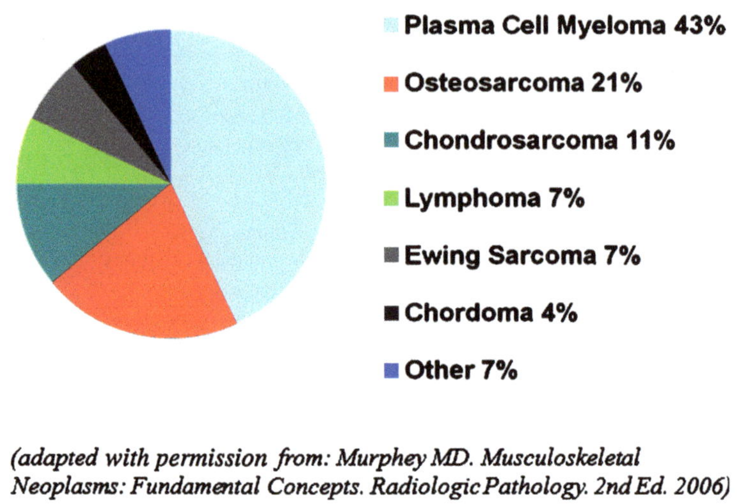

Fig. 1.2 Primary malignant bone tumors

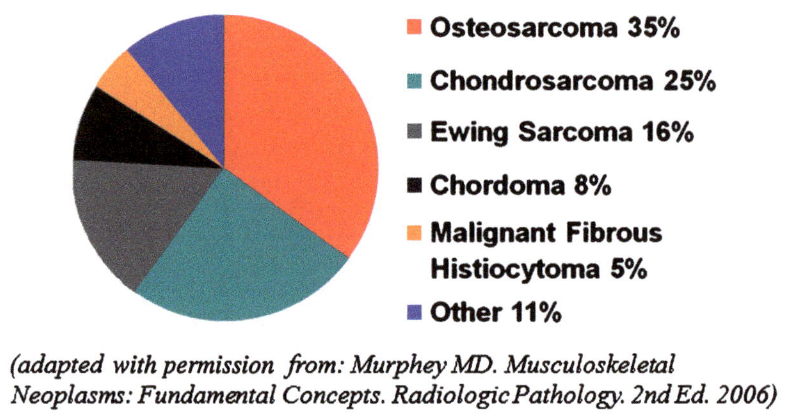

Fig. 1.3 Primary bone sarcomas

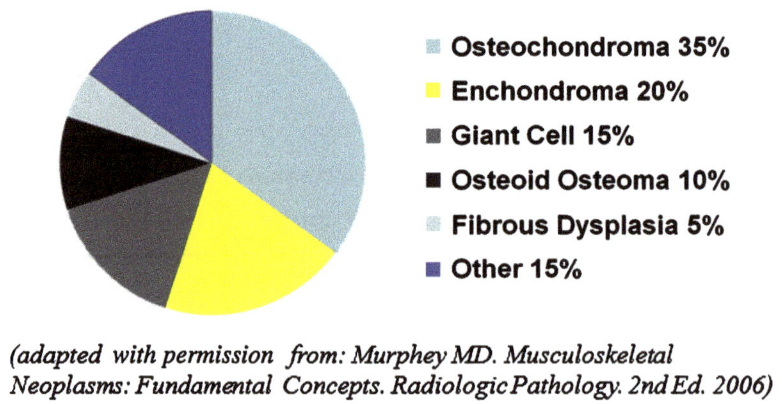

Fig. 1.4 Benign bone tumors

Value of Team Evaluation

Evaluation of a focal lesion in bone is best performed as a team effort by the clinician, radiologist, and pathologist (Fig. 1.5). All three team members have important roles that lead to the successful diagnosis and treatment of a patient with a bone lesion. The clinician provides data on the patient's history, physical examination, and laboratory values, and coordinates the patient's overall care. The radiologist performs the imaging studies and image-guided biopsy. Finally, the pathologist provides the tissue analysis which can include special stains, enzyme histochemistry, immunohistochemistry, electron microscopy, flow cytometry, and cytogenetics, leading to the identification of the lesion. Communication among all team members is vital in order to provide the best patient care.

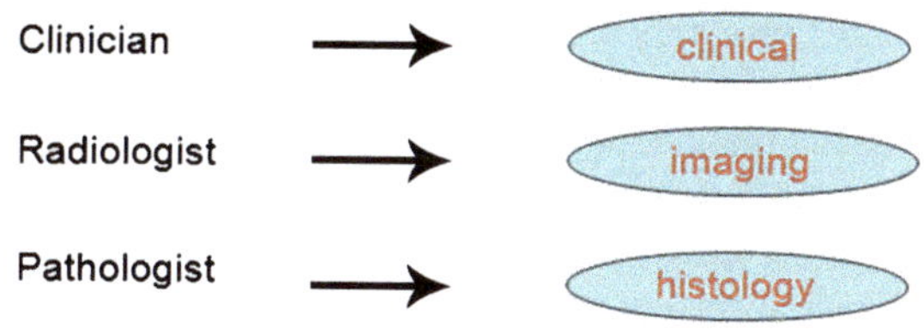

Fig. 1.5 Evaluation team

Clinical and Imaging Workup

The clinician is often the first to suspect a bone tumor. The patient may present with pain, swelling, limited mobility, weakness, and/or pathologic fracture, initiating the need for evaluation. Although pain can be nonspecific, it is invariably present with malignant tumors. Swelling occurs when the tumor enlarges and displaces adjacent tissue and often increases more rapidly with malignancies. However, both benign and malignant lesions can grow rapidly if there is bleeding or infection. Limited mobility can occur if the tumor develops around a joint. Lastly, any fracture may be the result of an underlying bone lesion. This is especially true if the degree of force is below the expected threshold to create a fracture or if the mechanism of injury is atypical. Children often present with pathologic fractures through benign lesions, such as non-ossifying fibromas (NOFs) and simple bone cysts. In some instances, the radiologist may be the first to discover the focal bone lesion, as an incidental finding. For instance, radiographs taken to exclude a foreign body in the soft tissues of the knee could reveal an enchondroma in the distal femur.

Once a focal bone lesion is discovered, it is important to decide if additional imaging is needed. Discussions between the clinician and the radiologist are important in order to determine the best imaging modality or modalities for arriving at the correct diagnosis. In cases where the clinician is not comfortable with the management of the bone lesion, she/he should consider referral of the patient to an orthopedic oncologist. The imaging workup typically begins with plain radiographs, as they are relatively inexpensive, easily to perform, and provide excellent assessment of the cortical features. CT can be useful to show that the lesion arises from the bone, to characterize internal matrix, and to determine the integrity of the cortex. MRI can be helpful in tumor characterization (showing the presence of fat or fluid–fluid levels); however, its main importance is in assessing the degree of tumor extension for staging and for identifying targets for biopsy. Bone scintigraphy and FDG-PET/CT can assess for multifocal disease and determine the osteoblastic and metabolic nature of the lesion, respectively. For some neoplasms such as multiple myeloma, a skeletal survey or whole-body MRI may be employed to assess for multifocal disease.

Management of the Focal Bone Lesion

After the imaging and clinical findings are gathered, the next step in clinical management is to determine whether the lesion requires tissue sampling to guide treatment (Fig. 1.6). There are three potential management recommendations: (1) do nothing; (2) perform follow-up imaging; or (3) perform biopsy/surgery. However, even lesions that are followed by imaging eventually either have to be left alone or biopsied. Practically speaking, only two real options really exist: (1) leave the lesion alone or (2) perform biopsy/surgery. Lesions can be categorized as "clearly benign," "indeterminate," or "clearly malignant." "Clearly benign" lesions such as a bone island or resolving fibroxanthomas are "don't touch" lesions that should be left alone. Lesions that are "clearly malignant" should undergo biopsy. This includes aggressive lesions with a high likelihood for malignancy, such as a large destructive tumor in a woman with invasive breast cancer. Lesions that are "indeterminate" can be further categorized into lesions that are "probably benign" or "suspicious for malignancy." "Probably benign" lesions, such as a large enchondroma with minimal endosteal scalloping, can be followed by imaging. Lesions that are "suspicious for malignancy" should go directly to biopsy; however, there can be biopsy decision factors that make imaging follow-up more practical. Recommendations for the interval and duration of imaging follow-up vary among lesions and between authors and are usually based on the degree of suspicion for malignancy generated by the imaging appearance of the lesion and the patient history. Typically, several years of stability is enough to suggest that the lesion is benign and argues against the need for additional imaging workup. "Indeterminate lesions" that show interval increase in lesion size and development of aggressive features such as cortical breakthrough, periosteal reaction, or soft tissue mass on follow-up imaging should raise the need for biopsy. Alternatively, on occasion, an indeterminate lesion may show changes on follow-up imaging that favor a benign entity, such as sclerosis seen in a resolving NOF.

Practically, the decision to go to biopsy is based not only on imaging features suspicious for malignancy (detailed in subsequent chapters) but also on other biopsy decision factors. Performing a biopsy may be the best management option for one patient, but not the appropriate course of action for another patient, even though the two lesions have identical imaging appearances. Factors such as known malignancy or severe pain at the site of the lesion can support the decision to biopsy. Conversely, factors such as medical comorbidities may make a biopsy risky to perform. In some instances, the lesion may be located adjacent to vital structures (nerves, vessels, lung, vital organs, and joint space), increasing the risk of procedure complications. Moreover, certain tumors and nonneoplastic conditions, such as infection, degenerative changes, ABC, SBC, and lymphoma, can have a relatively low diagnostic yield at core needle biopsy, suggesting that surgical biopsy would be a better option. In practice, patient anxiety can also have a major influence on the decision to biopsy. For some patients, a 10% risk of malignancy would be a compelling indication for biopsy, while, for others, a 10% risk of malignancy would be an indication for declining biopsy in favor of follow-up imaging. These decisions ultimately become a form of shared decision-making among the radiologist who evaluates the images and performs the percutaneous biopsy, the clinician caring for the patient, and the patient. However, it is important to understand that the radiologist's "recommendation" to perform or forego a biopsy should be based on the proper standard of medical care based on all the available information, while the final "decision" to actually perform or forego a biopsy must take into account patient preferences and other factors (Table 1.2).

Biopsy Considerations

Before a biopsy is undertaken, it is important for the radiologist and orthopedic oncologist to discuss the optimal approach to be used for percutaneous needle sampling and the specific biopsy technique. Percutaneous core needle biopsy (PCNB) with imaging guidance is performed by the radiologist and is the initial procedure to consider when tissue is required for pathologic diagnosis. PCNB can be performed on an outpatient basis utilizing CT, ultrasound, or fluoroscopy for image guidance and, when necessary, using conscious sedation for anesthesia. The procedure can be performed in less than an hour. Complications are rare, but can include hematomas, fractures, and injury to adjacent structures, such as pneumothoraces. Surgical biopsy is more invasive and is used when the percutaneous biopsy is nondiagnostic or when definitive resection is required. The benefits of surgical biopsy over PCNB are that the histologic samples are larger and small lesions can be completely resected (sometimes constituting definitive treatment). Fine needle aspiration (FNA) refers to a tissue sampling technique that uses a smaller size needle to sample a lesion than PCNB. FNA samples are sent for cytologic analysis (looking at cells), rather than histologic analysis (looking at tissue architecture). FNA can, at times, be helpful for lesions that are small and for lesions that carry a higher risk of complications if biopsied with a large core needle. However, the diagnostic yield with FNA is lower than with PCNB and most bone sarcomas cannot be adequately assessed with FNA alone.

Because of concerns related to possible seeding of tumor cells along the needle biopsy tract, the surgeon typically resects the needle tract at the time of definitive surgery. This is especially important for malignant primary tumors. Although technically appealing, biopsying along the shortest distance from the skin to the tumor may not always be the optimal trajectory. In general, one should avoid contamination of the neurovascular bundle, joint space, and certain muscles (e.g., partial resection of gluteus muscles and rectus femoris can lead to poor overall function). In addition, discussions with the pathologist prior to the biopsy are important for lesions that might require additional histologic and cytologic tests. In the majority of cases, samples can be submitted in formalin for histologic analysis. However, in cases where lymphoma is suspected, samples should be placed in Roswell Park Memorial Institute (RPMI) cell growth medium in order to perform flow cytometry.

Table 1.2 Non-imaging biopsy decision factors

Factor	Threshold to biopsy
Known malignancy	↓
Severe pain	↓
Comorbidities	↑
Risk of injury to adjacent structures	↑
Low diagnostic yield for certain lesions	↑
Patient anxiety	↑ or ↓

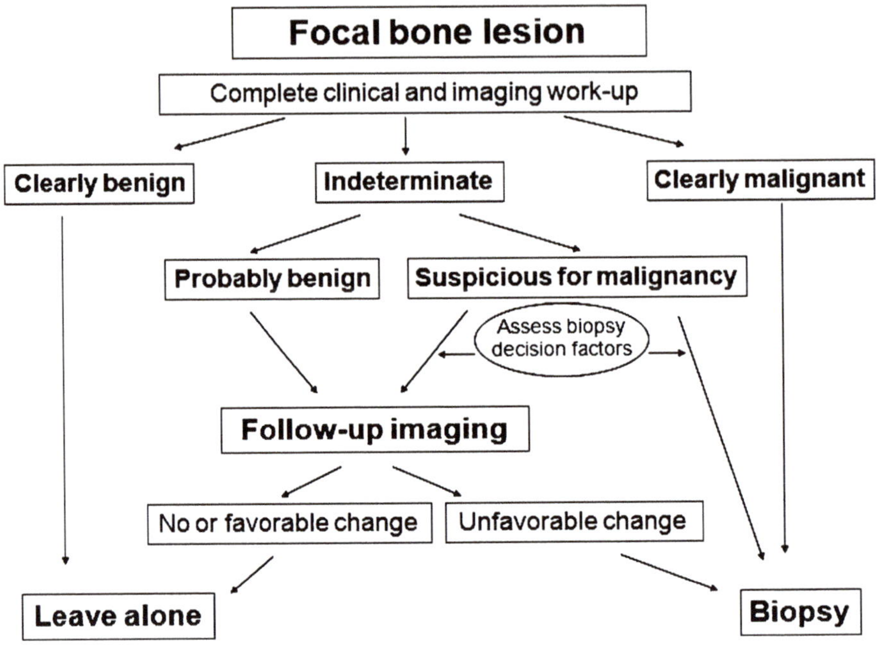

Fig. 1.6 Management of the focal bone lesion

Treatment

The treatment for each bone tumor depends on many factors, including whether the lesion is benign or malignant, the lesion location, the natural history of the disease entity, and the level of pain. Benign tumors that are asymptomatic often do not require treatment; however, benign lesions that are painful, injuring nearby anatomic structures, and/or at high risk for pathologic fracture, such as simple bone cysts, may require treatment. Curettage of the lesion followed by bone grafting or excisional biopsy can provide good results. However, these two treatment methods are inadequate for the treatment of malignant tumors, since residual tumors cells can remain at the margin of the lesion. Other nonsurgical treatment options exist for certain benign lesions. For instance, osteoid osteomas can be treated using radiofrequency ablation and Langerhans cell histiocytosis may resolve following steroid injections. Additionally, benign or malignant lesions that weaken the strength of the bone need to be stabilized with orthopedic hardware to prevent pathologic fracture.

Some malignant tumors, such as primary bone lymphoma, can be treated with chemotherapy or radiation without surgery. Other tumors will undergo treatment with radiation or chemotherapy in order to decrease the size of the tumor prior to definitive surgery, such as with a conventional osteosarcoma. Still other malignant processes can be treated with surgery alone. For instance, chondrosarcomas are typically low grade and do not respond well to chemotherapy, and in many instances, can be treated with surgery alone. Lastly, isolated metastatic lesions can be resected for potential cure. In general, surgery for bone metastases is reserved for preventing pathologic fracture, as the treatment is often limited to radiation and/or chemotherapy. Many malignant processes or aggressive benign processes can be treated with wide surgical resection, where a margin of normal tissue is resected along with the tumor. Others require radical resection, which involves removal of bone, muscle, or other tissues in the compartment along with the tumor.

Suggested Reading

1. Fletcher CD, Unni KK, Mertens F, editors. WHO classification of tumours: pathology and genetics of tumours of soft tissue and bone. Lyon, France: IARC; 2002.
2. Freiberger R. Thoughts on the diagnosis of bone tumors. Radiology. 1984;150:276.
3. Greenspan A, Jundt G, Remagen W. Differential diagnosis in orthopaedic oncology. 2nd ed. Philadelphia, PA: Lippincott Williams & Wilkins; 2007.
4. Ilaslan H, Schils J, Nageotte W, Lietman SA, Sundaram M. Clinical presentation and imaging of bone and soft-tissue sarcomas. Cleve Clin J Med. 2010;77 Suppl 1:S2–7.
5. Jaovisidha S, Subhadrabandhu T, Siriwongpairat P, Pochanugool L. An integrated approach to the evaluation of osseous tumors. Orthop Clin N Am. 1998;29:19–39.
6. Lietman SA, Joyce MJ. Bone sarcomas: overview of management, with a focus on surgical treatment considerations. Cleve Clin J Med. 2010;77 Suppl 1:S8–S12.
7. Miller TT. Bone tumors and tumorlike conditions: analysis with conventional radiography. Radiology. 2008;246:662–74.
8. Murphey MD. Fundamental concepts of musculoskeletal neoplasms: radiographs. Radiol Pathol. 2006;2:720–32.
9. O'Connor MI. Musculoskeletal imaging: what information is important to the orthopedic oncologist? Semin Musculoskelet Radiol. 2007;11:273–8.
10. Ofluoglu O, Boriani S, Gasbarrini A, De Iure F, Donthineni R. Diagnosis and planning in the management of musculoskeletal tumors: surgical perspective. Semin Interv Radiol. 2010;27:185–90.
11. Peabody TD, Gibbs Jr CP, Simon MA. Evaluation and staging of musculoskeletal neoplasms. J Bone Joint Surg Am. 1998;80:1204–18.
12. Pommersheim WJ, Chew FS. Imaging, diagnosis, and staging of bone tumors: a primer. Semin Roentgenol. 2004;39:361–72.
13. Resnick D, editor. Diagnosis of Bone and Joint Disorders. 4th ed. Philadelphia, PA: W.B. Saunders; 2002.

How to Evaluate a Bone Lesion

2

Using a systematic approach is key for evaluating a focal bone lesion. The ultimate goal should be to provide a definitive diagnosis; however, in many instances, this is not possible. Nonetheless, one should aim to provide a short, logical differential diagnosis and to comment on whether the lesion can be left alone as a "do not touch" lesion or whether additional workup is necessary. The analysis should begin with the patient's age and the location of the lesion, since these two factors play such a significant role in determining the differential diagnosis. Next, assessment of specific lesion characteristics can be used to help narrow the differential, i.e., the lesion's pattern of bone destruction and lesion margins and the presence of any matrix mineralization, periosteal reaction, or soft tissue component. If multiple lesions are present, that fact can help to refine the diagnosis even further. For example, the presence of multiple lytic lesions in an older individual would lead one to suspect metastatic disease or multiple myeloma. One should also search for relevant secondary findings, such as diffuse osteopenia in multiple myeloma or subperiosteal resorption and acro-osteolysis in hyperparathyroidism, and should consider relevant clinical information, such as a history of malignancy supporting a diagnosis of metastasis or fever and erythema supporting a diagnosis of osteomyelitis.

Factors to Consider

- Patient age
- Lesion location
- Lesion density
- Pattern of bone destruction and lesion margins
- Matrix and matrix mineralization
- Periosteal reaction
- Soft tissue component
- Single or multiple lesions

J.S. Wu and M.G. Hochman, *Bone Tumors: A Practical Guide to Imaging*,
DOI 10.1007/978-1-4419-0808-7_2, © Springer Science+Business Media, LLC 2012

Patient Age

Certain tumors tend to develop during specific age ranges (Tables 2.1 and 2.2). For example, most benign tumors occur before 30 years of age while lesions identified in persons over 40 years old are more likely to be metastases or multiple myeloma. Among benign lesions, non-ossifying fibroma, osteoid osteoma, simple (unicameral) bone cyst, Langerhans cell histiocytosis, and chondroblastoma occur in children or teenagers. However, giant cell tumor of bone almost always occurs in skeletally mature patients with closed physes and thus should not, for example, be mentioned in the differential diagnosis for a lytic lesion in a 10-year old. Among malignant bone lesions, metastases are by far the most common and should be considered high in the differential for patients over the age of 40 (especially if over 60 years of age). Among primary bone malignancies, osteosarcoma is the most common lesion biopsied in children and teenagers, while myeloma is the most frequent primary tumor of bone in adults (Fig. 2.1).

Table 2.1 Tumor and tumor-like lesions of bone: typical ages of patients

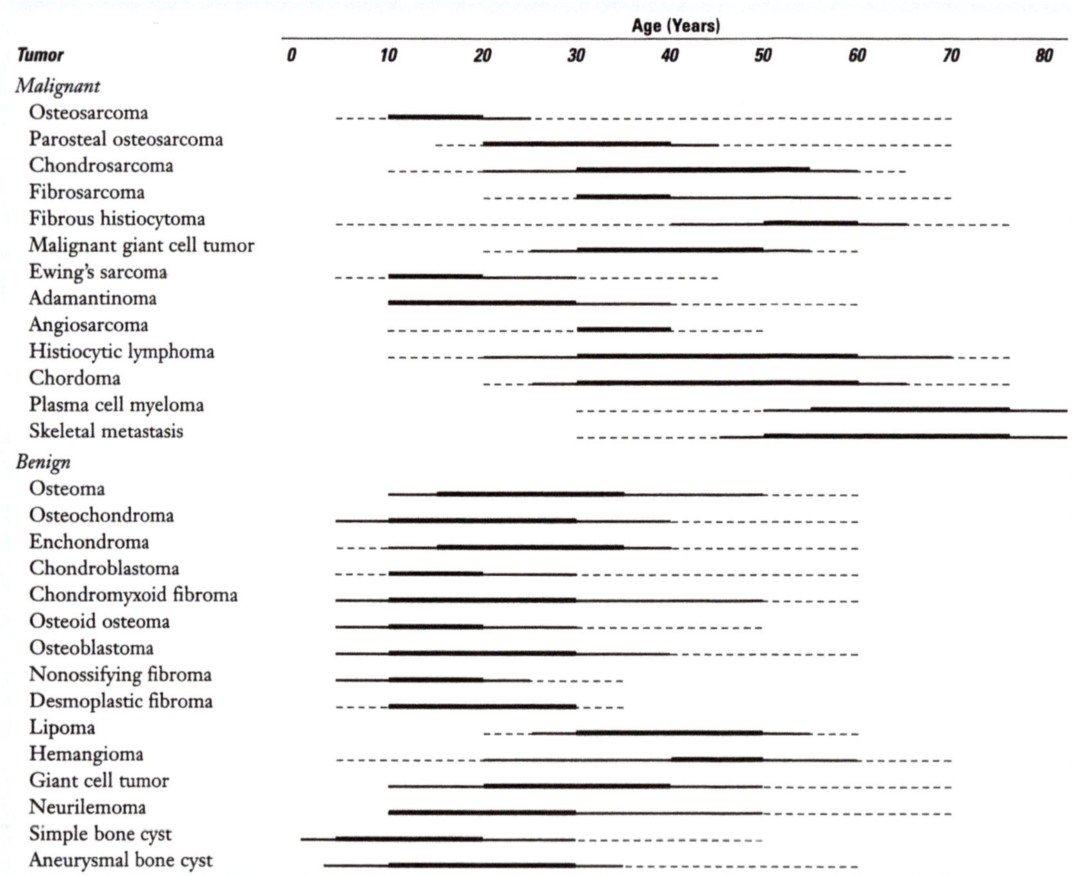

Reproduced with permission. This table was originally published in Bone and Joint Imaging, Third Edition, Donald Resnick, Michael Kyriakos, Guerdon G. Greenaway, Chapter 70: Tumor and Tumor-like Lesions of Bone: Imaging and Pathology of Specific Lesions, Donald Resnick, Mark J. Kransdorf, eds., pp. 112. Copyright Elsevier Saunders 2005

Table 2.2 Most likely tumors by age

Second decade	• Aneurysmal bone cyst (ABC) • Chondroblastoma • Ewing sarcoma • Langerhans cell histiocytosis • Osteosarcoma • Non-ossifying fibroma • Simple (unicameral) bone cyst
Third and fourth decades	• Giant cell tumor • Lymphoma • Parosteal osteosarcoma
Fifth to seventh decades	• Chondrosarcoma • Chordoma • Fibrosarcoma • Lymphoma • Metastases • Multiple myeloma

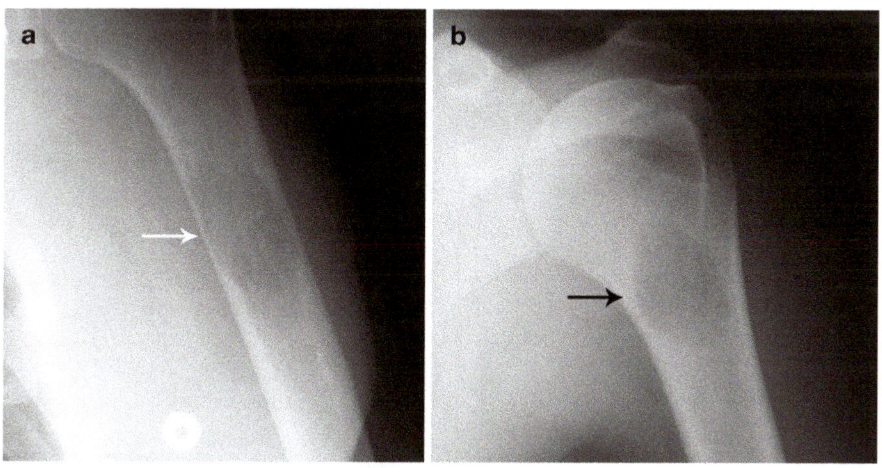

Fig. 2.1 Patient age plays a key role in shaping the differential diagnosis. Two different geographic, ovoid, lytic lesions in the humerus appear similar, but occur in patients of different ages and have very different diagnoses. (**a**) Sixty-eight-year-old man with a renal cell metastasis (*arrow*); (**b**) 17-year-old boy with Langerhans cell histiocytosis (LCH) (*arrow*)

Lesion Location

Some bone tumors and non-neoplastic bone lesions occur characteristically within specific bones or in specific locations within a bone. Bone tumors tend to develop near the ends of long bones, which are areas of rapid bone growth and remodeling. For example, osteosarcomas are commonly found about the knee in the distal femur or proximal tibia and in the proximal humerus, where rapid bone growth occurs. Non-ossifying fibromas tend to occur in these locations as well, probably for similar reasons. Enchondromas and osteochondromas, which are thought to arise from displaced cartilage that originates from the physis, tend to be associated with the metaphysis or metadiaphysis. The existence of a distinct relationship between a particular bone tumor and the anatomic site in which it typically arises has been described as the "field theory" of bone tumors: tumors of a particular cell type arise where the corresponding normal cells are most active, such that the composition of a tumor is related to the metabolic field in which it arises (Fig. 2.2). Additional factors contribute to the reproducibility of bone lesion locations. For example, seeding of either metastatic tumor or infection may occur in the metaphysis because of looping vessels and sinusoids which slow blood flow there. Round cell lesions tend to occur in areas of hematopoietic marrow and thus tend to be seen in the diaphysis or metadiaphysis. Because of differences in distribution of red marrow between children and adults, round cell tumors can occur in both the axial and appendicular skeleton in children, but are generally limited to the axial skeleton in adults. Chordomas, which arise from notochordal remnants, occur along the course of the spine, most often in the clivus and sacrum. Epidermoid inclusion cysts, which are thought to arise from implantation of epidermis into bone, tend to occur in the terminal phalanges and calvaria.

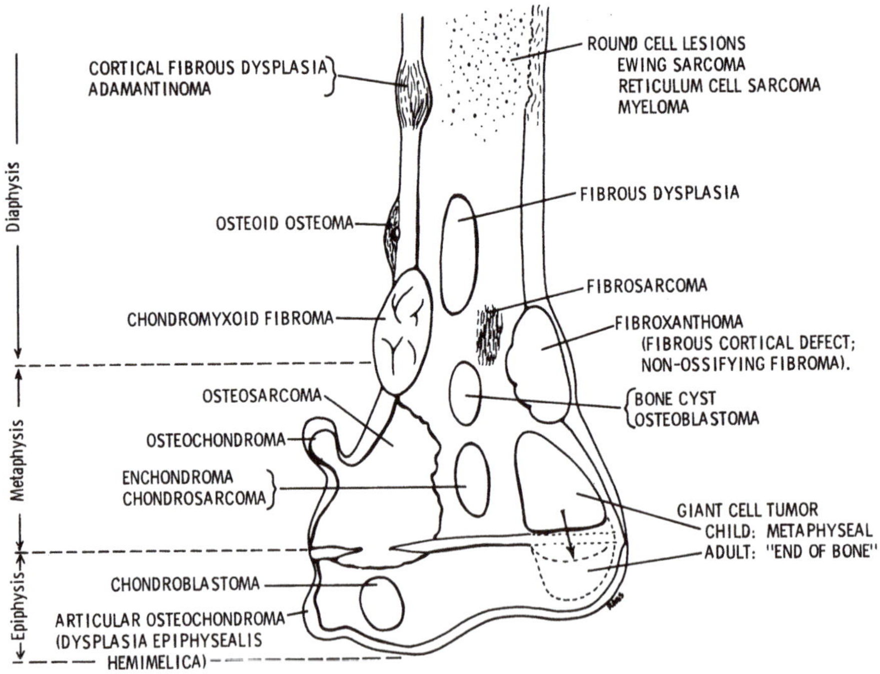

Fig. 2.2 Field theory of bone tumor locations. This diagram summarizes the most common location of various bone tumors within a long bone. For example, chondroblastoma tends to arise in the epiphysis, while osteochondromas and enchondromas tend to arise in the metaphysis and fibrous dysplasia, adamantinoma, osteofibrous dysplasia, and round cell lesions tend to arise in the diaphysis. In general, particular tumors tend to arise in the "field" where the corresponding cell type is normally most active. Adapted and reproduced with permission from Koeller KK, Levy AD, Woodward PJ, et al., editors, Radiologic-Pathology, Vol. 2: Musculoskeletal, Neuroradiologic, and Pediatric Radiologic Pathology Correlations, 3rd ed (2004) American Registry of Pathology, Armed Forces Institute of Pathology, Washington DC

Given the importance of location in generating a differential diagnosis, there are three key descriptors of location that should be included in every tumor description:

Three Descriptors of Tumor Location

- Which bone?
- Where along the bone?
- Where in axial plane?

Which Bone?

The specific bone involved can sometimes be used to help shape a preliminary differential diagnosis. In addition, a small number of lesions have an inordinately high tendency to occur in a specific location (Tables 2.3–2.8; Figs. 2.3–2.6). Examples of these include:

- Clivus, sacrum: chordoma
- Proximal femur: liposclerosing myxofibrous tumor
- Tibia: adamantinoma, osteofibrous dysplasia

Table 2.3 Skull lesions

- Metastases
- Myeloma
- Langerhans cell histiocytosis
- Epidermoid
- Sarcoid
- Paget disease
- Venous lake
- Leptomeningeal cyst
- Pitfall: postoperative defect

Table 2.4 Rib lesions

- Myeloma
- Metastasis
- Fibrous dysplasia
- Langerhans cell histiocytosis
- Chondrosarcoma (costochondral or costovertebral junction)
- Ewing sarcoma
- Lymphoma
- Osteosarcoma
- Pitfall: healing fracture

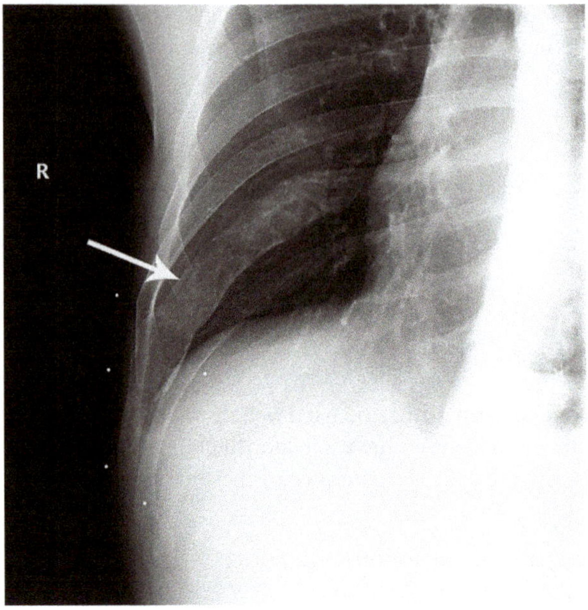

Fig. 2.3 Fibrous dysplasia. A long segment of a lower rib is expanded, with a hazy ground glass density (*arrow*). Fibrous dysplasia is the most common benign rib lesion

Table 2.5 Phalanx lesions

- Enchondroma
- Epidermoid inclusion cyst
- Foreign body granuloma
- Glomus tumor
- Metastases (lung, breast, and renal)
- Osteomyelitis
- Sarcoid
- Pitfalls: subchondral cysts and erosions (arthritis and gout)

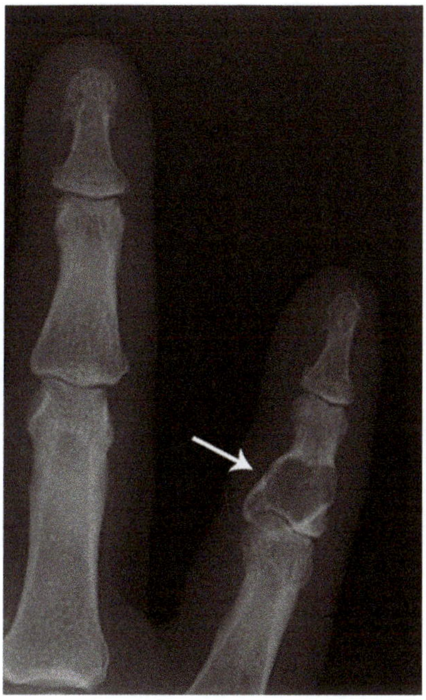

Fig. 2.4 Enchondroma. There is a slightly expansile, geographic, well-circumscribed lytic lesion (*arrow*) at the base of the middle phalanx of the small finger. Enchondromas are the most common lucent lesions in the phalanges. Note that enchondromas in the hands or feet, unlike enchondromas elsewhere in the body, can lack calcified matrix without raising concern for dedifferentiation

Table 2.6 Calcaneus lesions

- Intraosseous lipoma
- Simple (unicameral) bone cyst
- Aneurysmal bone cyst
- Giant cell tumor
- Chondroblastoma
- Pitfall: pseudotumor

Table 2.7 Spine lesions

- Vertebral body
  - Hemangioma
  - Myeloma
  - Metastasis
  - Lymphoma (HL and NHL)
- Vertebral posterior elements
  - Osteoblastoma
  - Osteoid osteoma
  - ABC
  - Metastases

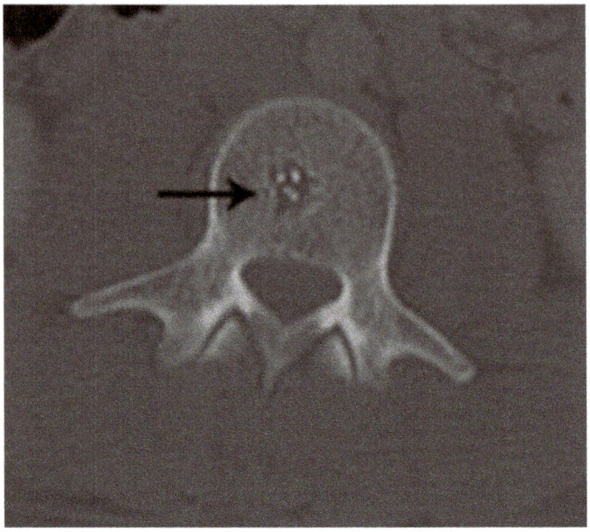

Fig. 2.5 Intraosseous hemangioma. Hemangiomas are the most common lucent lesion in the spine. They favor the vertebral body, as opposed to the posterior elements, and often demonstrate characteristic features, such as thickened vertical trabeculae (corduroy pattern) or fat content on CT or MRI

Table 2.8 Sacrum lesions

- Metastasis
- Plasmacytoma
- Chordoma
- Chondrosarcoma
- Giant cell tumor
- Pitfall: insufficiency fracture and Tarlov/perineural cyst

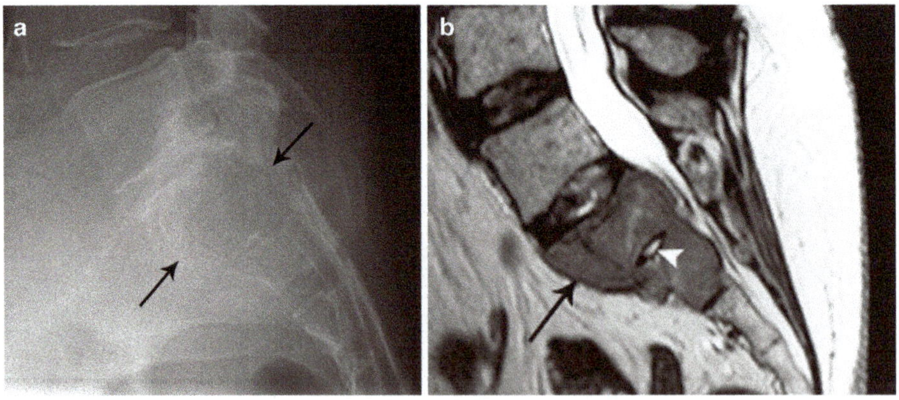

Fig. 2.6 Chordoma. Lateral radiograph (**a**) shows a lytic lesion (*arrows*) destroying the S1 vertebral body. Sagittal T2-weighted MRI (**b**) shows a low-signal soft tissue lesion (*arrow*) destroying and expanding S1 and S2. A limited number of lesions predilect to the sacrum. Sixty percent of chordomas, like the lesion depicted here, involve the sacrococcygeal spine. Chordomas arise from notochordal remnants and therefore usually occur along the axial spine in the midline, centered in the vertebral body. This lesion spares the disc space at S1/2 (*arrowhead*), a feature typical of chordomas

Where Along the Bone?

The location of a lesion along the longitudinal axis of a long bone is also very important for generating a differential diagnosis. As you proceed through the descriptions of the individual entities in the following chapters, you will notice that some lesions have characteristic locations in long tubular bones. These locations include the end of the bone (epiphysis), the region between the end of the bone and the shaft (metaphysis), and the shaft itself (diaphysis) (Tables 2.9 and 2.10; Figs. 2.7–2.10). The key descriptors are:

Location of Lesions Along Longitudinal Axis of Long Bones

- Epiphysis
- Metaphysis
- Diaphysis

Table 2.9 Characteristic site of lesions in a long bone

Benign	Malignant
Epiphysis (includes apophyses and epiphyseal equivalents)	
• Subchondral cyst (geode)	• Clear cell chondrosarcoma
• Erosion (inflammatory arthritis, PVNS, synovial osteochondromatosis)	
• Osteomyelitis (<18 months old; TB and fungus in adult)	
• Chondroblastoma (open physis)	
• Giant cell tumor (closed physis, extending from metaphysis)	
• Osteoid osteoma	
Metaphysis	
• Fibrous xanthoma (NOF and FCD)	• Metastases, myeloma (>40 years old)
• Enchondroma	• Lymphoma
• Giant cell tumor (extending to epiphysis)	• Osteosarcoma
• Simple (unicameral) bone cyst (central)	• Chondrosarcoma
• Aneurysmal bone cyst (eccentric)	
• Osteochondroma	
• Osteomyelitis, Brodie's abscess	
• Osteoid osteoma (cortical)	
Diaphysis	
• Fibrous dysplasia	• Metastases, myeloma
• Enchondroma	• Lymphoma, leukemia
• Simple (unicameral) bone cyst (late)	• Ewing sarcoma
• Osteofibrous dysplasia	• Adamantinoma

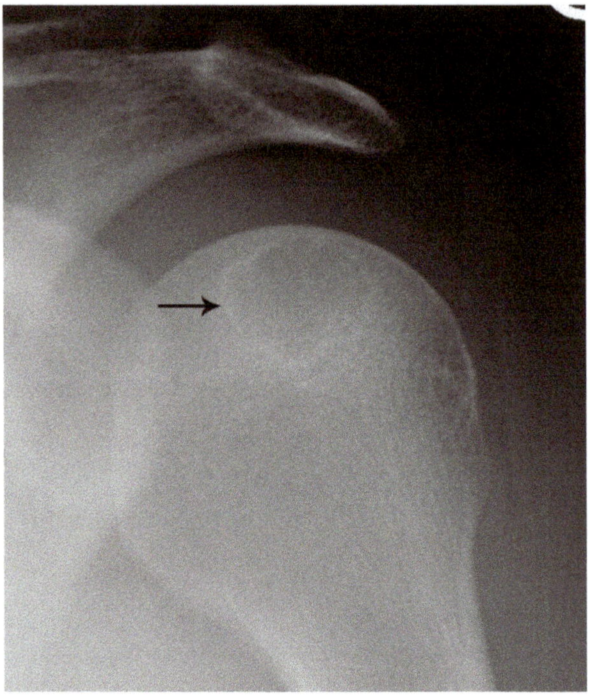

Fig. 2.7 Epiphyseal lesion. A geographic lucent lesion with a thin sclerotic rim, centered in the epiphysis of the proximal humerus (*arrow*), is a chondroblastoma, one of a limited number of lesions that arise in the epiphysis

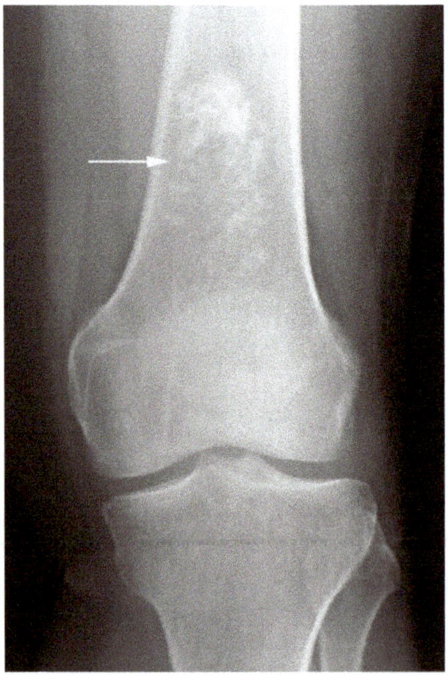

Fig. 2.8 Metaphyseal lesion. An ovoid enchondroma with dense chondroid matrix calcification is seen in the central metaphysis of the distal femur (*arrow*)

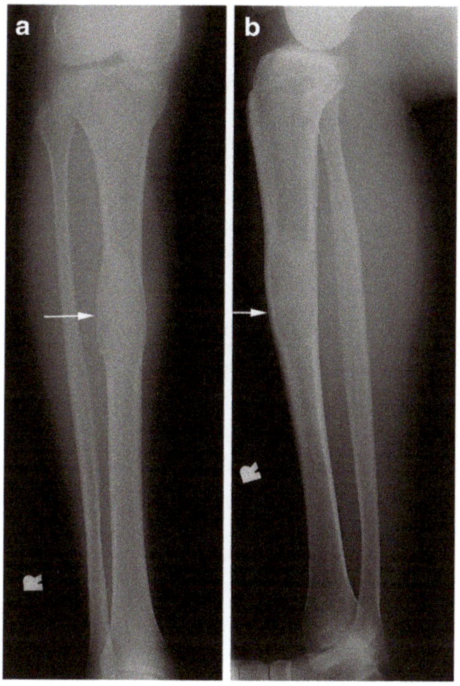

Fig. 2.9 Diaphyseal lesion. Classic appearance of fibrous dysplasia, seen as a "long lesion in a long bone," with ground glass density. Note that the lesion is slightly expansile

Table 2.10 Epiphyseal (end of bone) equivalent sites

- Ribs
- Greater and lesser tuberosities (humerus)
- Small bones of the wrist
- Acetabulum (fusion of triradiate cartilage)
- Greater and lesser trochanters (femur)
- Patella
- Tibial tubercle
- Calcaneus
- Small bones of the midfoot
- Any apophysis

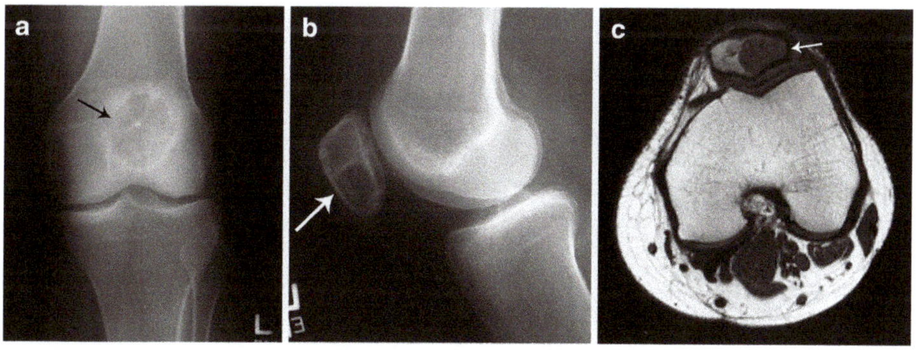

Fig. 2.10 Epiphyseal equivalent. This geographic lytic lesion in the patella is a giant cell tumor (*arrows*). Because the patella is an epiphyseal equivalent, lesions that tend to occur in the epiphysis can also be seen there. AP (**a**) and lateral (**b**) radiographs and axial T1-weighted MRI image (**c**)

Where in the Axial Plane?

The location of a lesion along the axial plane of a long bone provides additional important information for narrowing the differential diagnosis (Table 2.11, Figs. 2.11–2.14). For example, recognizing that a lesion arises from the surface of a bone significantly limits the differential diagnoses. The key descriptors related to position in the axial plane of long bone are:

Location of Lesions Along Axial Plane of Long Bones

- Central (intramedullary)
- Eccentric (intramedullary)
- Cortical
- Juxtacortical (periosteal and parosteal)*

* *Periosteal lesions arise from the deep layer of the periosteum and separate periosteum from cortex; parosteal lesions arise from the outer layer of periosteum and grow exophytically.*

Table 2.11 Location in axial plane of long bone

- Central
  - Enchondroma
  - Fibrous dysplasia
  - Simple (unicameral) bone cyst
- Eccentric
  - Giant cell tumor
  - Chondromyxoid fibroma
  - Fibrosarcoma
  - Non-ossifying fibroma
  - Enchondroma
  - ABC
- Cortical
  - Fibrous cortical defect
  - Osteoid osteoma (cortical)
  - Cortical metastases (lung, breast)
- Juxtacortical
  - Juxtacortical (periosteal) chondroma
  - Periosteal osteosarcoma
  - Parosteal osteosarcoma
  - Osteochondroma

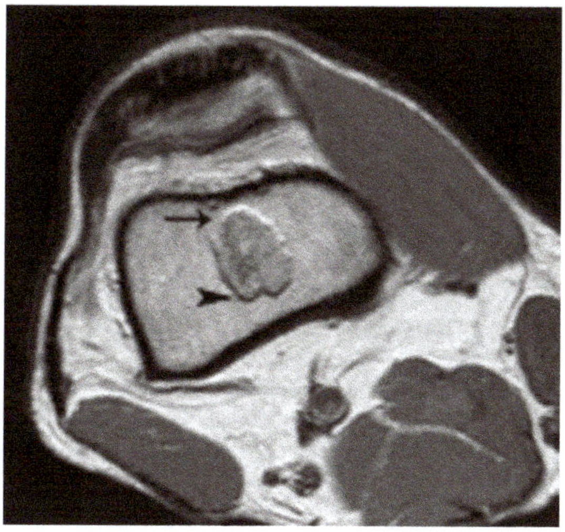

Fig. 2.11 Central lesion. Axial T1-weighted MR image showing an enchondroma located centrally in the medullary cavity of the distal femur. Incidentally noted is chemical shift artifact causing a high-signal line anteriorly (*arrow*) and a low-signal line posteriorly (*arrowhead*) at the interface of the lesion and the surrounding medullary fat. Although not pathognomonic for enchondroma, a peripheral rim of chemical shift artifact is a feature commonly seen in enchondromas

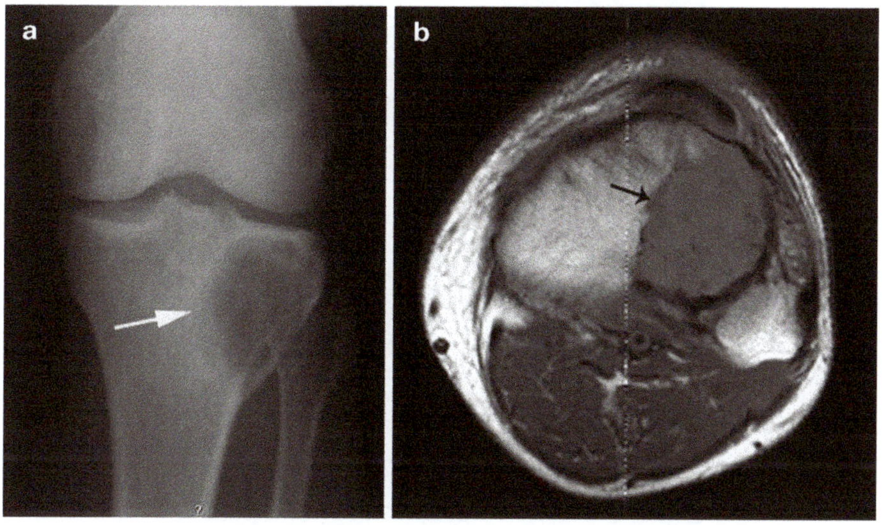

Fig. 2.12 Eccentric lesion. Giant cell tumor located eccentrically in the medullary cavity of the proximal tibia (*arrows*), seen on both the AP radiograph (**a**) and axial T1-weighted MRI image (**b**). Note that the lesion is centered in the metaphysis and extends to the subarticular surface. In this case, the lesion is also slightly expansile

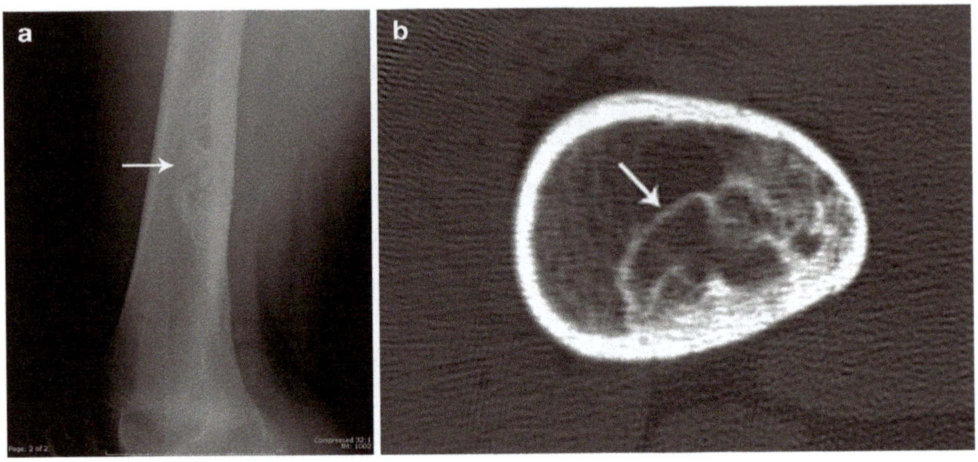

Fig. 2.13 Cortical lesion. Strictly speaking, a non-ossifying fibroma (*arrows*) is considered a cortical lesion because it is based in the cortex, though, when large, it appears to lie in an eccentric metaphyseal location, as seen on the lateral radiograph (**a**) and axial CT image (**b**) through the distal femur

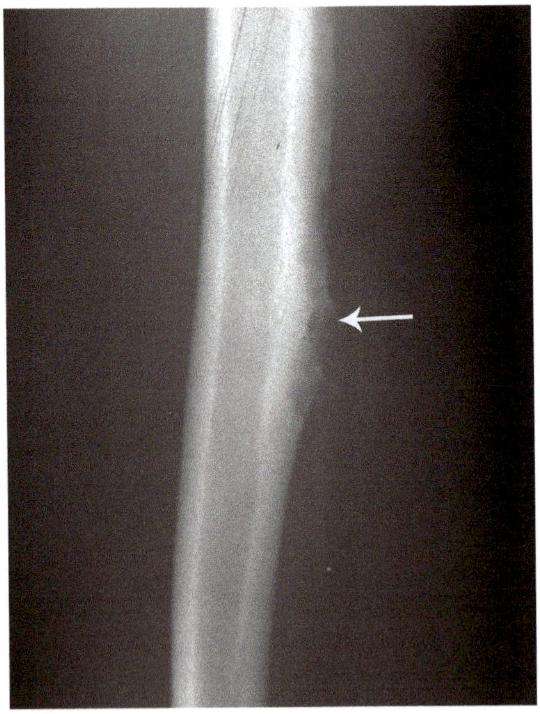

Fig. 2.14 Juxtacortical lesion. Juxtacortical chondroma (*arrow*) centered on the surface of the humeral cortex, with surrounding periosteal new bone formation. The lesion appears as a rounded radiolucency centered symmetrically in the periosteal new bone

Lesion Density: Lucent, Sclerotic, or Mixed

Focal bone lesions are visible on radiographs because they are abnormally lucent or dense or are a mixture of lucent and dense areas, relative to the surrounding bone. Lucent lesions are made up of any material that is not as dense as the surrounding bone, e.g., fluid, cartilage, fibrous tissue, myxoid tissue, woven bone, granulomatous material, or tumor cells. "Lucent" is a generic term for a lesion that is not as dense as the surrounding bone; "lytic" refers specifically to a lesion in which bone is known to be destroyed and represents a subset of lucent lesions. There are distinct differentials for lucent, sclerotic, and mixed lucent-and-sclerotic lesions (Tables 2.12–2.14; Figs. 2.15–2.18).

Of note, radiographs are not very sensitive for detection of bone destruction, particularly destruction of cancellous bone. Cancellous or trabecular bone is the lattice of interconnected bony spicules that are found in the marrow space. Although cancellous bone makes up the bulk of flat bones, in long bones it is found mainly in the epiphysis and metaphysis. This is in contrast to cortical bone, which is concentrated in the diaphysis and thins toward the ends of bone. Overall, perception of osteolysis on radiographs depends on the cancellous versus cortical structure of the bone in that location, the amount of bone loss, and the density of adjacent host bone, which provides a form of image contrast. A small amount of cortical bone destruction is more likely to be seen on a radiograph than a relatively large area of cancellous bone destruction. A sharply marginated lucent focus overlying a tubular bone should raise suspicion for cortical destruction and prompt careful scrutiny for confirmatory focal endosteal thinning on the orthogonal view. However, in order for a cortical lytic lesion to be visible on radiographs, at least 50% of the cortex must be destroyed. A given intramedullary lucent lesion is more likely to be visible in the metaphysis, where there is more cancellous bone than in the diaphysis, where cancellous bone is limited predominantly to the inner surface of the cortex. In addition, a lucent lesion is more likely to be visible in bone of normal density than in osteopenic or osteoporotic bone.

Table 2.12 Solitary lucent lesion

- Fibrous dysplasia
- Osteoblastoma in spine (though sclerotic in other locations)
- Giant cell tumor
- Myeloma, plasmacytoma
- Metastasis
- Aneurysmal bone cyst
- Chondromyxoid fibroma
- Chondroblastoma
- Langerhans cell histiocytosis
- Brown tumor (hyperparathyroidism)
- Osteomyelitis
- Fibrous xanthoma (non-ossifiying fibroma and fibrous cortical defect)
- Enchondroma in hands and feet
- Epithelial inclusion cyst
- Simple (unicameral) bone cyst

Table 2.13 Solitary sclerotic lesion

- Bone island
- Healing lesion (fracture, non-ossifying fibroma, metastasis, and Brown tumor)
- Osteoid osteoma (lucent nidus obscured by sclerosis)
- Osteoma
- Osteoblastic metastasis (prostate and breast)
- Osteosarcoma
- Ewing sarcoma (rare)
- Lymphoma (rare)
- Paget disease (blastic phase)
- Chronic osteomyelitis
- Bone infarct
- Heavily calcified enchondroma

Table 2.14 Mixed lytic and sclerotic lesion

- Adamantinoma
- Lymphoma
- Osteomyelitis
- Osteoid osteoma
- Fibrous dysplasia
- Langerhans cell histiocytosis
- Metastases

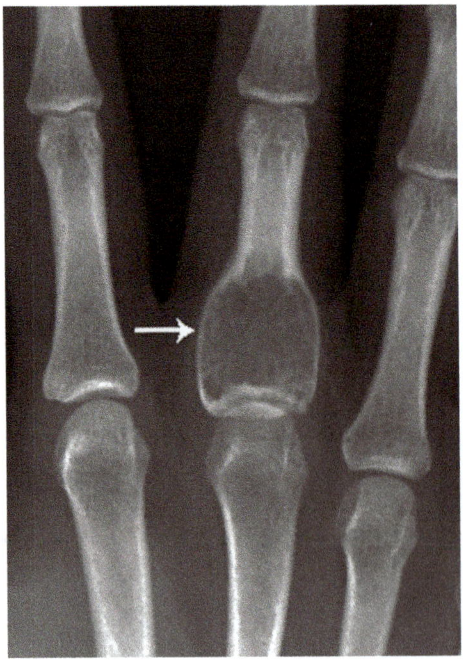

Fig. 2.15 Lucent lesion. Aneurysmal bone cyst (ABC) seen as an expansile lucent lesion in the proximal phalanx (*arrow*)

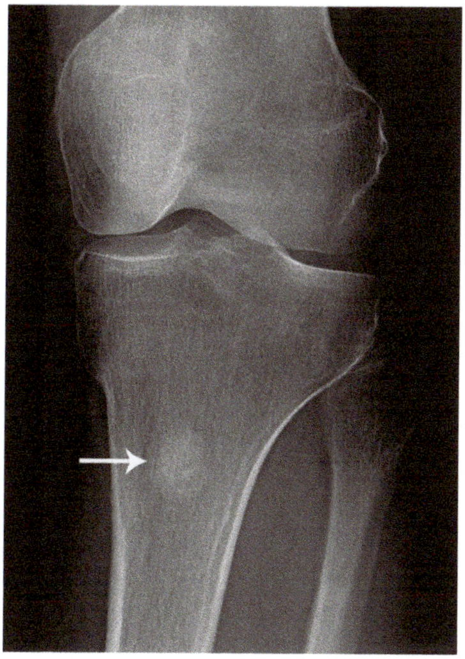

Fig. 2.16 Sclerotic lesion. Carcinoid metastasis seen as a focal sclerotic lesion in the proximal tibial metaphysis (*arrow*)

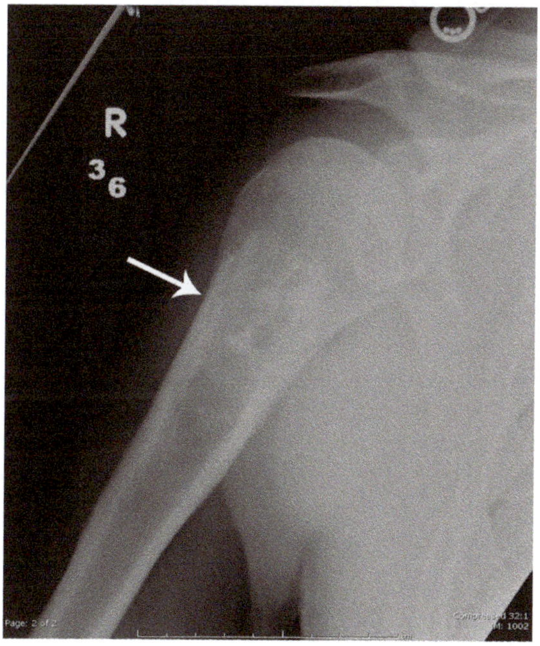

Fig. 2.17 Mixed lucent and sclerotic lesion. Fibrous dysplasia seen as a mixed lucent and sclerotic lesion in the proximal humeral metadiaphysis (*arrow*)

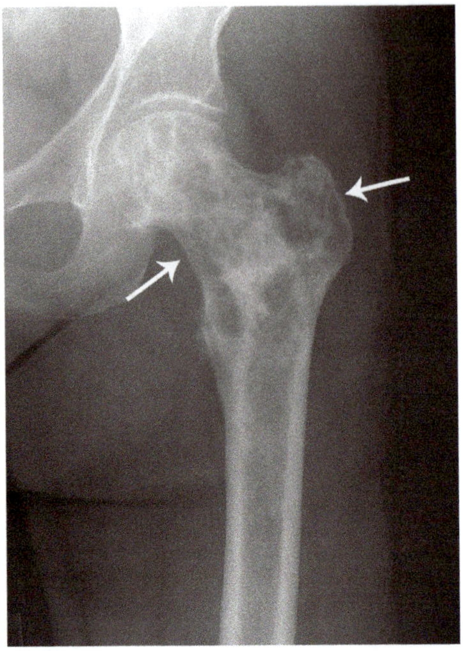

Fig. 2.18 Mixed lucent and sclerotic lesion. A breast cancer metastasis appears as a mixed lucent and sclerotic lesion in the proximal femur (*arrows*)

Pattern of Bone Destruction and Lesion Margins

The pattern of bone destruction and the margin formed between a lesion and the surrounding bone are often characteristic for specific lesions and can help generate a differential diagnosis. The pattern of bone destruction—geographic, moth eaten, or permeative—reflects the lesion growth rate. Geographic lesions tend to be nonaggressive and are often—but not always—benign. Moth-eaten and permeative lesions tend to be more aggressive and are often—but not always—malignant. The lesion margin reflects both the lesion growth rate and the response of the host bone and can be (1) sharply defined without a sclerotic margin, (2) sharply defined with a sclerotic margin, or (3) poorly defined. If present, the sclerotic border formed as a response by the host bone may be thin or thick. In some cases, the lesion itself actively stimulates an osteoblastic response from the host bone. The term "zone of transition" is a general descriptor that refers to how well or poorly demarcated a lesion is from the surrounding bone—the zone of transition can be either narrow (well-demarcated) or wide (poorly demarcated). Nonaggressive, slow-growing lesions tend to have well-defined margins while aggressive, fast-growing lesions tend to have poorly defined margins. However, it is very important to realize that aggressive borders do not necessarily imply a malignant lesion, since osteomyelitis and other benign entities, such as Langerhans cell histiocytosis, can appear aggressive.

Based on radiographic patterns originally proposed by Lodwick et al., lucent bone lesions can be described as follows (Fig. 2.19):

(1) Type I, ***geographic*** well-circumscribed lesion with or without a sclerotic border:
  IA: Well-defined, sclerotic border.
  IB: Well-defined, no sclerotic border.
  IC: Ill-defined.
(2) Type II, poorly delineated with a ***moth-eaten*** appearance.
(3) Type III, ***permeative*** and barely perceptible (Fig. 2.19).

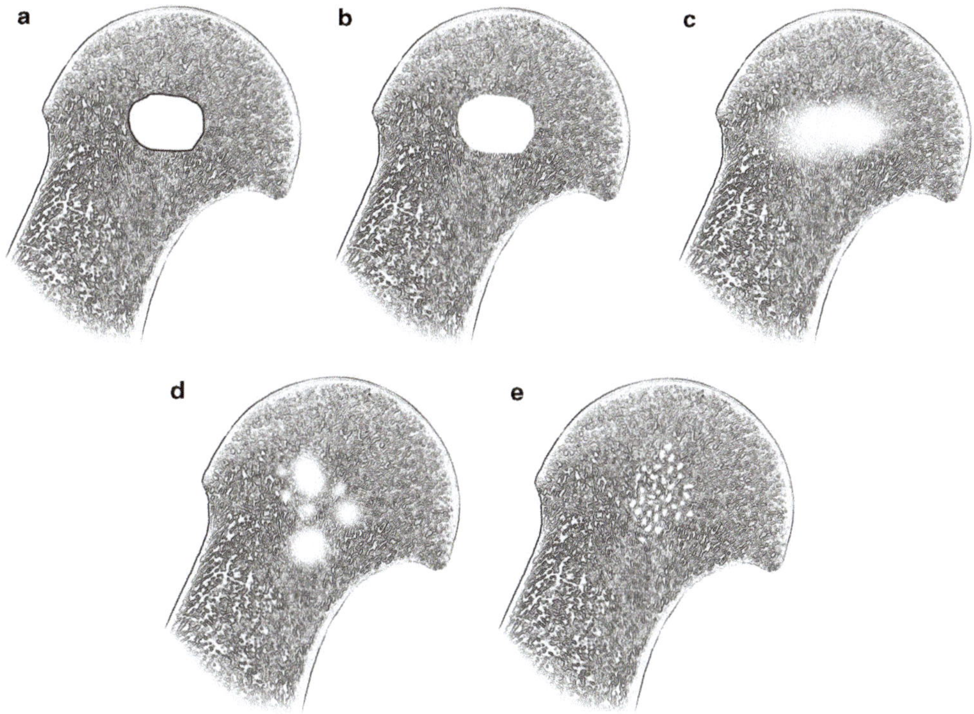

Fig. 2.19 Radiographic patterns of bone tumors. IA—geographic with well-defined border and sclerotic rim (**a**); IB—geographic with a well-defined border, but no sclerotic rim (**b**); IC—geographic, but with an ill-defined border(**c**); II—moth eaten (**d**); III—permeative (**e**). Courtesy of Michael Larson, Boston, MA

Geographic bone destruction describes a single discrete lytic lesion, often, but not always, with well-defined borders (Figs. 2.20–2.22). Moth-eaten bone destruction refers to multiple ill-defined focal lytic defects in the bone (Fig. 2.23). Permeative bone destruction can be a confusing term—it refers to bone lysis that permeates through the bone and is therefore near-imperceptible on radiographs. (Nonetheless, a permeative lesion might be readily visible on MRI) (Fig. 2.24). It is important to note that, in general, Type I lesions with a geographic pattern of destruction tend to be nonaggressive, and Type II and III lesions with moth-eaten or permeative patterns of destruction tend to be aggressive.

Lesions can be assessed according to their characteristic pattern of bone destruction and peripheral margin. For example, nonaggressive lesions, such as bone cysts, enchondromas, fibrous dysplasia, and chondroblastomas, tend to have a geographic pattern of bone destruction, whereas aggressive lesions, such as osteosarcoma, Ewing sarcoma, osteomyelitis, and Langerhans cell histiocytosis, tend to have a moth-eaten or permeative pattern of destruction. Although giant cell tumor and multiple myeloma are well-defined lesions, they typically do not have a sclerotic border. In contrast, enchondromas and simple cysts are well-defined lesions that typically have a thin surrounding sclerotic border, and the nidus of an osteoid osteoma often has a very thick rim of reactive bone. Note that some lesions appear under more than one category (Table 2.15).

Table 2.15 Lesion margins and patterns of bone destruction

IA—Geographic, well-defined, sclerotic rim	• Bone cyst • Brodie abscess • Chondroblastoma • Enchondroma • Fibroxanthoma (NOF and FCD) • Fibrous dysplasia • Intraosseous lipoma
IB—Geographic, well-defined, no sclerotic rim	• Bone cyst • Chondroblastoma • Enchondroma • Fibrous dysplasia • Giant cell tumor • Myeloma • Metastasis
IC—Geographic, not well-defined	• Chondrosarcoma • Enchondroma (active) • Fibrosacroma • Giant cell tumor • Osteosarcoma • Metastasis
II—Moth-eaten	• Small, round cell tumors • Ewing sarcoma • Fibrosarcoma • Langerhans cell histiocytosis • Malignant fibrous histiocytoma • Osteomyelitis • Osteosarcoma • Metastasis • Myeloma
III—Permeative	• Small, round cell tumors (especially lymphoma) • Ewing sarcoma • Fibrosarcoma • Langerhans cell histiocytosis • Leukemia • Lymphoma • Malignant fibrous histiocytoma • Metastasis • Myeloma • Osteomyelitis (acute) • Osteoporosis with intracortical tunneling • Osteosarcoma

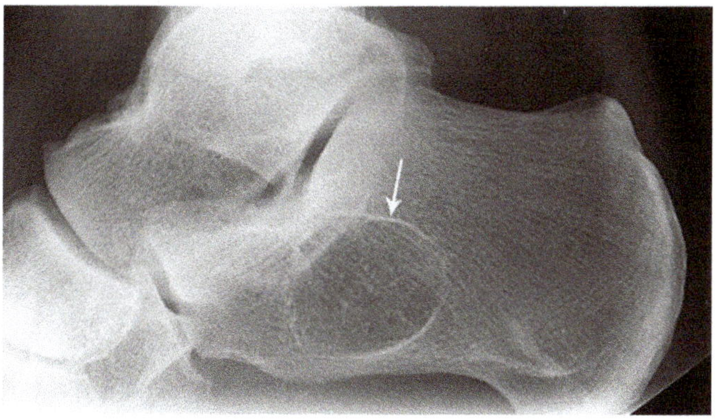

Fig. 2.20 Type IA geographic pattern. Intraosseous lipoma (*arrow*) shows characteristic Type IA features: it is geographic, well-circumscribed, and has a sclerotic rim

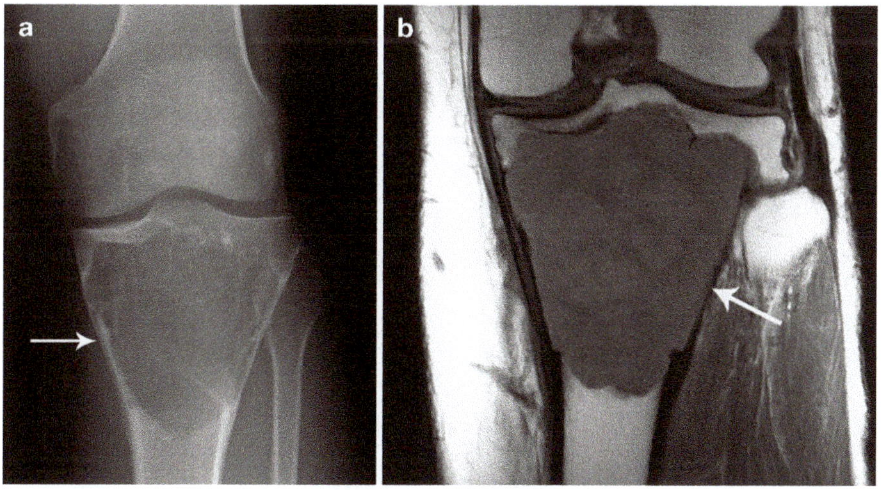

Fig. 2.21 Type IB geographic pattern. Giant cell tumor (GCT) in the proximal tibia (*arrows*) on radiograph (**a**) and coronal T1-weighted MRI (**b**). As shown here, the majority of GCTs are geographic and well-circumscribed, but do not have a sclerotic rim

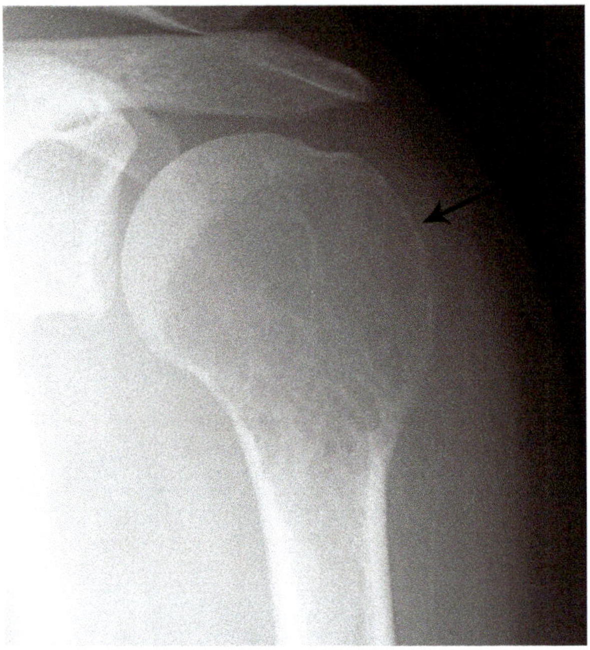

Fig. 2.22 Type IC geographic pattern. Giant cell tumor in the proximal humerus (*arrow*). In this case, the lesion is focal, but is not well-defined and does not have a sclerotic rim

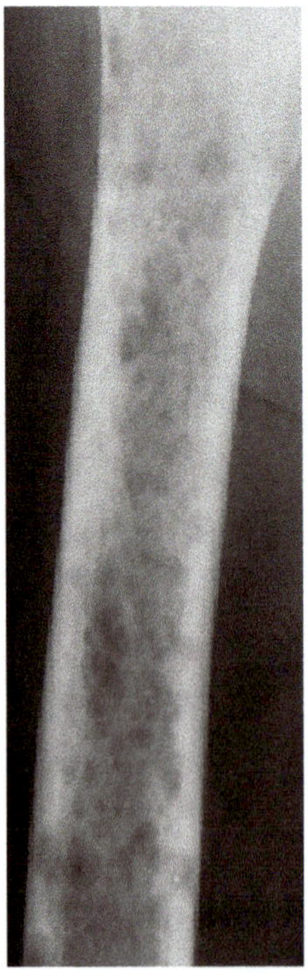

Fig. 2.23 Type II moth-eaten pattern. Lesions with a moth-eaten appearance, i.e., multiple discrete focal lytic lesions throughout the bone, tend to be aggressive lesions. Many of the lesions that present with this pattern are round cell tumors, in this case multiple myeloma

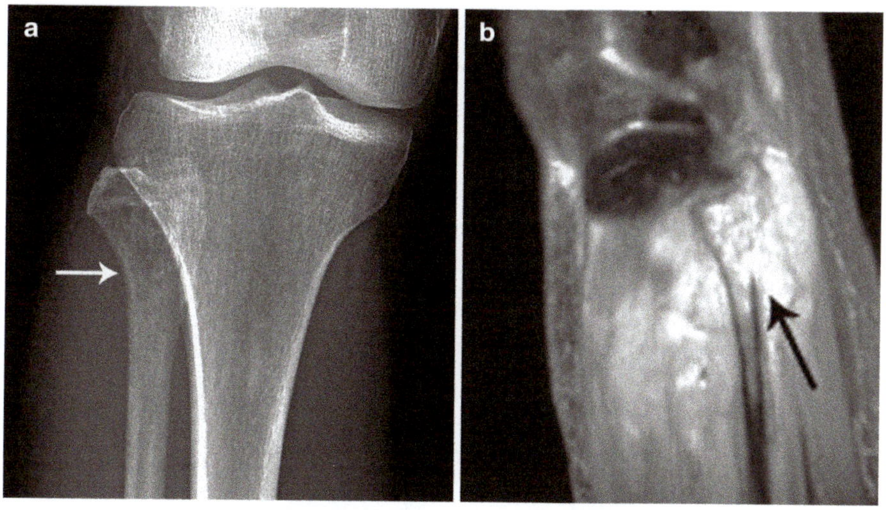

Fig. 2.24 Type III permeative pattern. The term "permeative" is used when the lesion permeates through the bone, but the pattern of bone destruction is so subtle as to be nearly invisible on radiographs. Permeative lesions tend to be aggressive and can be quite large, even though they are hard to detect on radiographs. Here, this plasmacytoma in the proximal fibula (*arrow*) is near-imperceptible on the radiograph (**a**), but it demonstrates extensive medullary involvement and soft tissue extension, seen as high signal on the sagittal fat-saturated T2-weighted MRI (**b**), and has even destroyed portions of the cortex (*arrow*)

The effect of the lesion on the surrounding cortex is also relevant to the diagnosis. Some lesions can cause endosteal scalloping of the cortex (thinning of the inner portion of the cortex) (Fig. 2.25). Endosteal scalloping is typical of enchondromas and other cartilaginous lesions and can also be seen with fibrous dysplasia. The depth of endosteal scalloping adjacent to an enchondroma is considered a sign of the lesion's aggressiveness: thinning of the cortex by >2/3 raises suspicion for a malignant cartilaginous lesion. Some lesions not only thin, but also bulge or expand the cortex (Fig. 2.26). Prominent, aneurysmal enlargement of the cortex with marked cortical thinning is characteristic for aneurysmal bone cyst (ABC), but mild bone expansion can also be seen in fibrous dysplasia or in slow-growing lesions occurring in small caliber bones, such as enchondroma, within a phalanx. In contrast, aggressive bone lesions demonstrate more aggressive cortical destruction, with marked cortical thinning and/or interruption (Fig. 2.27).

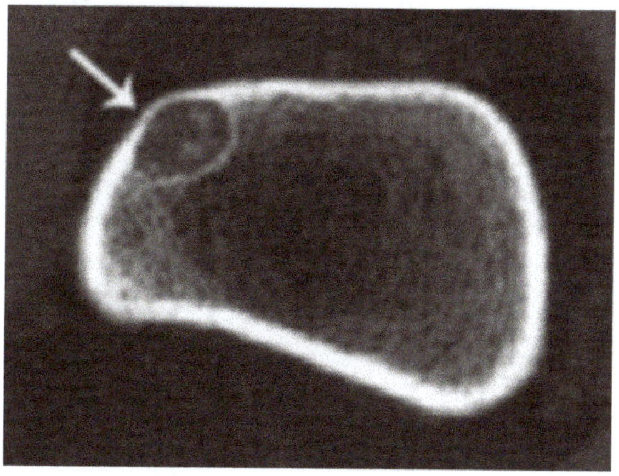

Fig. 2.25 Endosteal scalloping. Axial CT through an enchondroma, with overlying cortical thinning indicative of endosteal scalloping (*arrow*). Note chondroid matrix mineralization within the lesion

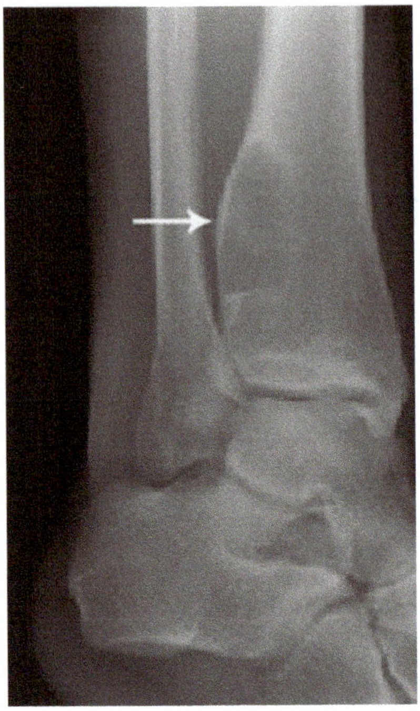

Fig. 2.26 Bone expansion and cortical thinning. Aneurysmal bone cyst (*arrow*) causing expansile remodeling of the distal tibia, with some thinning of the overlying cortex

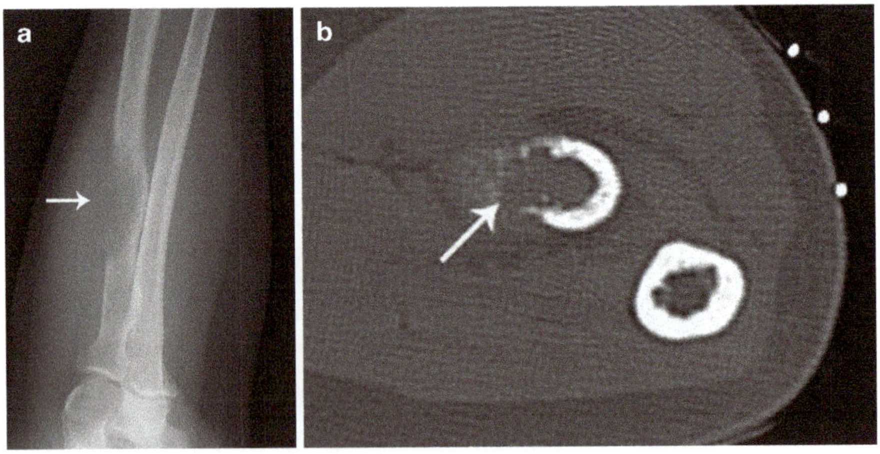

Fig. 2.27 Cortical destruction. Radiograph (**a**) and axial CT (**b**) depicting high-grade osteosarcoma (*arrows*) in the proximal radius causing frank cortical destruction

Matrix and Matrix Mineralization

The internal matrix of a bone tumor is material formed by the mesenchymal cells of the lesion itself. Lesion matrix can be osseous, cartilaginous, fibrous, or myxoid. Tumors—and their constituent mesenchymal cells—are typically named for the matrix they produce (e.g., osteosarcoma, chondroma, and fibroma). However, some bone lesions may not produce matrix (e.g., giant cell tumor and Ewing sarcoma) and others may contain fluid or fat. To further complicate matters, some lesions contain both matrix-producing and nonmatrix-producing components (e.g., ossifying lipoma) and other lesions can contain a mixture of matrix patterns (e.g., chondromyxoid fibroma, which has both chondroid and myxoid components; fibrous dysplasia, which can have both osseous and cartilaginous matrix).

At times, calcification and/or ossification may form in the lesion matrix, resulting in matrix mineralization. Matrix ossification may take the form of immature, woven bone or mature, lamellar bone. Depending on the circumstance, an osteosarcoma can form bony matrix that is more or less mature. When fibrous dysplasia forms bone, however, it is inevitably immature, woven bone. Woven bone in fibrous dysplasia is not as densely mineralized as mature lamellar bone, so it gives rise to the typical "ground glass" density associated with fibrous dysplasia. Matrix mineralization should not be confused with dystrophic calcification that forms in necrotic or degenerating tissue, callus or bone fragments from a pathologic fracture, or reactive sclerosis arising in non-neoplastic bone that surrounds the lesion.

Two main kinds of internal matrix can be distinguished (Tables 2.16 and 2.17; Figs. 2.28–2.30).

- ***Chondroid matrix mineralization***—arcs and rings; also stippled, flocculent—characteristic of lesions composed of cartilage, such as enchondromas.
- ***Osseous matrix mineralization***—cloudlike, fluffy, or ivory density—characteristic of bone-forming lesions, such as osteoarcomas.

Table 2.16 Lesions that can contain chondroid matrix mineralization

- Enchondroma
- Osteochondroma
- Juxtacortical chondroma
- Chondroblastoma
- Chondrosarcoma
- Chondromyxoid fibroma (less common)

Table 2.17 Lesions that can contain osseous matrix mineralization

- Osteosarcoma
- Parosteal osteosarcoma
- Ossifying fibroma
- Osteoma
- Osteoid osteoma
- Osteoblastoma

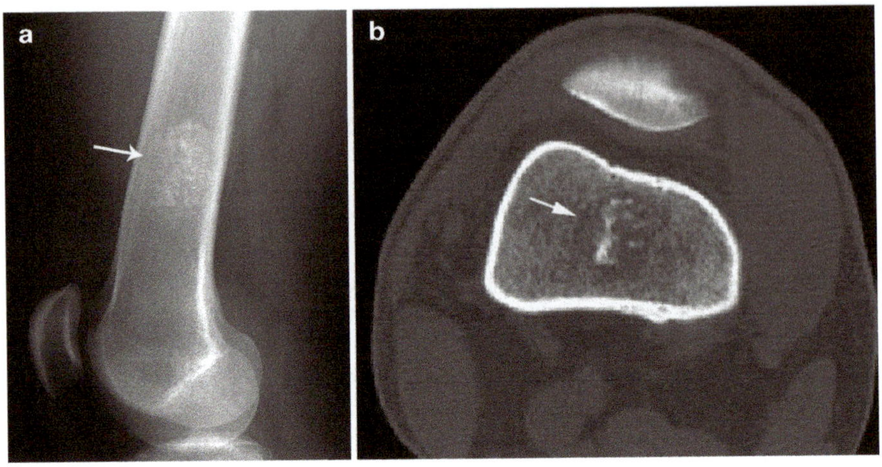

Fig. 2.28 Chondroid matrix mineralization. Lateral radiograph (**a**) of the knee shows a focal enchondroma with dense chondroid (cartilaginous) matrix mineralization (*arrow*), demonstrating the characteristic "arcs and ring" pattern. Axial CT (**b**) in a different patient shows a focal lucent lesion caused by the radiolucent hyaline cartilage of an enchondroma (*arrow*), with chondroid matrix mineralization, also in an "arcs and ring" configuration

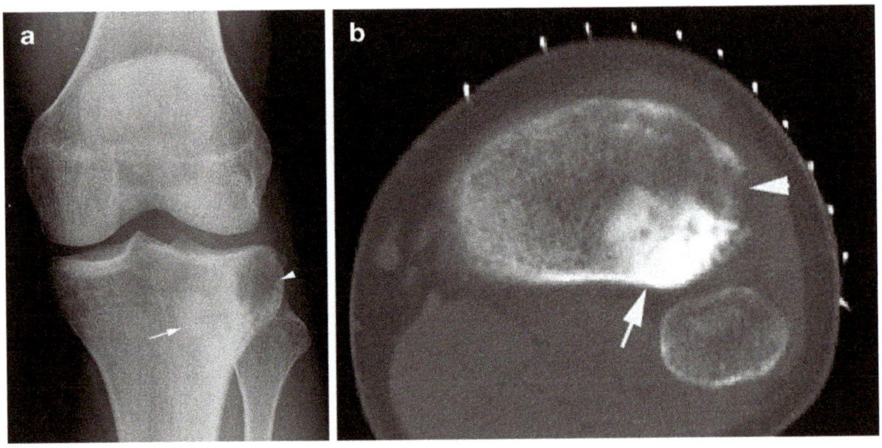

Fig. 2.29 Osseous matrix mineralization. AP radiograph (**a**) and axial CT (**b**) demonstrating cloud-like osseous matrix (*arrows*) within an osteosarcoma. Note adjoining areas of bony lysis and cortical destruction (*arrowheads*)

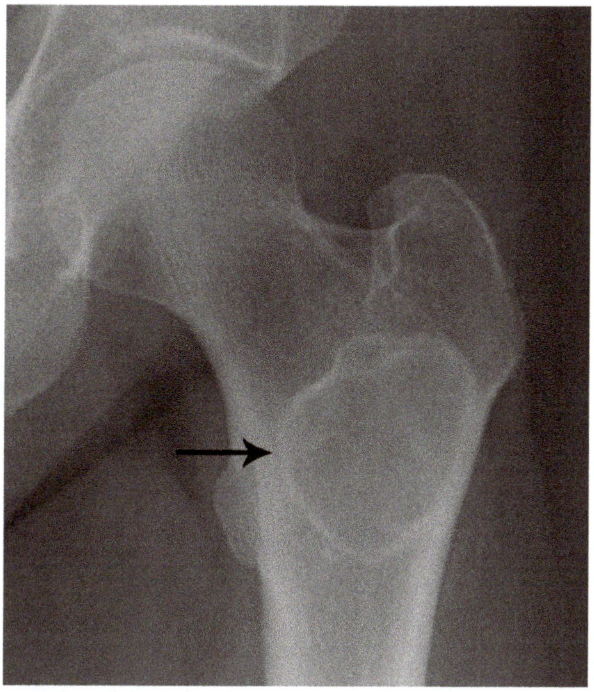

Fig. 2.30 Ground glass density. AP view of the proximal femur showing a focus of fibrous dysplasia (*arrow*). This is a common location and appearance for fibrous dysplasia. Although fibrous dysplasia is a lesion with fibrous matrix, it can contain immature woven bone, which tends to give it an intermediate "ground glass" density

Periosteal Reaction

Periosteal new bone formation is a nonspecific response of the periosteum to underlying "irritation." As periosteum is lifted up by an underlying bone lesion, it lays down new bone. The density of the new bone depends on whether the underlying process is expanding slowly or rapidly, with slow growth allowing for increased mineralization and greater density of the periosteal new bone. Nonaggressive periosteal reaction, in which a single line or lines of new bone can be traced in contiguity, suggests a slow-growing, nonaggressive process. Aggressive periosteal reaction suggests a fast-growing, aggressive process. Some authors use the term "uninterrupted" to refer to nonaggressive patterns of periosteal reaction and "interrupted" to refer to aggressive patterns of periosteal reaction. It is important to realize that aggressive-appearing periosteal reaction does not necessarily imply malignancy. Causes of nonaggressive periosteal reaction include vascular insufficiency and thyroid acropachy. Causes of aggressive new bone formation include not only malignancies such as osteosarcoma and Ewing sarcoma, but also aggressive benign processes, such as osteomyelitis and thalassemia (Table 2.18; Figs. 2.31–2.35).

Table 2.18 Periosteal new bone formation

Nonaggressive
• Thin
• Solid
• Thick, irregular
• Septated
Aggressive
• Laminated (onion skin)
• Spiculated
– Perpendicular/hair-on-end
– Sunburst
• Disorganized
• Codman triangle

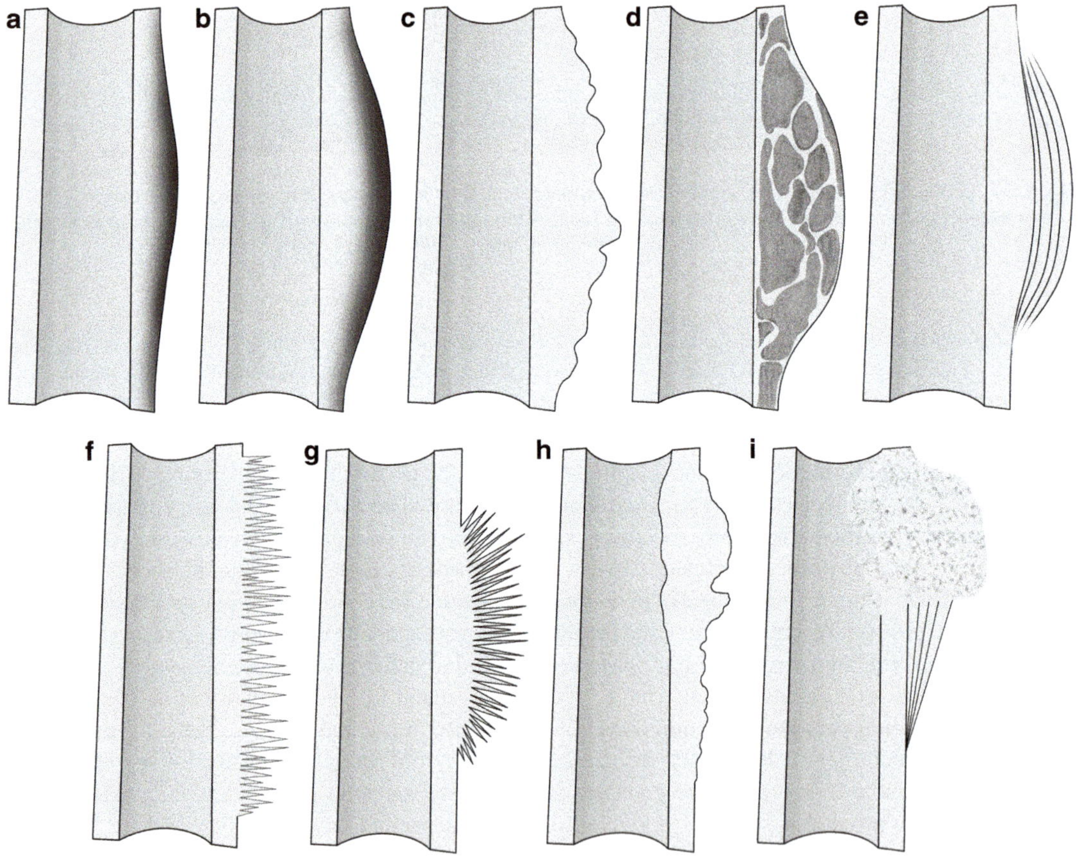

Fig. 2.31 Patterns of periosteal new bone formation. Nonaggressive forms are uninterrupted and include thin (**a**); solid (**b**); thick, irregular (**c**); and septated (**d**). Aggressive patterns are interrupted and include laminated or onion skin (**e**); spiculated in a perpendicular or hair-on-end pattern (**f**); spiculated in a sunburst pattern (**g**); disorganized (**h**); and Codman's triangle (**i**). Courtesy of Michael Larson, Boston, Massachusetts

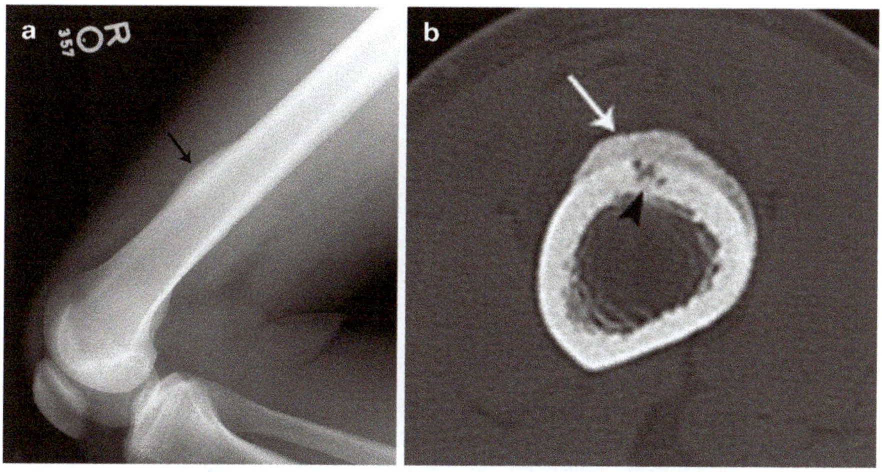

Fig. 2.32 Solid periosteal new bone (nonaggressive). Radiograph of the distal femur (**a**) shows a nonaggressive pattern of solid periosteal new bone formation along the distal femur anteriorly (*arrow*). Slow growth of the underlying process allows the bone matrix laid down by the periosteum time to completely mineralize, creating the uninterrupted, thickened pattern of periosteal new bone. Axial CT (**b**) in the same patient demonstrates the lucent nidus (*arrowhead*) of an osteoid osteoma centered in the cortex, as well as the reactive periosteal new bone (*arrow*) overlying the nidus. The solid periosteal new bone is homogeneously very dense, though not quite as dense as cortex

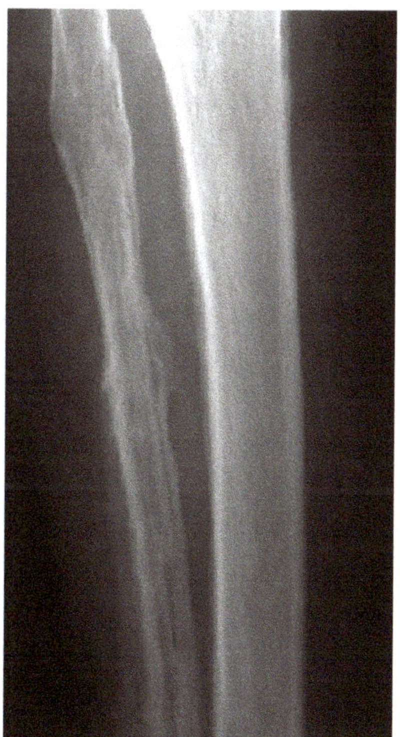

Fig. 2.33 Thick, irregular periosteal new bone (nonaggressive). Thick, irregular periosteal new bone along the fibula and, to a lesser extent, the tibia due to venous stasis

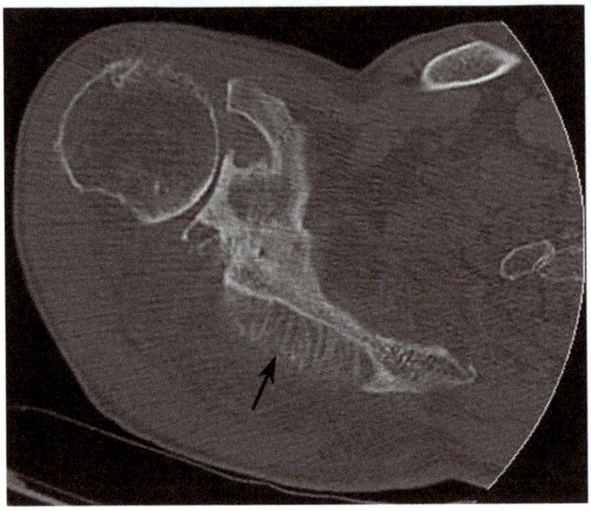

Fig. 2.34 Perpendicular or "hair-on-end" form of spiculated periosteal new bone (aggressive). Axial CT image shows classic "hair-on-end" periosteal reaction (*arrow*) associated with acute on chronic osteomyelitis in the scapula (Image courtesy of Dr. Lee Katz, New Haven, connecticut)

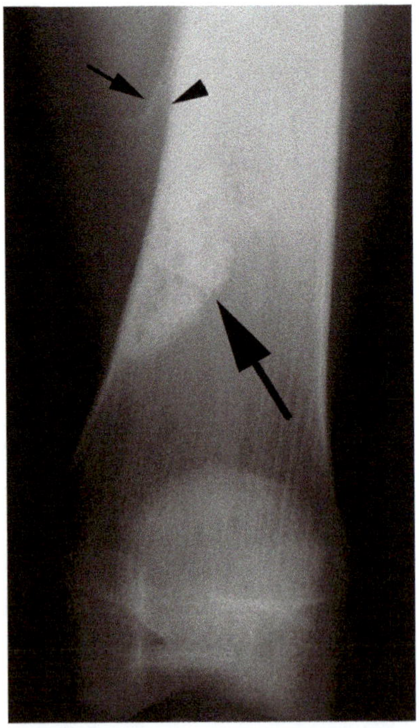

Fig. 2.35 Codman's triangle (aggressive). AP radiograph shows an osteosarcoma (*large arrow*) located eccentrically in the distal femoral metaphysis, seen as a predominantly sclerotic lesion. A radiolucent soft tissue component is lifting the periosteum and creating a Codman's triangle (*arrowhead* and *arrow*), an aggressive pattern of periosteal new bone formation

Soft Tissue Component

A soft tissue component extending outside bone typically indicates an aggressive lesion. However, some benign lesions can also have an associated soft tissue mass, e.g., osteomyelitis, GCT, ABC, and desmoplastic fibroma. Soft tissue extension from a bone lesion is probably not visible on radiographs, unless it is calcified or ossified or it distorts fat and muscle planes (Figs. 2.36–2.38). Nonetheless, soft tissues should be assessed for (1) density (e.g., fat, fluid, or air); (2) presence of calcification or ossification; and (3) secondary changes in the bone adjacent to a soft tissue abnormality. When possible, soft tissue calcification should be distinguished from ossification. In mature ossification, distinct cortical and medullary components are evident. This feature can be seen, for example, in myositis ossificans. However, this corticomedullary distinction is not expected in ossification associated with osteosarcomas—indeed, ossification associated with osteosarcomas tends to be more dense centrally and less dense peripherally. The morphology of calcifications should also be evaluated—similar to internal matrix mineralization, calcifications in areas of soft tissue extension may have an "arcs and rings" pattern characteristic of chondroid lesions or may have a cloud-like or amorphous pattern more typical of osseous lesions.

It can sometimes be difficult to determine whether a bone lesion is invading soft tissues or a soft tissue mass is invading bone. The geographic center of the soft tissue mass—bone versus soft tissue—often indicates its site of origin. The relative size of the lesion components and the location of the center of the process can also help: a large bone lesion with a small soft tissue component is more likely to originate in the bone while a large soft tissue component with a small bone lesion is more likely to originate in the soft tissues. One exception is Ewing sarcoma, which is a bone lesion that can be associated with a disproportionately large soft tissue mass. The presence of periosteal reaction can also help to determine the center of origin of a mass, since periosteal reaction is typically a feature seen with bone lesions that are centered in the bone and expanding out from it.

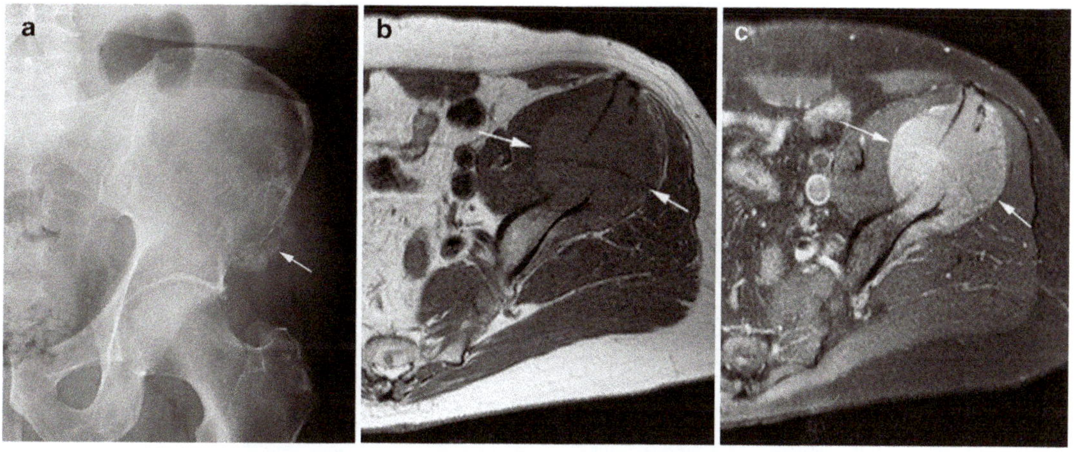

Fig. 2.36 Soft tissue extension. Pelvic radiograph (**a**) demonstrates a lytic lesion in the left iliac bone (*arrow*), somewhat difficult to discern due to overlying soft tissues. Corresponding axial T1-weighted (**b**) and postcontrast, fat-saturated T1-weighted (**c**) MR images show a large, enhancing soft tissue mass centered in the bone and expanding symmetrically outward, representing a plasmacytoma (*arrows*)

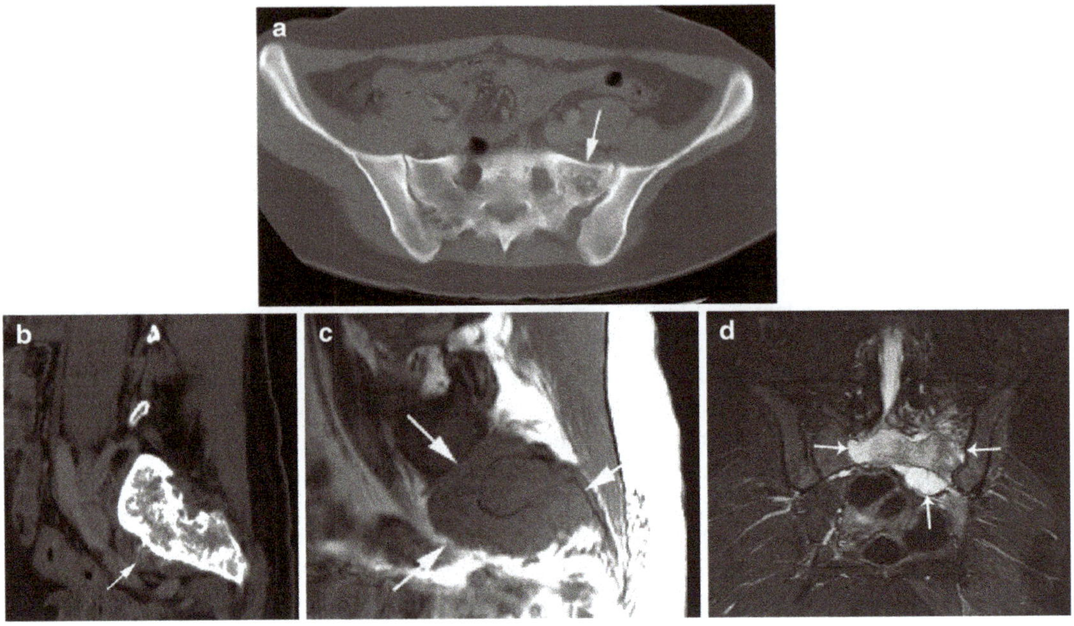

Fig. 2.37 Soft tissue extension. Axial CT image in bone windows (**a**) shows abnormal heterogeneous density in the left sacrum (*arrow*). Sagittal reformat CT (**b**) shows that there is a mass extending into the soft tissues anterior to the right sacrum (*arrow*), with aggressive hair-on-end periosteal new bone formation. Sagittal T1-weighted (**c**) and coronal fat-saturated T2-weighted (**d**) images show that the mass is continuous with the signal abnormality in the bone (*arrows*). Note that the periosteal new bone formation is more difficult to appreciate on the MR images

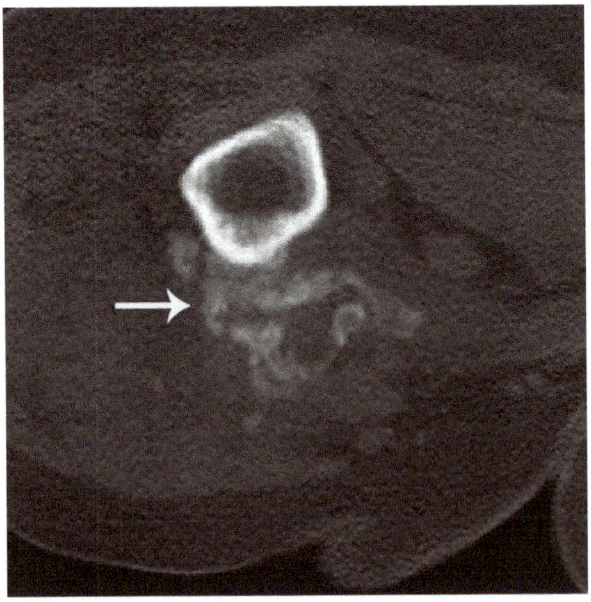

Fig. 2.38 Axial CT showing ossification in the soft tissues adjacent to the femur (*arrow*), related to myositis ossificans. The pattern of increased density peripherally (zoning) is characteristic of mature lamellar bone in the soft tissues. This pattern helps distinguish benign myositis ossificans from parosteal osteosarcoma, which is classically more densely mineralized in its central portion and near its bony attachment and less densely mineralized peripherally

Single or Multiple Lesions

When multiple lesions are present, the differential diagnosis for a bone lesion is shorter and more specific (Tables 2.19 and 2.20). In patients over 40 years old, multiple lucent lesions are highly suggestive of metastases or multiple myeloma (Figs. 2.39 and 2.40). In a child with constitutional symptoms, hematogenous spread of osteomyelitis or Langerhans cell histiocytosis should be considered. Multiple lucent lesions can also be seen in certain syndromes (e.g., polyostotic fibrous dysplasia in McCune–Albright syndrome and multiple enchondromas in Maffuci's or Ollier's syndromes). In contrast, primary bone tumors tend to be solitary.

A nuclear medicine bone scan is usually used to search for multiple bone lesions. However, a bone scan is typically only positive for lesions that cause reactive bone formation because the usual radionuclide agent employed—technetium-99m pertechnetate—is adsorbed onto newly deposited hydroxyapatite that has formed in response to the lesion itself. When lesions are predominantly lytic, then a radiographic skeletal survey is preferred. Skeletal surveys are typically used for assessment of multiple myeloma and other purely lytic lesions, such as renal cell carcinoma and thyroid carcinoma. In addition, PET and whole-body MR imaging can play a role in demonstrating lytic metastases. PET shows lytic metastases that are metabolically active and therefore take up the FDG radionuclide tracer. MRI shows lytic metastases because the tumor cells replace normal marrow and is most effective when the background marrow is comprised of fat.

Table 2.19 Multiple lytic lesions (mnemonic: FEEMHIS)

- Fibrous dysplasia
- Enchondroma
- EG (Langerhans cell histiocytosis)
- Metastasis, myeloma
- Hyperparathyroidism (Brown tumors)
- Infection (osteomyelitis)
- Sarcoid

Table 2.20 Multiple sclerotic lesions

- Blastic metastases
  - (breast, bladder, carcinoid, lung, medulloblastoma, prostate)
- Treated metastases
- Treated brown tumors
- Osteopoikilosis
- Multiple osteomas (Gardner syndrome)
- Melorheostosis
- Congenital stippled ephiphyses (chondrodystrophia calcificans congenita)
- Mastocytosis
- Tuberous sclerosis

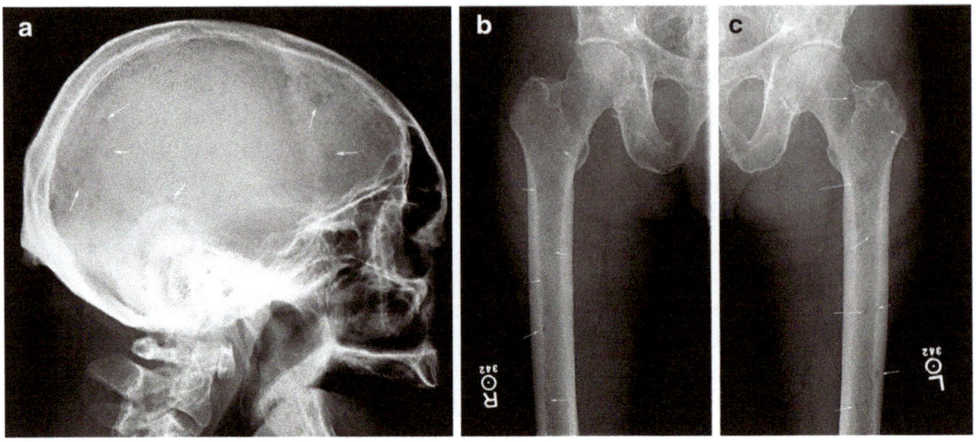

Fig. 2.39 Skeletal survey in multiple myeloma. Radiographs of skull (**a**) and both femurs (**b**, **c**) demonstrate multiple lytic lesions (*arrows*). In a patient over 40 years old, the presence of multiple lytic lesions would be highly suggestive of metastases or, as in this case, multiple myeloma

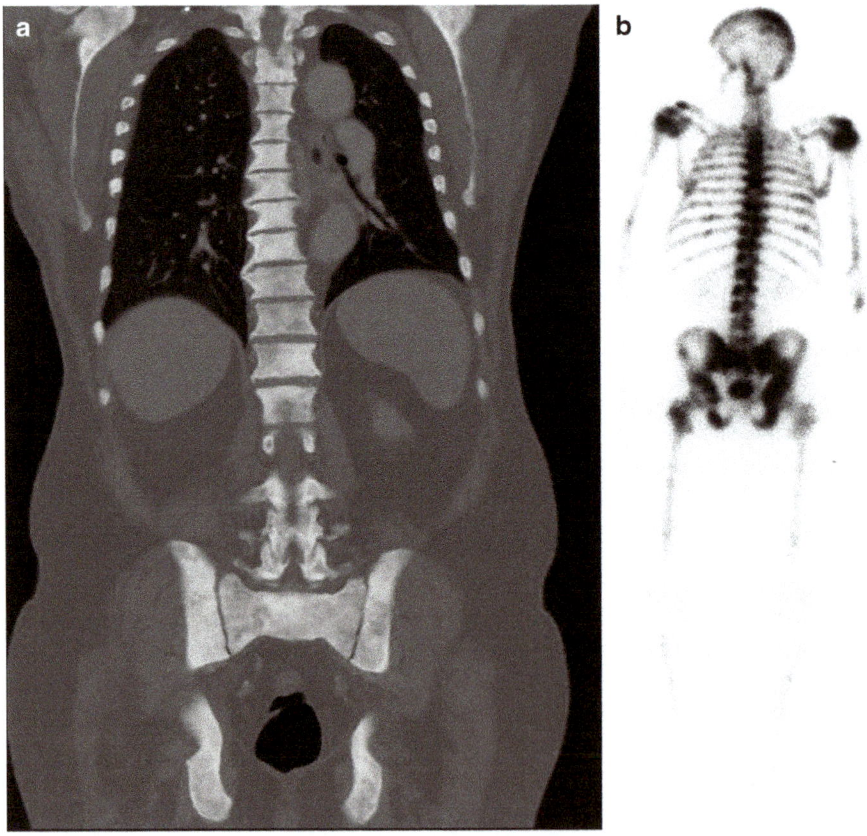

Fig. 2.40 Bone scan in metastatic prostate carcinoma. Coronal CT image (**a**) demonstrates diffuse sclerotic areas throughout the pelvis, spine, ribs, and scapula. Whole-body static image from technetium-99m bone scintigraphic exam (**b**) shows multiple areas of increased activity throughout the skeleton. Note the lack of uptake in the kidneys and soft tissues indicating a "superscan" appearance

Aggressive or Nonaggressive

It may not be possible to determine whether a lesion is benign or malignant, based on its imaging appearance. However, it is important to characterize a lesion as aggressive or nonaggressive, because aggressive lesions almost always warrant additional workup and may require biopsy. Aggressive features include ill-defined margins with a wide zone of transition, cortical breakthrough, aggressive forms of periosteal reaction, and a soft tissue component. In general, a grouping of aggressive features favors a malignant diagnosis, while nonaggressive features favor a benign diagnosis, but there is definitely overlap. Some benign processes can have a deceptively aggressive appearance, e.g., fracture, osteomyelitis, Langerhans cell histiocytosis, and giant cell tumor. On the other hand, some malignant processes can appear nonaggressive, e.g., low-grade chondrosarcomas and osteosarcomas and many metastases (Table 2.21; Figs. 2.41–2.44).

Table 2.21 Aggressive versus nonaggressive features of bone lesions

Aggressive features

- Moth-eaten or permeative pattern of bone destruction
- Indistinct margins/wide zone of transition
- Cortical breakthrough
- Aggressive periosteal reaction
  - Laminated (onion skin)
  - Spiculated
    - Perpendicular/hair-on-end
    - Sunburst
  - Disorganized
  - Codman triangle
- Soft tissue mass

Nonaggressive features

- Geographic pattern of bone destruction
- Well-defined margins/narrow zone of transition
- Sclerotic margins
- Intact cortex
- Nonaggressive or no periosteal reaction
  - Thin
  - Solid
  - Thick, irregular
  - Septated

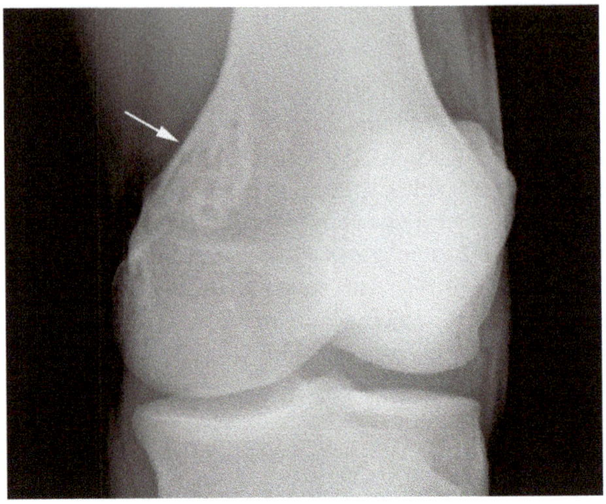

Fig. 2.41 Benign lesion with nonaggressive features. A mixed lucent and sclerotic lesion in the proximal tibia (*arrow*) demonstrates several nonaggressive features: well-defined with narrow zone of transition, sclerotic margins, intact cortex, lack of periosteal new bone formation, and lack of a soft tissue component. Diagnosis: non-ossifying fibroma

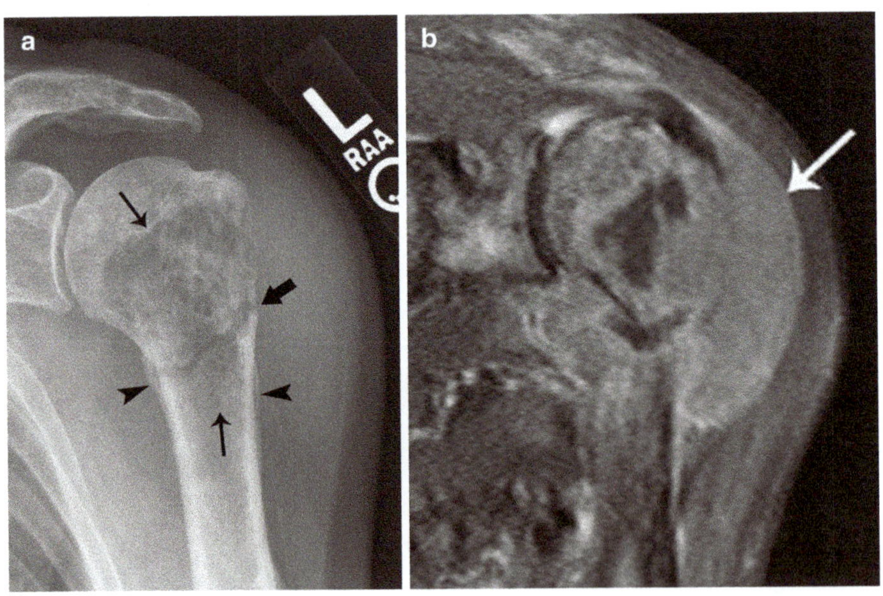

Fig. 2.42 Malignant lesion with aggressive features (B-cell lymphoma). Shoulder radiograph (**a**) shows a lytic lesion in the left proximal humerus (*arrows*), with pathologic fracture (*thick arrow*). There is periosteal reaction (*arrowhead*) related to the fracture. Although the lesion is geographic, it has aggressive features, including ill-defined borders with a wide zone of transition and cortical thinning and penetration. The coronal fat-saturated T2-weighted MR image (**b**) shows a large soft tissue mass extending out through the lateral humeral cortex. Pathologic fractures can occur in both benign and malignant lesions and are not specific for aggressive lesions

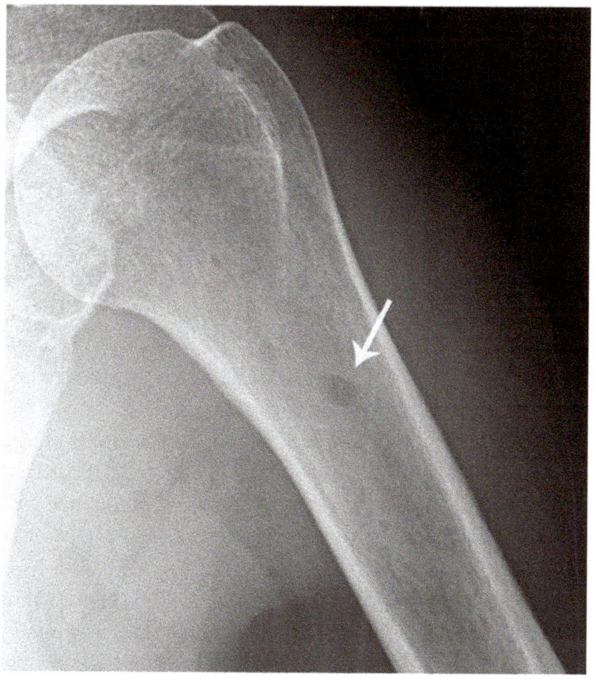

Fig. 2.43 Malignant lesion with nonaggressive features. Occasionally, a malignant lesion can have a deceptively non-aggressive appearance. Here, a focus of myeloma in the proximal humerus (*arrow*) does not demonstrate aggressive features. In a patient over 40 years old, myeloma should nonetheless be considered and appropriate lab work should be performed. (Potential pitfall: Iatrogenic bone defect due to biceps tenodesis should be excluded in this location!)

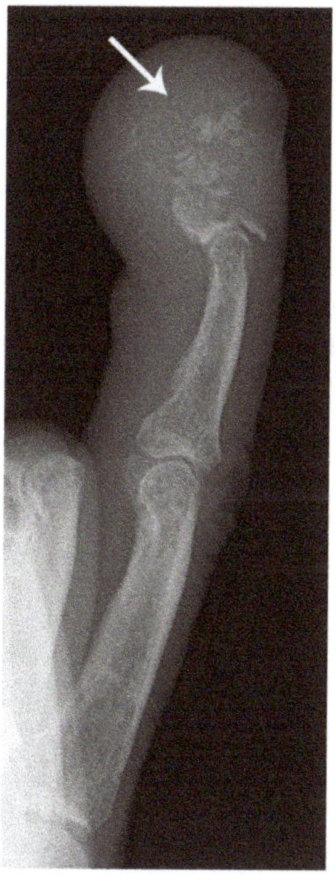

Fig. 2.44 Benign lesion with aggressive features. There is extensive osteolysis of the distal phalanx of the thumb (*arrows*), with aggressive features, such as indistinct margins and wide zone of transition, cortical destruction, and abnormality in the surrounding soft tissues. Some benign lesions, such as osteomyelitis (the diagnosis here) and Langerhans cell histiocytosis, should also be considered in the differential diagnosis of aggressive lesions

In Summary: Reporting the Bone Lesion

In summary, when reporting an imaging study that shows a bone lesion, you should make use of all available information, including the patient's age, clinical presentation, lesion location, and the lesion's imaging features. The description of the lesion should include a discussion of lesion density (lucent, sclerotic, or mixed); pattern of bone destruction (geographic, moth-eaten, and permeative); lesion margin (well- or ill-defined) and zone of transition (narrow or wide); the presence, absence, and thickness of any sclerotic reaction in the surrounding bone; available information regarding the lesion composition, e.g., fluid or fat; the presence, absence, and type of any internal matrix mineralization (chondroid and osseous) or of ground glass density; the presence and degree of any endosteal scalloping (and indicate whether it is less than or greater than 50% of cortical thickness); the presence and extent of any cortical penetration or interruption; the presence and degree of any bony enlargement (mildly expansile or aneurysmal enlargement); the presence and nature of any periosteal reaction (aggressive or nonaggressive); and the presence of a soft tissue mass (including nearby soft tissue calcifications, lucency indicative of nearby soft tissue fat, or saucerization of bone). A pathologic fracture should be searched for and, if present, reported, since it can cause findings that might confuse the picture (e.g., periosteal new bone formation or marrow edema pattern on MRI). If multiple lesions are present, that should be included. If the differential includes bone lesions that might be related to a systemic process, then pertinent secondary signs should be searched for and reported, e.g., bone resorption or rugger jersey spine in hyperparathyroidism; characteristic chest findings in sarcoid. On CT studies, reporting Hounsfield Units, indicative of lesion density, can suggest lesion composition (fat, fluid, soft tissue, or mineralized matrix). On MRI studies, the presence of high T2 signal edema pattern in the bone marrow and soft tissue should be reported, since it can be characteristic of certain lesions and can be absent in others (e.g., not seen in simple enchondromas, but seen in some giant cell tumors due to prostaglandin effects). On both CT and MRI studies, the presence and characteristics of any contrast enhancement should be described (slight, moderate, and marked; rapid/delayed; homogeneous/heterogeneous; peripheral, nodular, cystic, or necrotic). In addition, it is extremely important to assess change in the lesion over time by comparing with prior imaging studies. Lesions that are stable in appearance and size for several years are more suggestive of a benign process. Pertinent negatives are important to include, if they can effectively exclude certain diagnoses.

Using this information, you should be able to characterize a lesion as aggressive, nonaggressive, or indeterminate. Even if there are several nonaggressive features present, the most aggressive feature should be the determining one. Ultimately, you should provide a brief differential diagnosis, indicating the rationale for your choices. For aggressive lesions, recommendations for additional workup, including biopsy, when appropriate, should be included. Some nonaggressive lesions also warrant additional imaging, as detailed in the chapters that follow (Table 2.22).

Table 2.22 Reporting a bone lesion on an imaging study

Consider

- Patient age
- Clinical presentation
- Additional available imaging studies

Describe

- Lesion location
  - Which bone?
  - Where in the bone? Epiphysis/metaphysis/diaphysis
  - Where in the axial plane? Central/eccentric/cortical/juxtacortical
- Margin, pattern of destruction
  - Pattern of bone destruction—geographic/moth eaten/permeative
  - Zone of transition—well-defined/ill-defined
  - Sclerotic rim—none/thin/thick/incomplete
- Lesion composition
  - Fluid density on CT or cystic nonenhancement on MRI
  - Fat on CT or MRI
- Internal matrix mineralization
  - Chondroid
  - Osseous
  - Ground glass density (e.g., metaplastic woven bone in fibrous dysplasia)
- Cortical integrity
  - Endosteal scalloping— >50% thickness?
  - Cortical penetration or interruption
- Bone expansion, if present
  - Mildly expansile
  - Aneurysmal enlargement
- Periosteal reaction
  - Nonaggressive—thin, solid, thick, irregular, septated
  - Aggressive—laminated (onion skin), spiculated (perpendicular/hair on end; sunburst), disorganized, Codman triangle
- Soft tissue component
  - Soft tissue calcifications
  - Soft tissue fat
  - Cortical saucerization
- Single or multifocal
- Additional findings—e.g., osteoporosis, subperiosteal resorption, and acro-osteolysis
- If CT—Hounsfield units, enhancement pattern (e.g., slight, moderate, and marked; rapid/delayed; homogeneous/heterogeneous; peripheral, nodular, cystic, or necrotic)
- If MRI—edema-like signal in surrounding marrow or soft tissue, enhancement pattern

Provide conclusions

- Diagnosis, if possible
- If not, aggressive versus nonaggressive—most aggressive feature rules
- Brief relevant differential diagnosis with rationale
- Any previous data that helps establish the chronicity of the lesion
- Recommendations for additional workup or follow-up, including biopsy, if appropriate

Suggested Reading

1. Johnson LC, Vinh TN, Sweet DE. Bone tumor dynamics: an orthopedic pathology perspective. Semin Musculoskelet Radiol. 2000;4(1):1–15.
2. Kricun MR. Parameters of diagnosis In: Kricun, Morrie E, editors. Imaging of bone tumors. Chap. 1. Philadelphia: W.B. Saunders Company; 1993. p. 2–45.
3. Lodwick GS, Wilson AJ, Farrell C, et al. Determining growth rates of focal lesions of bone from radiographs. Radiology. 1980;134:577–83.
4. Madewell JE, Ragsdale BD, Sweet DE. Radiologic and pathologic analysis of solitary bone lesions. I. Internal margins. Radiol Clin N Am. 1981;19:715–48.
5. Madewell JE, Ragsdale BD, Sweet DE. Radiologic and pathologic analysis of solitary bone lesions. II. Periosteal reactions. Radiol Clin N Am. 1981;19:749–83.
6. Madewell JE, Ragsdale BD, Sweet DE. Radiologic and pathologic analysis of solitary bone lesions. III. Matrix patterns. Radiol Clin N Am. 1981;19:785–815.
7. Miller TT. Bone tumors and tumor-like conditions: analysis with conventional radiography. Radiology. 2008;246:662–74.
8. Priolo F, Cerase A. The current role of radiography in the assessment of skeletal-tumors and tumor-like lesions. Eur J Radiol. 1998;Suppl 1:S77–85.
9. Rana RS, Wu JS, Eisenberg RL. Periosteal reaction. Am J Roentgenol. 2009;193:W259–72.
10. Resnick D, Kransdorf MJ. Bone and joint imaging. 3rd ed. Philadelphia: Elsevier Saunders; 2005.

3 Imaging Modalities

When imaging bone tumors, the primary aims are to (1) identify the presence of a lesion; (2) characterize the lesion; and (3) delineate the location and extent of the lesion for staging and treatment. In these respects, each imaging modality has characteristic strengths and weaknesses. Certain modalities highlight features of a lesion better than others, contributing to an accurate diagnosis. Radiographs continue to be the best imaging modality to begin the workup and offer excellent assessment of the effects of the tumor on the host bone. CT and MRI can help troubleshoot certain features of the tumor and help in assessing the best targets for biopsy. Bone scan and PET/CT can establish the activity of the lesion and the distribution of disease. Often, the "workup" of a bone tumor or tumor-like lesion includes the use of several complementary imaging modalities. The utility of different imaging modalities for the workup of bone lesions is summarized below.

Radiographs

- Used in the initial evaluation of suspected or known bone tumor
- Guide the differential diagnosis by determining location, mineralization, and margins
- Best overall modality for characterizing a primary bone tumor
- Limited assessment of soft tissue component

Computed Tomography (CT)

- Confirms osseous origin when radiographs are ambiguous
- Demonstrates lesion features that may be subtle on radiograph: margins, internal matrix, mineralization, cortical destruction, and periosteal reaction

Magnetic Resonance Imaging (MRI)

- Good for assessing size and location of marrow and soft tissue extension
- Not very sensitive for detection of calcification or periosteal reaction
- In general, not specific for diagnosis, but can characterize some lesions based on certain appearances
- Aids preoperative planning, including assessment of neurovascular and joint involvement
- Routine targeted exams do not allow for detection of remote metastases, but additional sequences can detect skip lesions within a particular bone and can provide whole-body imaging
- Allows for assessment of tumor vascularity and helps target areas amenable to biopsy
- Can be useful in monitoring response to therapy and recurrence

J.S. Wu and M.G. Hochman, *Bone Tumors: A Practical Guide to Imaging*,
DOI 10.1007/978-1-4419-0808-7_3, © Springer Science+Business Media, LLC 2012

Bone Scintigraphy (radionuclide bone scan)

Can demonstrate many radiographically occult bone lesions

Specificity limited, as both benign and malignant processes can demonstrate increased activity

Allows for whole-body imaging that can demonstrate polyostotic lesions and aid in staging

Demonstrates distribution of disease that can aid in characterization or biopsy planning

Can help in monitoring response to therapy

Flouro-deoxy-glucose Positron Emission Tomography (FDG-PET)

Limited experience to date for primary bone tumors

Is useful for detection of metastatic disease for a variety of nonosseous malignancies

Has a promising potential role in the diagnosis, staging, and follow-up of bone tumors with radiopharmaceuticals, including FDG and NaF

Ultrasound

Negligible role in imaging of bone tumors due to shadowing from cortex

Can be used to biopsy bone tumors when prior CT or MRI demonstrates extraosseous soft tissue component

Radiographs

Radiographs should be the initial study performed in the evaluation of a suspected or known bone lesion. In most instances, radiographs are the most effective modality for demonstrating the key features that are used to characterize bone lesions. By providing information regarding lesion location, internal matrix, margins, and associated periosteal reaction, radiographs play a central role in guiding the differential diagnosis. Assessment of soft tissue extension on radiographs is usually limited, unless there are characteristic soft tissue calcifications or the mass is predominantly fatty. Often, a soft tissue mass is not apparent radiographically, even when large, unless it causes significant distortion of tissue planes.

Questions to Answer When Assessing Radiographs

- Is there a lesion?
- Is there mineralized internal matrix and, if so, what kind?
- What are the lesion margins and effect on surrounding cortex?
- Is there periosteal reaction?

Is There a Lesion?

Bone lesions become visible on radiographs because they (1) replace normal marrow; (2) replace or distort the normal trabecular structure; (3) create reactive sclerosis or resorption in the surrounding bone; or (4) cause thinning, scalloping, bulging, or disruption of the cortex. The ability to detect a bone lesion on radiographs depends on the degree to which the normal structure is altered in these ways. For example, infiltrative lesions may permeate through the bone without much disruption of trabeculae and may be difficult to detect on radiographs. These infiltrative lesions are often better demonstrated on MRI. Bone-forming lesions, such as an osteosarcoma or prostate metastasis, replace normal marrow with osseous material. Visibility is directly related to the amount of bone loss or bone formation. For example, in order for a cortical lytic lesion to be visible on radiographs, at least 50% of the cortex must be destroyed. The ability to detect a lesion is also dependent on good radiographic technique so that bone contrast is optimally displayed and bony anatomy is optimally visualized.

Is There Mineralized Matrix and, If So, What Kind?

Radiographs can demonstrate the presence and quality of matrix mineralization, which can help narrow the differential: matrix mineralization in an "arcs and rings" pattern indicates a chondroid lesion (Fig. 3.1) while matrix mineralization in a "cloud-like" pattern is suggestive of an osseous lesion. "Ground glass" density within a lesion is seen with immature, woven bone and is suggestive of fibrous dysplasia.

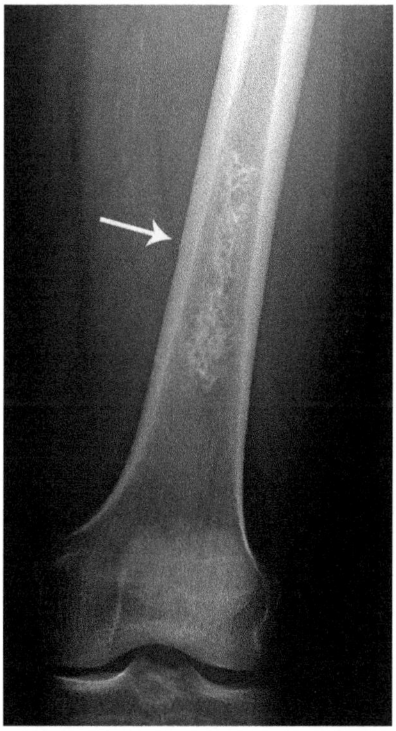

Fig. 3.1 Enchondroma (*arrow*) with chondroid matrix calcifications

What Are the Lesion Margins and the Effect on Surrounding Cortex?

Lesions with well-defined margins (narrow zone of transition) tend to be less aggressive; lesions with poorly defined margins (wide zone of transition) tend to be more aggressive. In some areas of complex bony anatomy, a tomographic technique, such as CT or magnetic resonance imaging (MRI), may be required to better define lesion margins. Some lesions may elicit a sclerotic reaction from the surrounding bone, which suggests that the lesion is indolent, growing slowly enough that the surrounding bone has time to form reactive bone (Figs. 3.2 and 3.3). For example, a benign enchondroma has well-defined margins with a thin sclerotic rim, while aggressive lesions, like Ewing sarcoma or acute osteomyelitis, tend to have poorly defined margins without sclerotic borders. If the lesion abuts the cortex, the presence of endosteal scalloping, bony expansion, or cortical penetration can be observed (Fig. 3.4).

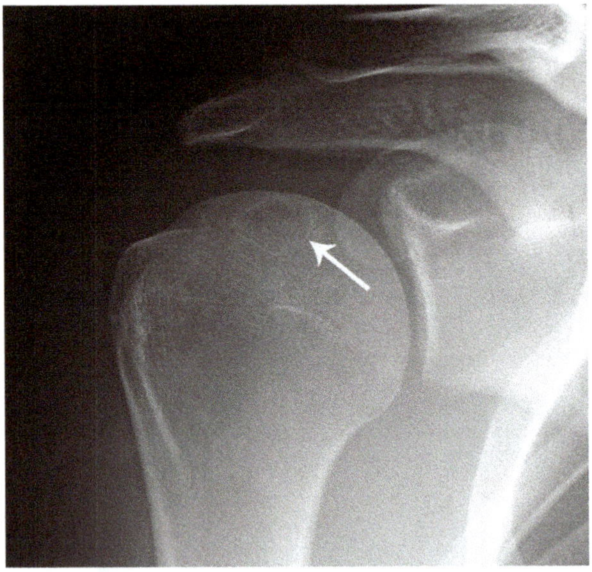

Fig. 3.2 Chondroblastoma. A round, lucent lesion in the epiphysis (*arrow*) has well-defined margins, consistent with a nonaggressive lesion. It has a thin, sclerotic rim, which represents a reactive response formed by the surrounding bone to the lesion. When present in a geographic lesion, the sclerotic rim can be an indication of slow lesion growth rate

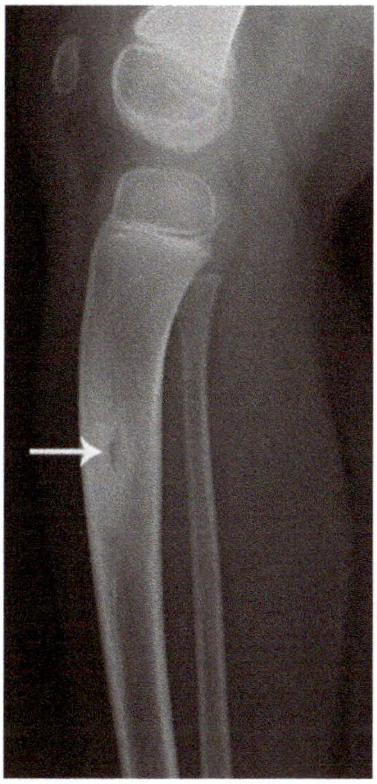

Fig. 3.3 Osteoid osteoma. A small, rounded lucency (*arrow*) has elicited a large area of reactive sclerosis in the surrounding bone. This pattern is characteristic of an osteoid osteoma, though this could also be seen in Brodie's abscess

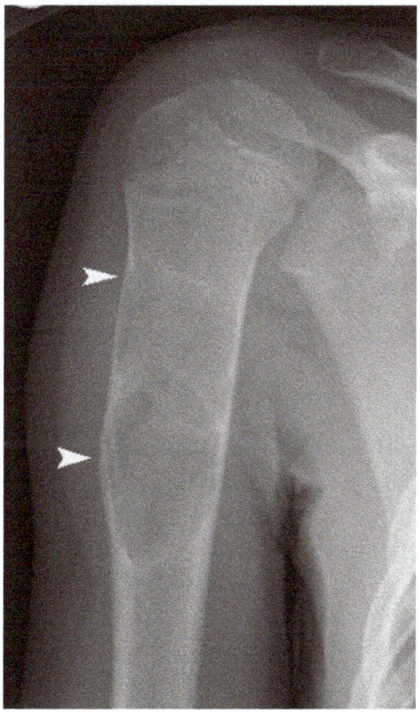

Fig. 3.4 Simple (unicameral) bone cyst. An elongated lucent lesion extends across the entire width of the proximal humerus. The overlying cortex is thinned and the lateral cortex is remodeled, creating a slightly expansile contour (*arrowheads*). The expansile cortex and remodeling around the lesion indicate a slow rate of lesion growth. In contrast, faster growing, aggressive lesions tend to break through the cortex, without time for cortical remodeling (image courtesy of Dr. Daniel Siegal, Detroit, Michigan)

Is There Periosteal Reaction?

Radiographs can demonstrate the presence of periosteal reaction and characterize it as aggressive or nonaggressive. Flat or wavy, uninterrupted, periosteal new bone is associated with a nonaggressive process. Lifted-up and discontinuous periosteal reaction is associated with an aggressive process, either benign or malignant. Lesions such as simple bone cysts, aneurysmal bone cysts, non-ossifying fibromas, and enchondromas are not associated with periosteal reaction, unless they are complicated by fracture. Lesions such as osteosarcoma, Ewing sarcoma, and lymphoma, often demonstrate aggressive periosteal reaction (Fig. 3.5). Acute osteomyelitis, although benign, is another entity that can demonstrate aggressive periosteal reaction.

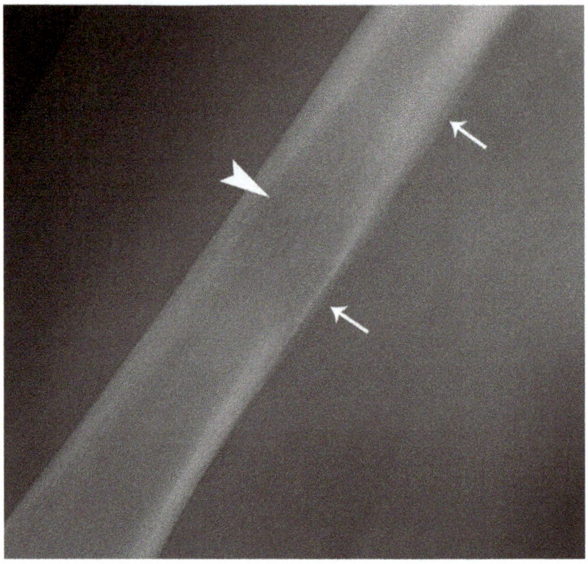

Fig. 3.5 Melanoma metastasis. There is irregular, discontinuous, periosteal new bone formation along the posterior femoral cortex (*arrows*), indicating an aggressive process. Note the lytic lesion (*arrowhead*) in the medullary cavity with poorly defined margins and cortical thinning

Computed Tomography

CT is a useful second-line modality when it is difficult to determine whether a lesion actually arises from the bone or when a more detailed look at typical "radiographic" features (internal mineralization, lesion margins, cortical features, and periosteal reaction) is required. For areas that are difficult to evaluate because of overlapping structures, such as the pelvis or midfoot, CT's tomographic capability can be used to better visualize the lesion and its "radiographic" features. The ability to generate reformatted images in any plane from the helically-acquired CT image sets is particularly helpful. CT also plays an important role in image-guided biopsy. In the future, rapid-acquisition, dual-energy CT, a recently introduced technique, may contribute to the evaluation of bone tumors. Dual-energy CT is based on acquiring two datasets from the same anatomic location using different kVps (usually, 80 and 140 kVp). Early musculoskeletal applications include differentiation of uric acid and calcium crystals (gout versus pseudogout), reduction of metal artifact, CT arthrography, and detection of bone marrow edema and infiltration.

Questions to Answer When Assessing CT Studies

- Does the lesion arise from bone?
- Is there characteristic internal content (fat, fluid, fluid levels, and matrix mineralization)?
- What are the marginal, cortical, and periosteal features (lesion borders, surrounding sclerosis, endosteal scalloping, cortical breakthrough, and periosteal reaction)?

Does the Lesion Arise from Bone?

While it may seem that localizing a lesion to the bone would be easy from a radiograph, it can often be very difficult due to complex anatomy and the inability to visualize the interface between the lesion and underlying bone in true profile. CT can address this problem through the use of tomographic imaging. Multiplanar-reformatted images can provide high spatial resolution and high contrast depiction of high-density structures, such as cortical bone and internal mineralization. The differential diagnosis of an ossified lesion in the soft tissues is highly dependent on determining whether the abnormality is located entirely in the soft tissues (favoring, e.g., myositis ossificans) or arising from the underlying bone (suggesting a surface lesion, such as an osteochondroma or parosteal osteosarcoma) (Fig. 3.6).

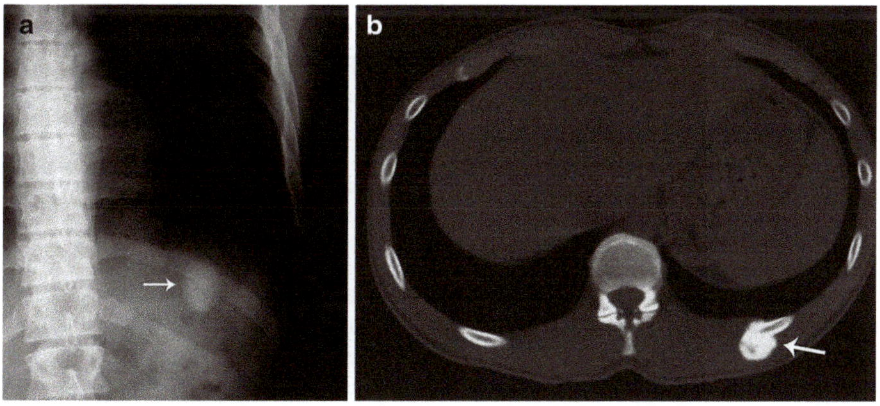

Fig. 3.6 Based on the radiograph (**a**), this ossified mass (*arrow*) could either arise from the rib or soft tissue or from organs anterior or posterior to the rib. The axial CT (**b**) shows that the lesion arises from the surface of the rib (*arrow*), consistent with the diagnosis of parosteal osteosarcoma

Is There Characteristic Internal Content?

CT provides quantitative data, in terms of Hounsfield units, to aid in characterizing the internal content of a lesion. Typical Hounsfield values are fat −70 to −130 HU, simple fluid 0 to +12, hematomas and proteinaeous fluid +20 to +70, muscle and similar soft tissues +40 to +60, and dense bone +1,000 to +2,000. CT can help to demonstrate fluid levels in simple (unicameral) and aneurysmal bone cysts and to show fallen fragments within a simple bone cyst. CT also serves an important complementary role to radiographs in characterizing matrix mineralization of a bone lesion. On some occasions, matrix may not be evident or well-seen on radiographs. In these instances, CT images can be used to demonstrate the characteristic "arcs and rings" chondroid mineralization seen in cartilage lesions, the dense, "cloud-like" osteoid mineralization of an osseous lesion, or the absence of internal matrix mineralization in a giant cell tumor or other lesion, thereby helping to narrow the differential diagnosis (Fig. 3.7).

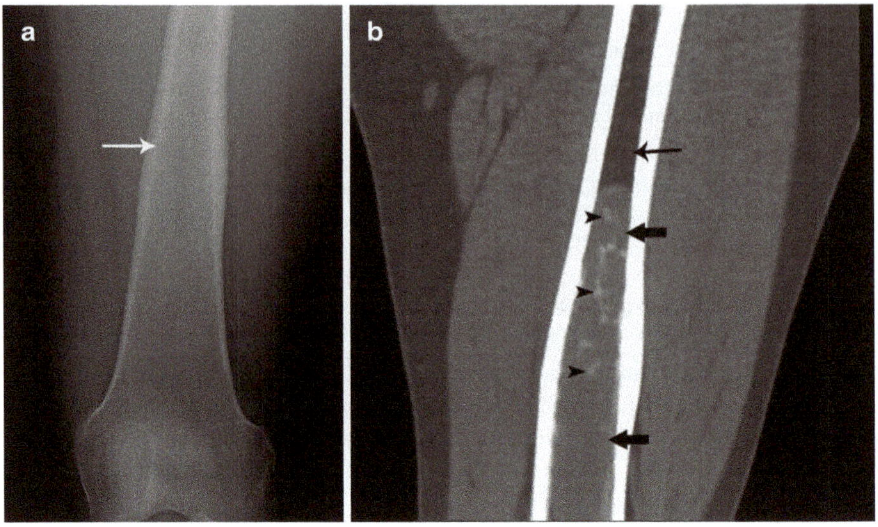

Fig. 3.7 Enchondroma. Chondroid matrix (*arrow*) is not well-seen on the radiograph (**a**), but is well-demonstrated on the coronal CT image (**b**). Note the difference in density between the normal fatty marrow (*thin arrow*) and the enchondroma (*thick arrows*). Cartilage calcifications (*arrowheads*) appear as areas of increased density within the lesion

What Are the Marginal, Cortical, and Periosteal Features?

CT provides a more detailed look at the "radiographic" features of a bone lesion. When lesion margins or reactive bone sclerosis is obscured on radiographs due to surrounding bone or overlapping anatomy, these features can be exquisitely demonstrated using computed tomography. CT can also aid in assessment of the cortex, a crucial step in the evaluation of bone lesions. The appearance of the cortex can help guide the differential diagnosis, with aggressive patterns of cortical destruction increasing suspicion for aggressive processes, such as malignant tumors or infection. Accurate assessment of cortical destruction is also important for prognosis: destruction of more than 50% of the cortex increases the risk of pathologic fracture (especially in a weight-bearing bone, such as the femur) and should be reported as an urgent finding to the referring physician.

CT is the ideal modality for the assessment of the cortex. Radiographs may show evidence of cortical destruction, but may miss areas of abnormality if the cortical change is small or subtle or if the X-ray beam is not optimally oriented with respect to the site of abnormality. MRI depicts normal cortex as low signal on all sequences. However, the "baseline" thickness and position of normal cortex on MRI are distorted by susceptibility and chemical shift artifacts and, as such, are highly dependent on the sequence and sequence parameters. As a result, subtle areas of cortical thinning or destruction can be obscured.

CT is particularly well-suited for imaging lesions that arise within the cortex. Intracortical lesions, such as osteoid osteoma, stress fracture, and Brodie's abscess, can be associated with cortical thickening that obscures the underlying lesion on radiographs. CT can help demonstrate the underlying lesion and identify key distinguishing features: the small rounded radiolucent nidus of an osteoid osteoma, linear lucency of a stress fracture, or lucencies associated with a cloaca or intracortical Brodie abscess in osteomyelitis. CT can also help to detect the intramedullary form of osteoid osteoma, which can be completely obscured by reactive sclerosis on radiographs (Figs. 3.8–3.10).

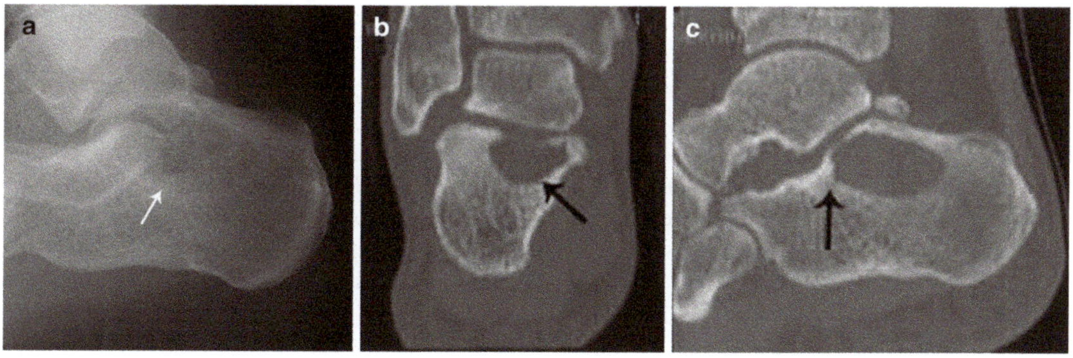

Fig. 3.8 Calcaneal chondroblastoma. Radiograph (**a**) of the hindfoot shows a well-defined ovoid lucency in the calcaneus (*arrow*), but the relationship of the lesion to the subtalar cortex is not well-seen. CT images (**b**, **c**) better depict the extent of juxta-articular cortical thinning. They also confirm the absence of matrix mineralization

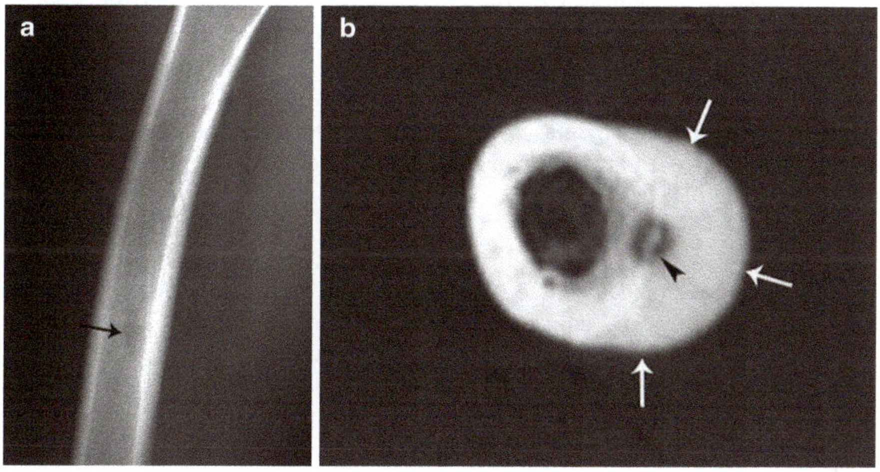

Fig. 3.9 On the femur radiograph (**a**), there is a small lucent lesion in the femur (*arrow*), but the margins are obscured by reactive sclerosis. Axial CT image (**b**) provides direct visualization of the lesion (*arrowhead*) and its borders, allowing for a definitive imaging diagnosis of periosteal osteoid osteoma. CT also demonstrates the mature, nonaggressive, periosteal new bone formation (*arrows*) elicited by the lesion

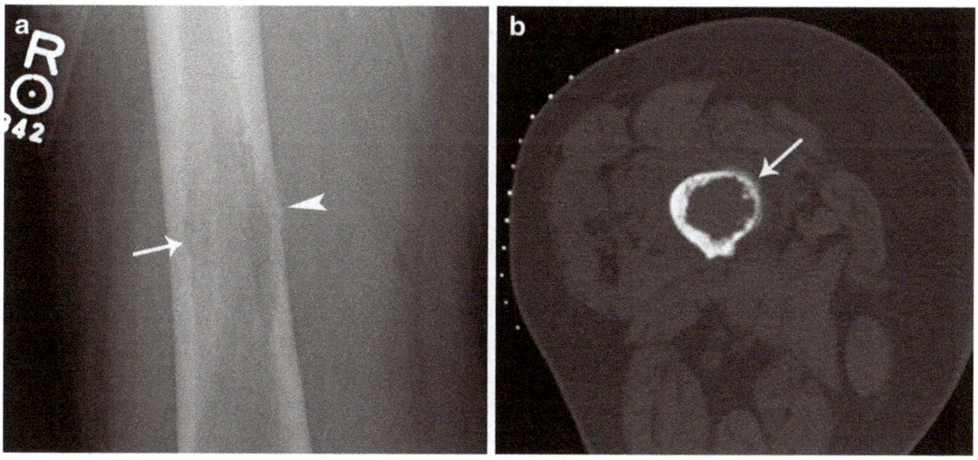

Fig. 3.10 Radiograph (**a**) shows a subtle lytic metastasis in the femoral diaphysis, with thinning of the cortex (*arrow*) and very subtle periosteal new bone (*arrowhead*). Axial CT image (**b**) through the femur better depicts the extent of cortical destruction, including areas of cortical fenestration and overlying periosteal reaction (*arrow*)

Magnetic Resonance Imaging

In general, radiographs or CT are used to characterize bone lesions while MRI is used to determine lesion extent for treatment and surgical planning. MRI is very sensitive for detection of bone marrow involvement, including marrow changes that may be occult on radiographs or CT. MRI is also the preferred study for demonstrating soft tissue extension because of its high intrinsic soft tissue contrast.

Although sensitive for detection of an abnormality, MRI findings are often nonspecific in appearance and require correlation with clinical history and radiographic appearance for improved lesion characterization. In a subset of cases, MRI can demonstrate additional features that may aid in tumor characterization, such as fat in a hemangioma or intraosseous lipoma or fluid-fluid levels in an aneurysmal bone cyst. The radiologist should be aware that several very important features of bone lesions may be very difficult to appreciate on MR images. These features include calcifications within the lesion, sclerotic reaction surrounding the lesion, small cortical defects, and periosteal new bone formation. Contraindications to MRI include ferromagnetic aneurysm clips, metallic foreign bodes in the orbits, pacemakers, cochlear implants, insulin pumps, and other electronic implants. Hardware creates susceptibility artifact that can limit assessment of nearby marrow and soft tissue. The degree of metal artifact varies with the type of metal and with the sequence and sequence parameters; however, various hardware artifact-reducing techniques can be employed. Orthopedic hardware can also, albeit rarely, be a contraindication to MRI and can sometimes cause patient tissue heating.

When reviewing a bone tumor on MRI, key features to assess and report on are the size and signal characteristics of the bone lesion; the presence, size, and characteristics of any soft tissue components; gadolinium enhancement characteristics, including any solid areas amenable to biopsy; extension into any other anatomic compartments; involvement of surrounding structures, such as the joint space, neurovascular structures, and surrounding muscles, tendons, or ligaments; and, when appropriate, the presence of skip metastases. Relationship to important anatomic landmarks should also be described.

Questions to Answer When Assessing MR Images

- What is the extent of marrow involvement?
- Is there soft tissue extension?
- Are there MRI features that that can help with further characterization?
- Is there involvement of neurovascular structures, joint space, or other anatomic compartments?
- Are there skip lesions within the bone?
- How vascular is the lesion? Where is the best place to biopsy?
- Has there been a response to treatment?

What Is the Extent of Marrow Involvement?

MRI is highly sensitive for detection of marrow abnormality and can demonstrate marrow involvement by tumor, even when radiographs, CT, and bone scan are negative (Figs. 3.11 and 3.12). It is the most accurate modality for assessing bone lesion extent and for quantifying lesion volume. However, MRI can overestimate bone lesion extent when there is surrounding peritumoral “reactive” marrow edema (Fig. 3.13). On the other hand, when the marrow signal is normal, MRI carries a very high negative predictive value.

Normal marrow signal varies depending on its fatty or erythropoietic composition, which, in turn, varies with patient age and medical status. Normal fatty marrow is high signal on T1, intermediate to high signal on T2-weighted images, and low signal on fat-saturated T2-weighted (FS T2W) and STIR images. Bone lesions are usually readily visible as an alteration in the typical signal pattern, on T1-weighted (T1W), FS T2W images, or both. Normal erythropoeitic marrow is lower signal than fat, but slightly higher in signal intensity than normal muscle or normal intervertebral disc on T1W images and intermediate signal intensity—i.e., similar to muscle—on FS T2W and STIR images. On T2W images, particularly those obtained with fast/turbo spin echo technique, fatty and erythropoeitic marrow may be difficult to distinguish. Patients who are anemic or have chronic illnesses may demonstrate reconversion from fatty to erythropoietic marrow. Normal marrow can have some heterogeneous patterns that can appear striking, but are nonetheless normal, and it is useful to become familiar with these patterns to avoid potential pitfalls.

Bone lesions appear as alterations of the normal marrow pattern. Replacement of normal bone marrow by osteoid, cartilage, fibrotic material, neoplastic, granulomatous or inflammatory cells, or edema alters the normal MRI appearance of the tissue. Sclerotic bone tends to be low signal on T1- and T2-weighted images while areas of bone tumor infiltration associated with increased interstitial fluid tend to have high signal on T2W or FS T2W images. The MR signal intensity of the lesion may reflect a mix of low- and high-signal components. For example, hyaline cartilage is notably bright on T2W images, but, when the matrix is calcified, includes corresponding areas of low T2 signal intensity. High T1 signal may reflect the presence of hemorrhage, fat, or proteinaceous fluid. The specificity of abnormal bone marrow signal around a tumor is limited; however, bone marrow edema-like signal can be seen within uninvolved marrow adjacent to tumor so that the extent of MR signal abnormality can overestimate the extent of bone marrow involvement by tumor. However, the negative predictive value of normal-appearing marrow is high.

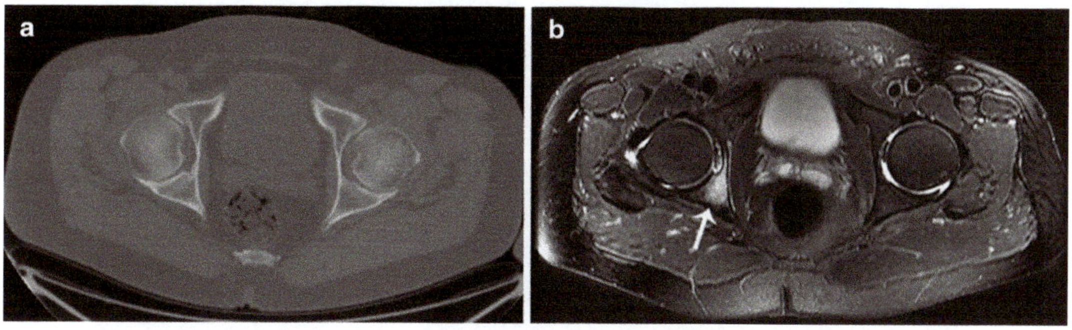

Fig. 3.11 The patient presented with right hip pain, but no lesion, was detected on the CT scan (**a**). The axial fat-saturated T2-weighted MR image (**b**) shows focal abnormal high signal in the posterior column (*arrow*). Biopsy revealed metastatic melanoma

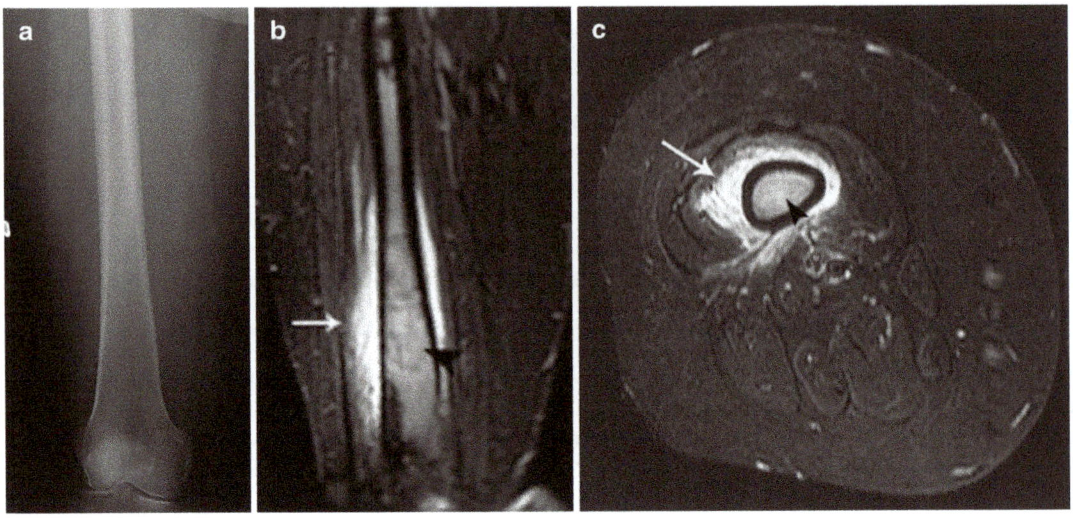

Fig. 3.12 48-Year-old man with leg pain and normal appearing femur radiograph (**a**). Coronal (**b**) and axial (**c**) fat-saturated T2-weighted MR images show extensive abnormally elevated marrow signal throughout the femur (*arrowheads*) and edema in the surrounding soft tissues (*arrows*), in this patient with biopsy-proven lymphoma. Infiltrative lesions can permeate the bone while remaining near-imperceptible on radiographs or CT

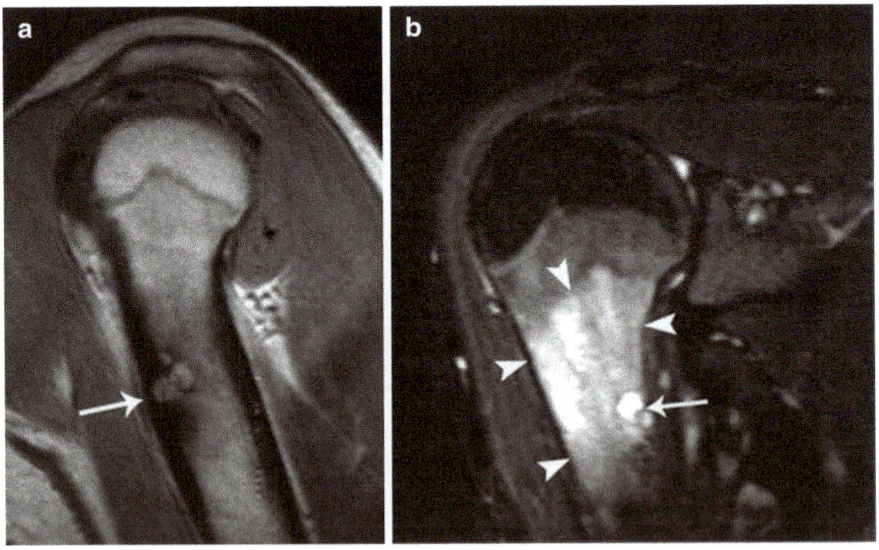

Fig. 3.13 Sagittal proton density MRI image (**a**) shows a small focal cortically based lesion in the medial proximal humerus (*arrow*). Fat-saturated T2-weighted MR image (**b**) shows that the lesion (*arrow*) is surrounded by profuse-reactive marrow edema (*arrowheads*), involving a much larger area of the bone. In this case, the extent of the marrow abnormality overestimates the size of the lesion. The differential diagnosis includes osteoid osteoma and Langerhans cell histiocytosis

Is There Soft Tissue Extension?

MRI is the method of choice for identifying the presence of soft tissue extension of bone tumors due to its high intrinsic soft tissue contrast (Figs. 3.14 and 3.15). Although CT can also demonstrate soft tissue extension from bone tumors, particularly when contrast is employed, the abnormalities are typically more readily detected on MRI. Soft tissue extension is best depicted on axial MR images, and is often assessed on T2-weighted, fat-saturated T2-weighted, or contrast-enhanced images. As with the intraosseous component, peritumoral soft tissue edema may be present and may lead to overestimation of the size of the soft tissue mass. IV gadolinium contrast helps to demonstrate areas of cyst formation or necrosis within the bone and soft tissue components and can also help in delineating borders of the soft tissue component. Presence of soft tissue extension is considered an aggressive feature and can aid in differential diagnosis. However, both benign and malignant lesions can demonstrate soft tissue extension, e.g., osteomyelitis, Langerhans cell histocyosis, osteosarcoma, and Ewing sarcoma. Some lesions characteristically show no soft tissue extension, e.g., fibrous dysplasia and osteoid osteoma. In some cases, the presence of soft tissue extension indicates a more aggressive form of the index lesion, e.g., giant cell tumor and adamantinoma.

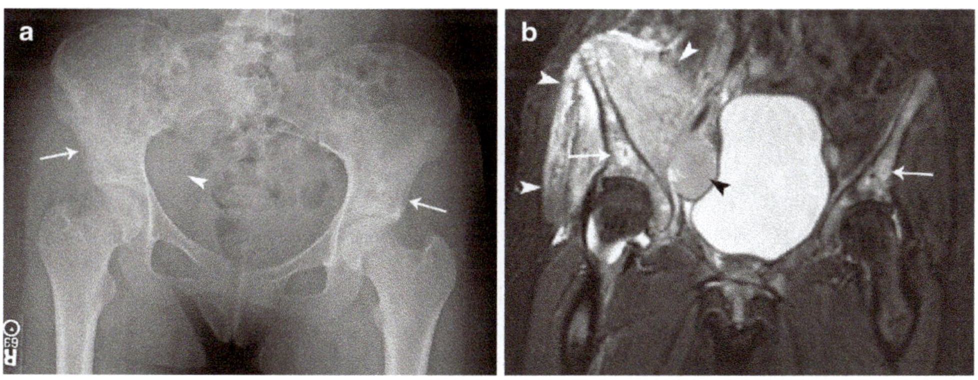

Fig. 3.14 Radiograph (**a**) shows irregular mineralization in both the right and left iliac bones (*arrows*), but no cortical destruction or gross soft tissue abnormality. On careful scrutiny, subtle distortion of a fat plane (*arrowhead*) and displacement of bowel gas can be seen medial to the right iliac bone, suggesting a soft tissue mass. Coronal fat-saturated T2-weighted MRI image (**b**) shows diffusely abnormal signal throughout both iliac bones (*arrows*) and readily demonstrates a large mass extending outward from the right iliac bone (*arrowhead*) in this patient with lymphoma

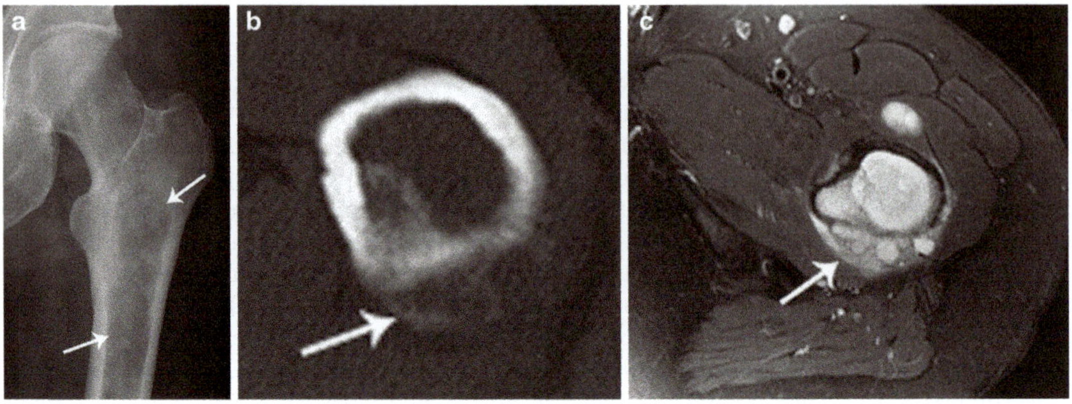

Fig. 3.15 Chondrosarcoma. AP radiograph (**a**) shows an ill-defined area of abnormal lucency and sclerosis in the proximal femur. Axial CT (**b**) shows cortical thinning and abnormal mineralization in the intramedullary cavity and periosteal reaction (*arrow*). Axial fat-saturated T2-weighted MR image (**c**) not only shows the intramedullary lesion, but also demonstrates the contiguous soft tissue extension (*arrow*). Note that the cortical abnormalities and periosteal reaction are better depicted by CT, but the marrow abnormalities and soft tissue mass are better seen on the MRI

Are There Lesion Features that Can Help with Further Characterization?

In general, radiographs and CT remain the methods of choice for characterization of bone tumors. However, MRI can help to demonstrate features that aid in characterization. For example, bone infarcts may mimic enchondromas or create nonspecific bone density on radiographs, but they have a pathognomonic appearance on MRI. In general, high T1 signal on MRI can indicate fat, methemoglobin from hemorrhage, proteinaceous fluid, melanin, or gadolinium enhancement. However, intraosseous lipomas can be readily diagnosed on MRI because macroscopic fat in the lipoma decreases in signal on T1W images obtained with frequency-selective fat saturation. In-and out -of- phase MR sequences can demonstrate microscopic fat, which can help in the diagnosis of intraosseous hemangioma (Fig. 3.16). MRI can demonstrate fluid–fluid levels, suggesting a diagnosis of primary or secondary aneurysmal bone cyst (Fig. 3.17). High T2 signal can indicate fluid in a cyst or necrotic area, hyaline cartilage in an enchondroma, or myxoid tissue. Low T2 signal can be seen with fibrosis, calcification, hemosiderin, and densely cellular tissues. It should be noted that some benign lesions appear deceptively aggressive on MRI and correlative imaging with radiographs is important. For example, large amounts of reactive edema can be associated with osteomyelitis, Langerhans cell histiocytosis, and osteoid osteoma. Because detection of matrix, periosteal new bone, cortical bone, and soft tissue calcification is limited on MRI, radiographs, and occasionally CT, remain important adjuncts.

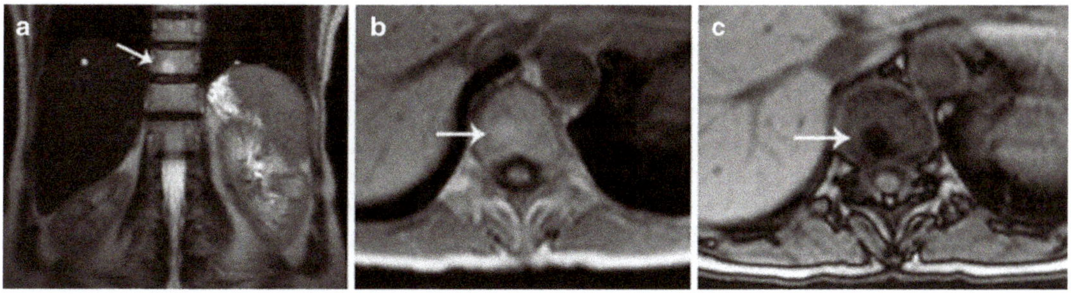

Fig. 3.16 Coronal single shot fast spin echo (HASTE) image (**a**) shows a rounded high-signal lesion in the T12 vertebral body (*arrow*). The differential diagnosis includes metastasis and benign intraosseous hemangioma. Axial in-phase (**b**) and out-of-phase (**c**) T1-weighted gradient echo MR images confirm the presence of intravoxel fat, supporting a diagnosis of hemangioma. The lesion is high signal on the in-phase image (*arrow*), but loses signal (gets darker) on the out-of-phase image (*arrow*) due to the presence of microscopic fat (images courtesy of Dr. Suzanne Long, Philadelphia, PA)

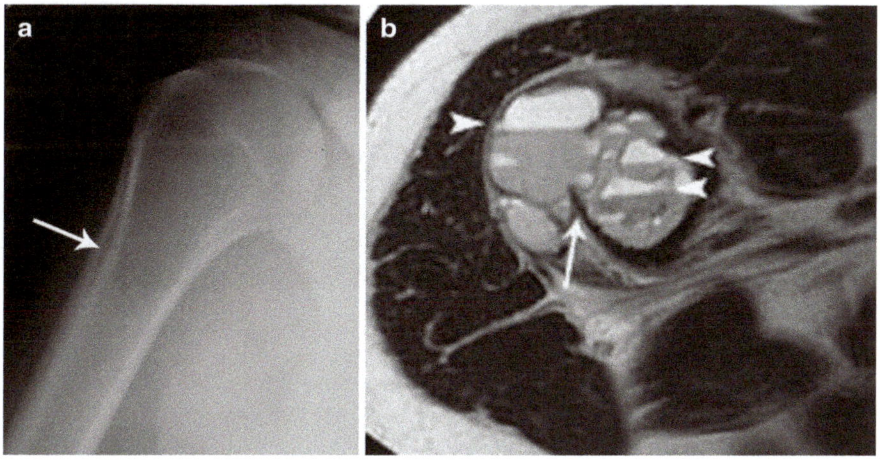

Fig. 3.17 AP radiograph of the proximal humerus (**a**) shows a faint lucent lesion in the proximal humerus (*arrow*). Axial T2-weighted MRI image (**b**) through the same patient shows multiple fluid-fluid levels (*arrowheads*), with non-dependent higher signal representing simple fluid and dependent lower signal representing proteinaceous fluid and debris. The presence of multiple fluid levels is highly suggestive of ABC, but can be seen in either primary or secondary ABC and, as a secondary ABC, can occur in both benign and malignant lesions. Note that there is soft tissue extension (*arrow*) through a breach in the cortex

Is There Involvement of Neurovascular Structures, Joint Space, or Other Anatomic Compartments?

MRI plays an extremely important role in local staging of a bone lesion and in preoperative planning because of its ability to demonstrate the involvement of critical surrounding structures, including invasion or encasement of neurovascular structures, extension into a joint, muscle invasion, and extension into an adjoining anatomic compartment. These areas must be carefully evaluated and reported. Relationship to any surgically relevant anatomic landmarks should also be described. Axial T1W and T2W images are essential for assessment of compartmental anatomy and neurovascular involvement.

Coronal, sagittal, or oblique images can help to evaluate articular involvement and can also help to demonstrate the relationship to neurovascular structures (Fig. 3.18). Unless a fat plane can be demonstrated between the tumor and overlying neurovascular structures, involvement of the vessel or nerve cannot be excluded. Nonetheless, when the tumor is draped over or displaced by a tumor and no fat plane is detected, it may still not be infiltrated by tumor and it may be possible to "peel off" the vessels or tumor at surgery. IV contrast can sometimes help to delineate tissue planes and help evaluate for tumor infiltration. However, nontumoral reactive enhancement may also occur, leading to overestimation of tumor extension. In the future, diffusion tensor imaging may play a role in evaluation nerve infiltration.

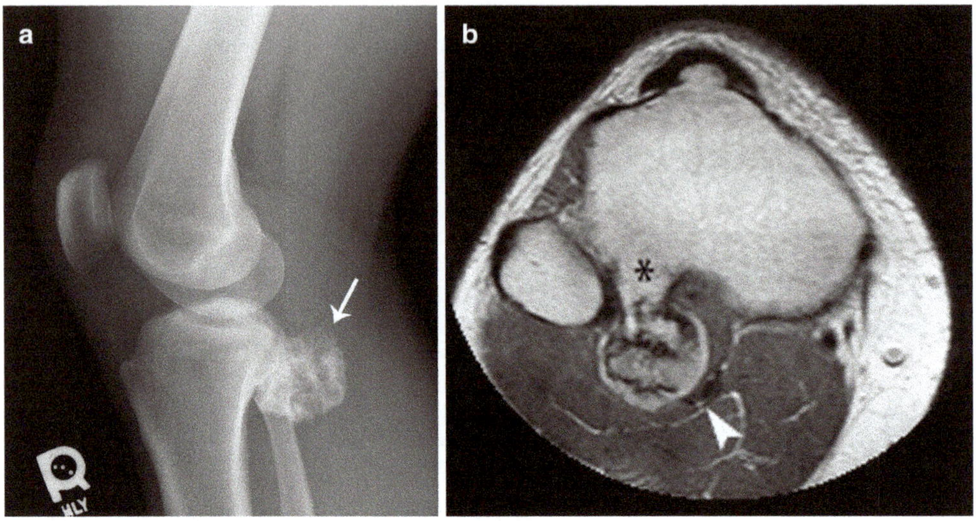

Fig. 3.18 Lateral radiograph of the knee (**a**) demonstrates a pedunculated osetochondroma arising from the posterior proximal tibia. Note "arcs and rings" chondroid calcifications in the cartilage cap (*arrow*). Axial PD-weighted MRI image (**b**) shows that the osteochondroma is displacing and compressing the popliteal neurovascular bundle (*arrowhead*). Note the contiguity of the marrow cavities between the lesion and host bone (*asterisk*)

Are There Skip Lesions Within the Bone?

In most cases, an MRI examination is targeted to a specific location and a small field of view is employed in order to maximize spatial resolution in the area of interest. In general, assessment for distant metastases would be performed by a bone or PET scan or, in some institutions, by whole-body MRI. However, for tumors with a propensity to form skip metastases in the same bone, an additional sequence with a larger field of view that encompasses the entire bone should be performed (Fig. 3.19). Osseous skip metastases are most often associated with osteosarcoma, but may also be seen with Ewing sarcoma. Recently, techniques for large field of view "whole-body" MRI imaging for detection of remote metastases have been described. Bone or PET scans remain the modalities of choice for whole-body imaging, but MRI may play an important adjunct role for lytic lesions that are not well-demonstrated on bone scans and for which PET scan is not indicated.

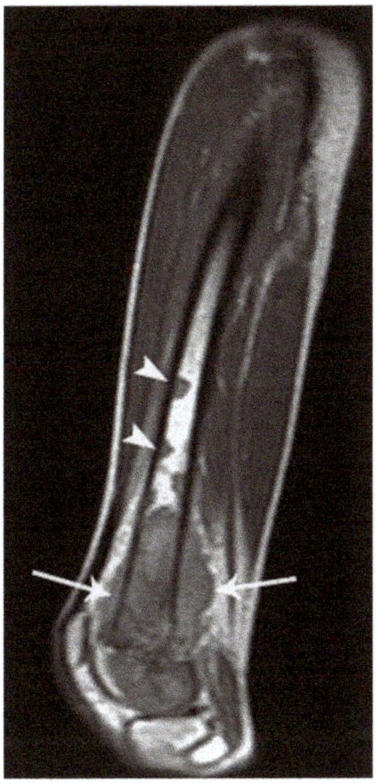

Fig. 3.19 Sagittal T1-weighted MRI shows an osteosarcoma centered in the distal femur, with anterior and posterior soft tissue extension (*arrows*). Additional small "skip" metastases (*arrowheads*) are seen more proximal in the femoral diaphysis, separated from the index lesion by normal high T1 signal marrow fat. (Image courtesy of Dr. Megan Anderson, Boston, MA.)

How Vascular is the Lesion? Where Is the Best Place to Biopsy?

Most bone tumors are visible on MRI without the use of intravenous contrast due to signal alterations on the T1W and/or T2W images. Though intravenous contrast is of limited utility in characterizing lesions on MRI, it does help to distinguish cystic from solid lesions, particularly when the lesion is high signal on T2W. Cystic lesions show only a thin rim of peripheral enhancement without internal enhancement. This can be highlighted by subtracting pre- and postcontrast images. Two important pitfalls are: (1) When comparing pre- and postcontrast images, images must be obtained with the exact same technique and parameters, preferably in sequential order and without changing the transmit gain between the two image sets. (2) Chondroid lesions also typically demonstrate peripheral enhancement, with limited internal enhancement, and should not be mistaken for cysts, even though they may be very high signal on T2W images. IV contrast can also distinguish cystic and solid areas *within* a lesion and, as such, can help identify solid nodules within a tumor that are amenable to biopsy. Contrast can also help guide biopsies of solid lesions, as areas that enhance are more likely to yield diagnostic material at biopsy (Fig. 3.20).

IV contrast can sometimes help with staging by helping to delineate tumor involvement of joint, muscle, and overlying neurovascular structures. It is important to be aware that not all areas that enhance with contrast represent tumor—edema, inflammation, and vascularized fibrosis can also enhance.

Postcontrast images obtained with non-dynamic technique can provide a very rough assessment of tumor vascularity, but, in fact, non-dynamic enhancement within a lesion reflects a complex composite of tumor vascularity, vessel permeability, and interstitial space. The early phases of dynamic-enhanced images can provide a more quantitative assessment of lesion vascularity and can demonstrate the lesion's relationship to feeder and draining vessels. As noted above, the use of dynamic gadolinium enhancement to evaluate response of sarcomas to chemotherapy and to demonstrate tumor recurrence has also been described.

Although anaphylactic reaction to gadolinium contrast is quite rare, there are new concerns about the role of certain types of gadolinium contrast as a cause of nephrogenic systemic fibrosis (NSF), the risk of which is increased in the setting of renal failure. For this reason, a current creatinine value is often required prior to contrast-enhanced MRI, if there is reason to think that the patient may have diminished renal function.

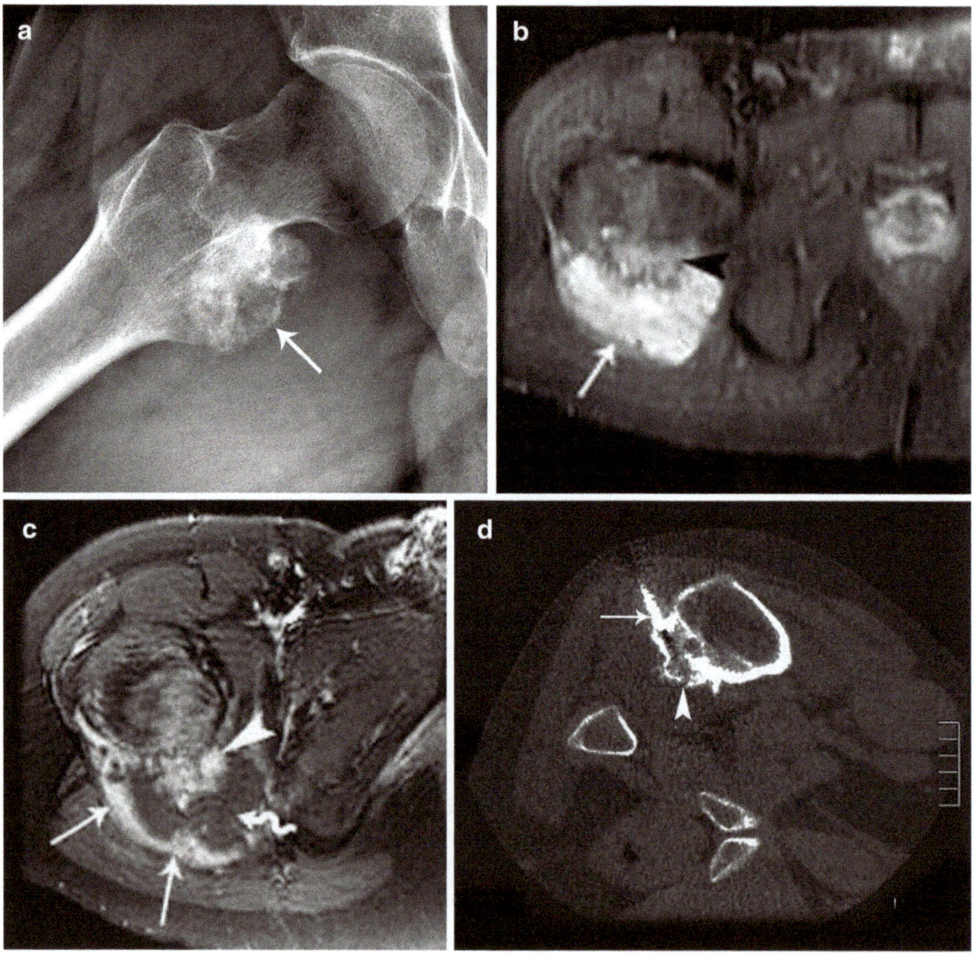

Fig. 3.20 Frog leg lateral view of the hip (**a**) shows a sessile osteochondroma arising from the greater trochanter (*arrow*). Axial fat-saturated T2-weighted MRI image (**b**) demonstrates high signal representing an enlarged cartilage cap (*arrow*), with marrow edema pattern in the bony component of the osteochondroma. Axial postcontrast subtraction MRI image (**c**) shows thick, irregular rim enhancement (*arrows*), lack of central enhancement (*wavy arrow*) from necrosis, and a cortically based enhancing soft tissue component (*arrowhead*) which would be the best area to target on the biopsy. Axial image from the CT-guided biopsy (**d**) shows the needle (*arrow*) in the cortically based component seen on the MRI. The biopsy revealed malignant degeneration of an osteochondroma to a chondrosarcoma

Has There Been Response to Treatment?

MRI is often used to assess tumor response to treatment, but its utility for this is limited. In lesions being treated with chemotherapy or radiation, the tumor may decrease in size and areas of high T2 signal may convert to lower T2 signal. Alternatively, new high T2 areas may develop due to hemorrhage and necrosis (Fig. 3.21). Gadolinium enhancement may also decrease and new nonenhancing areas may develop due to necrosis, hemorrhage, or cyst formation. The use of dynamic contrast enhancement, which allows for quantitative assessment of enhancement slope and amplitude for assessing response to therapy, has been described in osteosarcoma and Ewing sarcoma. However, the presence or absence of viable tumor cells is not conclusively assessed by MRI. In addition, some tumors may enlarge after treatment, even though they are responding, because of internal hemorrhage. MRI is also used to monitor for recurrence status post surgery and other treatment. In these cases, early assessment can be difficult due to postoperative edema, seroma, fibrosis, callus, and enhancing fibrovascular tissue, as well as due to artifact from any hardware placed at surgery. Acquisition of a baseline study can help as a reference for future follow-up studies. Tumor recurrence may manifest as a change in marrow or soft tissue signal intensity, a new soft tissue mass, or new or increased contrast enhancement (Fig. 3.21).

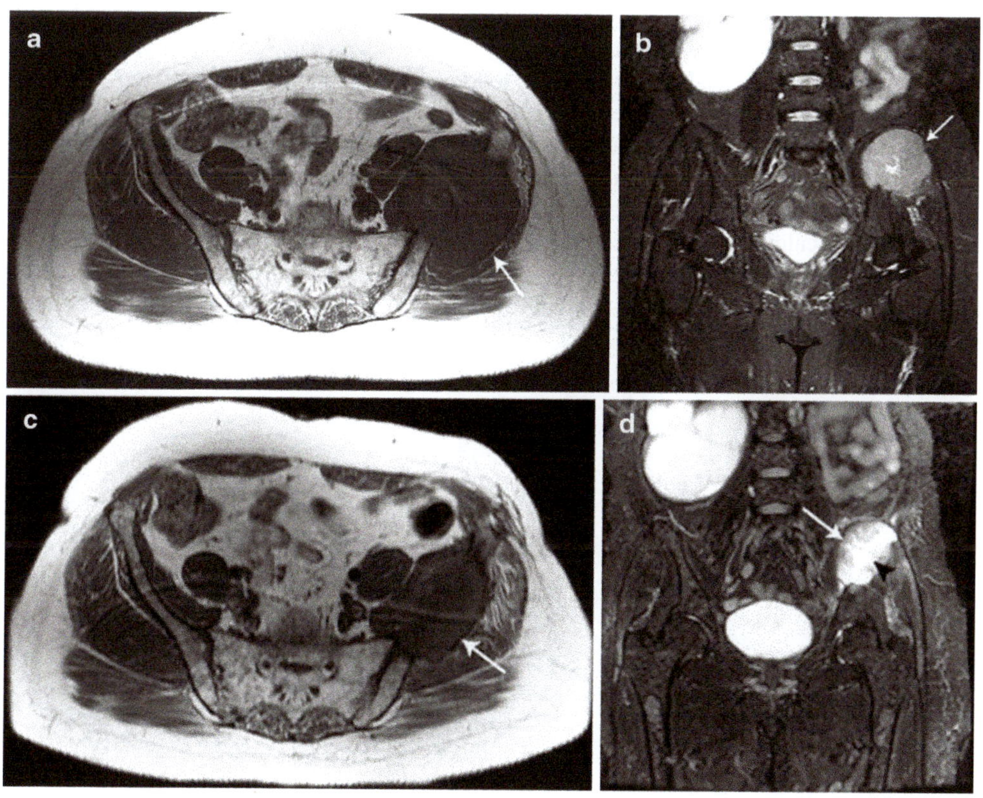

Fig. 3.21 Axial (**a**) T1-weighted and coronal (**b**) fat-saturated T2-weighted MR images of the pelvis show a large plasmacytoma centered in the left iliac bone (*arrows*). Corresponding MR images (**c**, **d**) obtained after treatment show that the lesion (*arrows*) has decreased in size and there is now an area of high T2 signal (*arrowhead*) in the lesion, reflecting post-treatment necrosis

Bone Scintigraphy (Radionuclide Bone Scan)

A bone scintigraphy exam demonstrates increased activity in lesions that cause reactive bone formation because the usual radionuclide agent employed—technetium-99m pertechnetate—is adsorbed onto newly formed hydroxyapatite that is laid down by osteoblasts in response to the bone destruction. The main roles of radionuclide bone scan in evaluation of bone tumors are to assess the degree of activity in a lesion, often discovered on another imaging modality, and, most importantly, to "survey" the skeleton for the presence and distribution of additional sites of bony disease. Of course, bone scintigraphy is also used to detect osseous metastases in patients with nonosseous primary malignancies. Bone scans can also be used to monitor lesions for response to therapy, but, in many instances, this role is being taken over by PET/CT scanning.

Bone scans have several important limitations with regard to the workup of bone lesions. Although scintigraphy can be highly sensitive for detection of bone lesions and can identify lesions that are occult on radiographs and CT, it has limited ability to characterize bone lesions, to determine the intraosseous extent of bone lesions, or to demonstrate extraosseous soft tissue extension. Moreover, extremely lytic lesions lacking significant hydroxyapatite formation may not be detected on bone scan. For this reason, radiographic skeletal surveys are preferred for assessment of multiple myeloma and other purely lytic lesions, such as renal cell and thyroid carcinoma. Radiotracer-avid lesions may not be well-demonstrated on routine planar bone scintigraphy due to overlap or attenuation, unless single photon emission computed tomography (SPECT) is used (Figs. 3.22 and 3.23).

Bone scans do not provide accurate assessment of the intraosseous extent of a bone lesion in part because of issues related to camera resolution, but also because the size of the lesion may be artifactually augmented in areas of hyperemia and edema adjoining the tumor. For example, giant cell tumors can show activity in an adjacent bone or joint due to hyperemia rather than tumor extension. Moreover, in the small bones of the hands and feet, it may be difficult to precisely localize the site of increased activity, particularly if pinhole collimation views are not obtained. Soft tissue components of bone lesions are not effectively evaluated on bone scans. The soft tissue component of the lesion does not demonstrate uptake on delayed phase bone scans, unless the soft tissue abnormality is hyperemic or it contains areas of calcification or ossification. An example of the latter phenomenon is activity in osteogenic pulmonary metastases in osteosarcoma (Fig. 3.24). On occasion, the soft tissue component of a bone tumor may be visible during the angiographic or blood pool phases of a triple phase bone scan because of its intrinsic neovascularity.

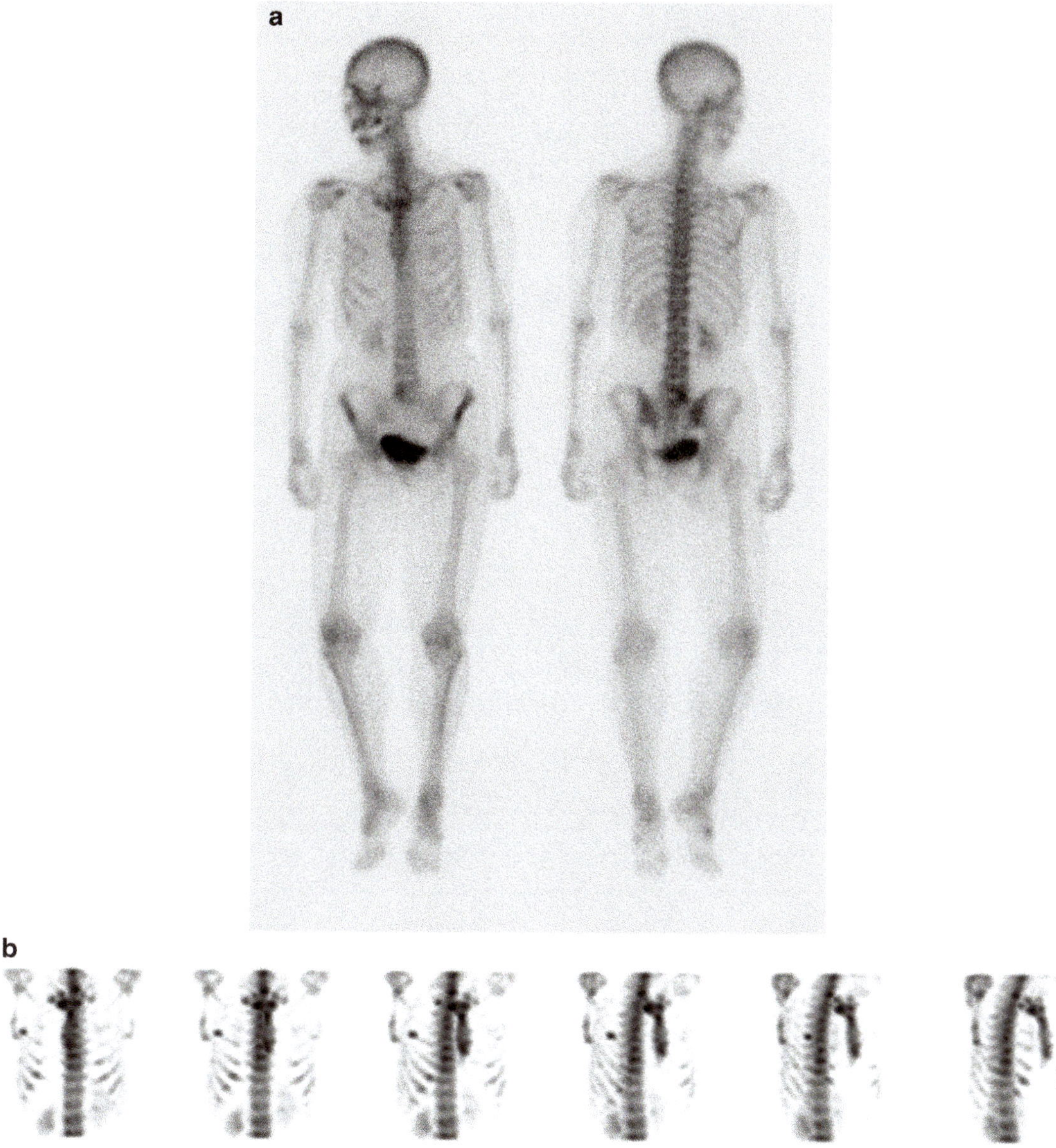

Fig. 3.22 Breast cancer metastases. Planar bone scan images (**a**) show no significant areas of radiotracer uptake. Selected SPECT images (**b**) help to accurately localize lesions to the right fifth rib, C7 vertebral body, and manubrium

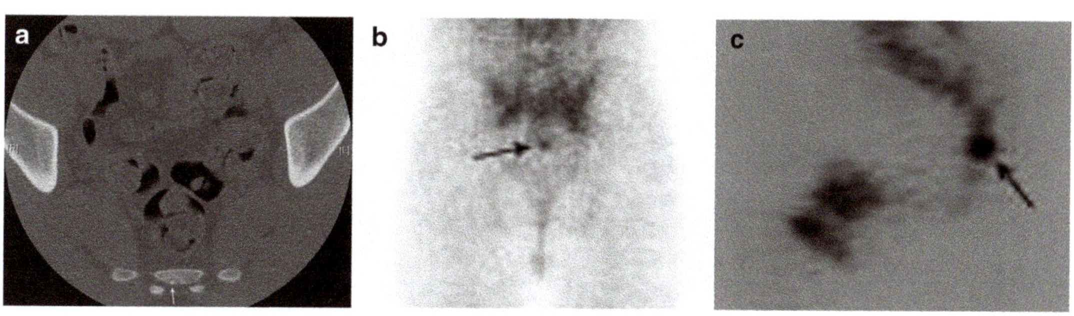

Fig. 3.23 Axial CT image (**a**) shows a small lucent lesion in the coccyx (*arrow*), with a central calcification, consistent with an osteoid osteoma. Coronal blood pool image (**b**) indicates hyperemia in the osteoid osteoma (*arrow*). The sagittal SPECT image (**c**) helps to confirm that the area of increased activity is in the coccyx

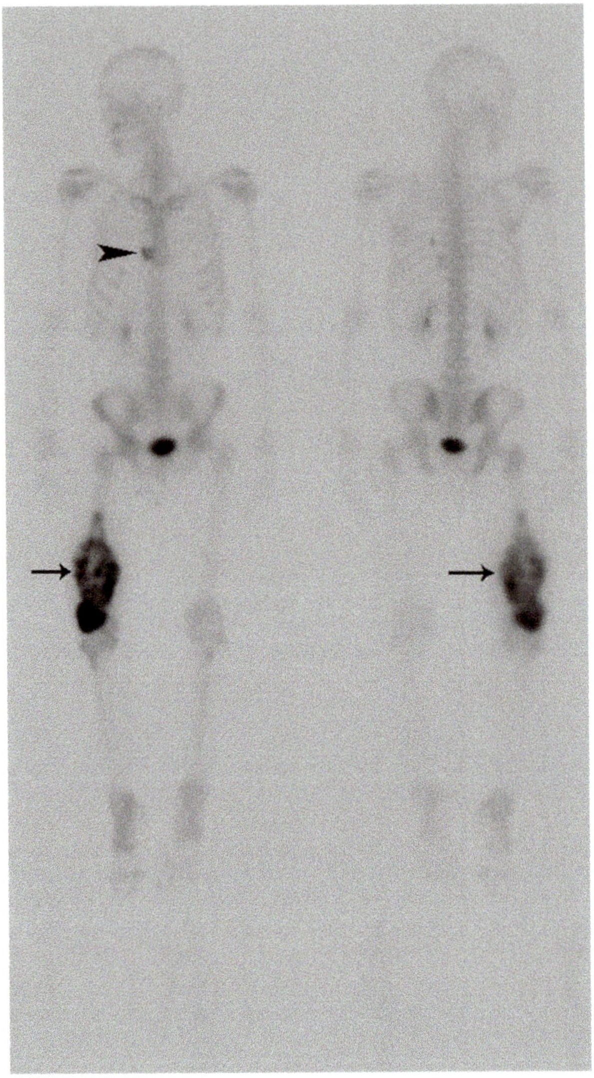

Fig. 3.24 Osteosarcoma. Static whole-body bone scan images show increased activity not only in the femur, but also in the surrounding soft tissue (*arrows*). Soft tissue activity reflects radionuclide uptake in bone that has formed within the extraosseous soft tissue mass. Note the focus of increased activity overlying the thorax (*arrowhead*) which corresponds to a pulmonary metastasis

Questions to Answer When Assessing a Bone Scintigraphy Scan

- Is the lesion active on bone scan and, if so, how active?
- Is there more than one bone lesion?
- Does lesion appearance or the distribution of lesions suggest a particular diagnosis?
- Has there been a change in the number or activity of lesions over time?

Is the Lesion Active on Bone Scan and, If So, How Active?

In general, benign and malignant lesions cannot be distinguished on the basis of their bone scan activity. Radionuclide uptake in bone is a nonspecific finding, reflecting processes as varied as increased metabolic bone turnover, new bone formation within a bone tumor, reactive new bone formation surrounding a benign or malignant bone lesion, and localized uptake in bone due to localized increased blood flow. Thus, Paget disease, osteosarcoma, osteomyelitis, and healing fractures can all show increased activity on bone scintigraphy. However, malignant processes tend to have higher activity than benign processes. Paget disease and fibrous dysplasia are important exceptions—they are both benign processes that can have intense bone scan activity. On occasion, bone scans can help to evaluate a sclerotic or partially sclerotic lesion that is visible on radiographs, but of uncertain clinical significance, possibly residua from a "burnt out" process, such as a non-ossifying fibroma or healed intraosseous abscess. If there is no correlative activity on bone scan, then the lesion is unlikely to represent an active benign or malignant process. An important caveat applies for lytic lesions, such as multiple myeloma or renal cell metastases, that do not generate significant reactive bone formation. These types of osteolytic lesions cannot be reliably detected by bone scan and, therefore, should be assessed by skeletal survey (radiographs). New techniques, such as whole-body MRI and PET/CT scans, may play a role in this setting (Fig. 3.25).

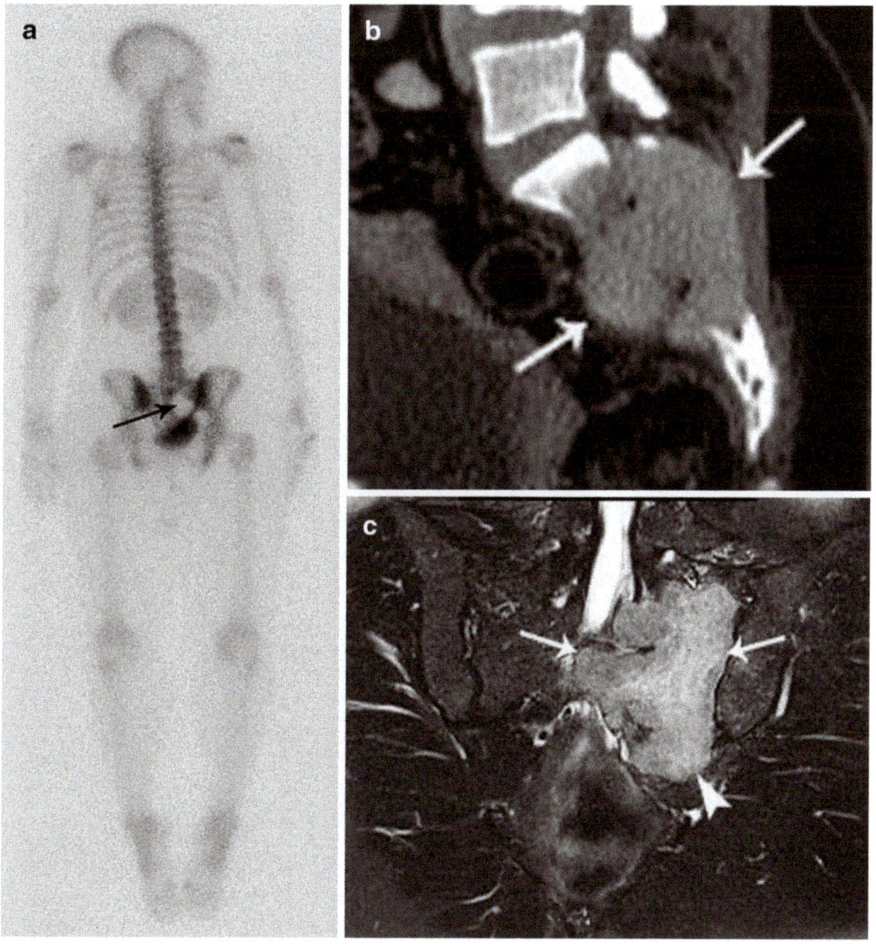

Fig. 3.25 Plasmacytoma. There is a photopenic area (*arrow*) in the left sacrum on the bone scan (**a**). In this case, the lesion is so large that it becomes visible as a "cold spot." The majority of plasma cell myeloma lesions do not show increased activity on bone scan and are, therefore, best followed by skeletal survey radiography, FDG PET/CT or whole-body MRI. Sagittal CT-reformatted image (**b**) depicts the tumor and associated bone destruction (*arrows*). Coronal T2-weighted MR (**c**) shows the marrow replacement (*arrows*) and soft tissue extension (*arrowhead*)

Is There More Than One Bone Lesion?

The main role of bone scintigraphy in assessment of bone tumors and tumor-like lesions is to image the entire skeleton in order to detect the presence or absence of polyostotic disease. Bone scans can aid in the detection of synchronous bone lesions accompanying a primary bone tumor (e.g., "skip" metastases in osteosarcoma) (Fig. 3.26); multiple bone lesions associated with a metastasis that present deceptively as a solitary bone lesion; and polyostotic forms of benign processes (Fig. 3.27), such as fibrous dysplasia and Paget disease. In this way, bone scans provide information that is complementary to MRI or CT for the purposes of bone tumor staging. Because bone scans provide whole-body imaging, they can be used to detect additional sites of involvement that may be more amenable to diagnostic biopsy. In assessing bone scans for polyostotic disease, care must be taken to recognize a superscan, i.e., abnormal, elevated bone uptake that is so diffuse that it can be mistaken for normal skeletal activity. To avoid this pitfall, the reader must check to ensure that normal renal and soft tissue activity is visible. Although bone scans are still the most commonly used modality for whole-body imaging of bone lesions, there is growing interest in the use of newer techniques, such as whole-body MRI and FDG PET/CT scans, for this purpose.

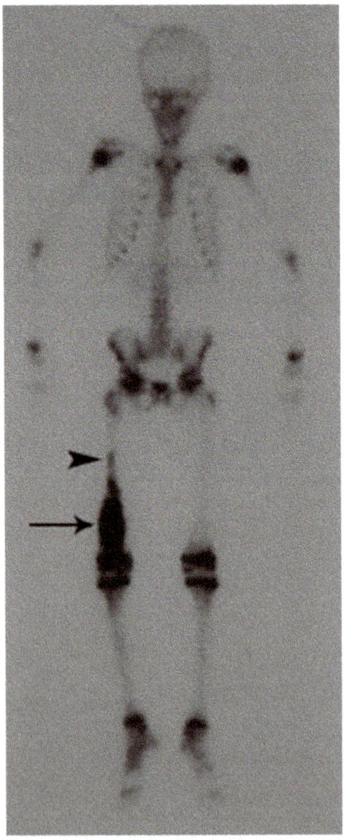

Fig. 3.26 Child with osteosarcoma (*arrow*) seen as area of increased activity and bone enlargement in the distal right femur. There is a small separate focus of increased activity in the right femoral diaphsysis (*arrowhead*) that represents a pathologically proven "skip" metastasis. Note that the physes and calcaneal apophyses show increased uptake, which is a normal finding in this skeletally immature individual. (Image courtesy of Dr. Mark Gebhardt, MD, Boston, MA.)

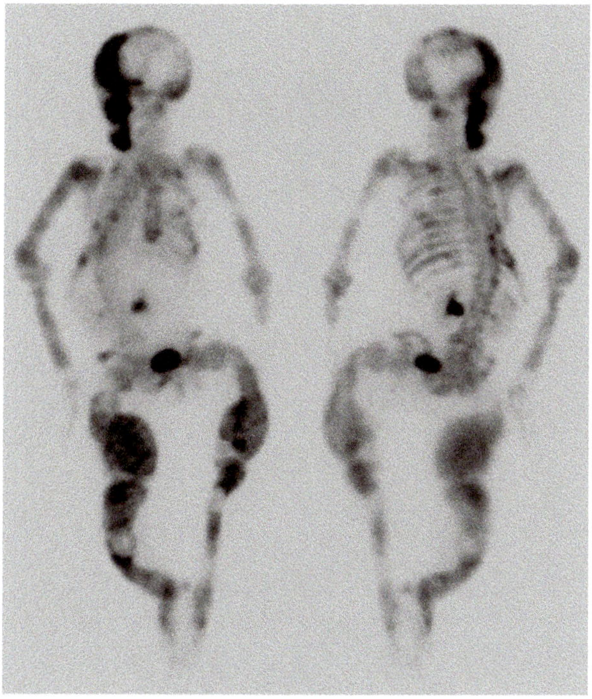

Fig. 3.27 Bone scan demonstrates the extent and distribution of bony involvement in this patient with polyostotic fibrous dysplasia. Involvement of the calvarium, ribs, and extremities is in keeping with the diagnosis. Note the long lesions in the ribs and also the bony deformity due to insufficiency fractures

Does Lesion Appearance or the Distribution of Lesions Suggest a Particular Diagnosis?

As noted above, radionuclide uptake in bone is generally a nonspecific finding. On occasion, however, a distinctive pattern of radionuclide activity can aid in lesion characterization, e.g., a "double-density" pattern of activity in osteoid osteoma, evidence of bone enlargement in Paget disease (Fig. 3.28), or anatomic distribution in the cranium and ribs suggestive of fibrous dysplasia. Bone lesions that are cystic or that do not take up radionuclide may appear as a "cold spot," a pattern seen in bone infarcts, among others. Some lesions, such as giant cell tumors, have a "donut" pattern, with a rim of higher activity surrounding a central area of lower activity (Fig. 3.29). These patterns can be suggestive of a specific diagnosis, but are not pathognomonic.

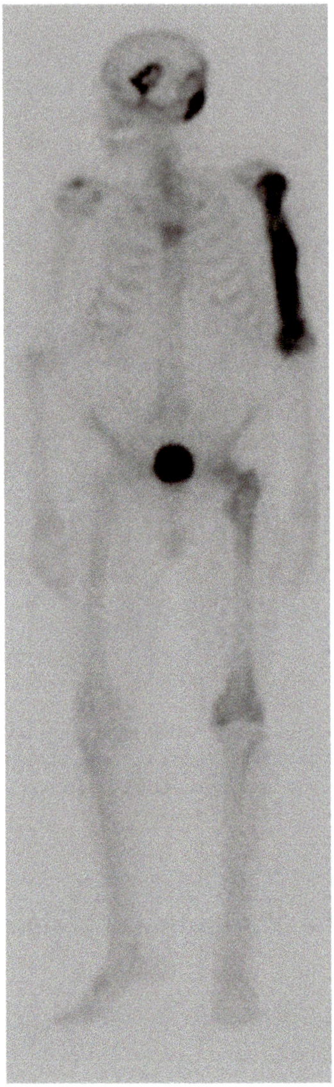

Fig. 3.28 Whole-body AP view demonstrates increased activity in the skull, left humerus, and left femur. This activity extends from the end of the bone and the humerus and femur appears diffusely enlarged. This distribution and these features are consistent with Paget disease

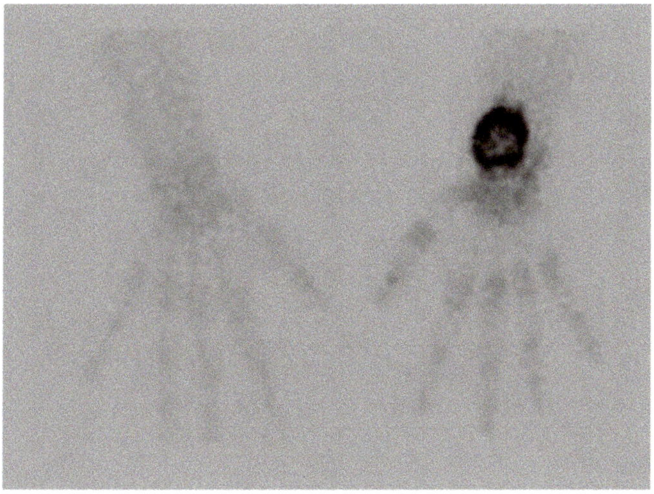

Fig. 3.29 Pinhole collimation PA view of the hands and wrists demonstrates a characteristic "donut" pattern of increased activity in a distal radius giant cell tumor. Note the relative increased activity in the carpal bones, remote from the tumor, reflecting hyperemia, rather than tumor extension

Has There Been a Change in the Number or Activity of Lesions Over Time?

Bone scans have traditionally been used to follow treatment response in patients with skeletal metastases, e.g., prostate, lung, and breast cancers. Response to treatment is seen as a decrease in the number, extent, or intensity of activity of bone lesions that were originally demonstrated on a pretreatment scan (Fig. 3.30). Stability of bone scan findings does not necessarily indicate unfavorable treatment response. A "flare phenomenon" of increased activity in metastatic lesions that are actually responding to therapy sometimes can be observed due to hyperemia and/or increased hydroxyapatite turnover and should not be mistaken for a sign of progression. At present, the use of FDG PET/CT scans—which can demonstrate both soft tissue and skeletal metastases—to monitor response to treatment is becoming more important.

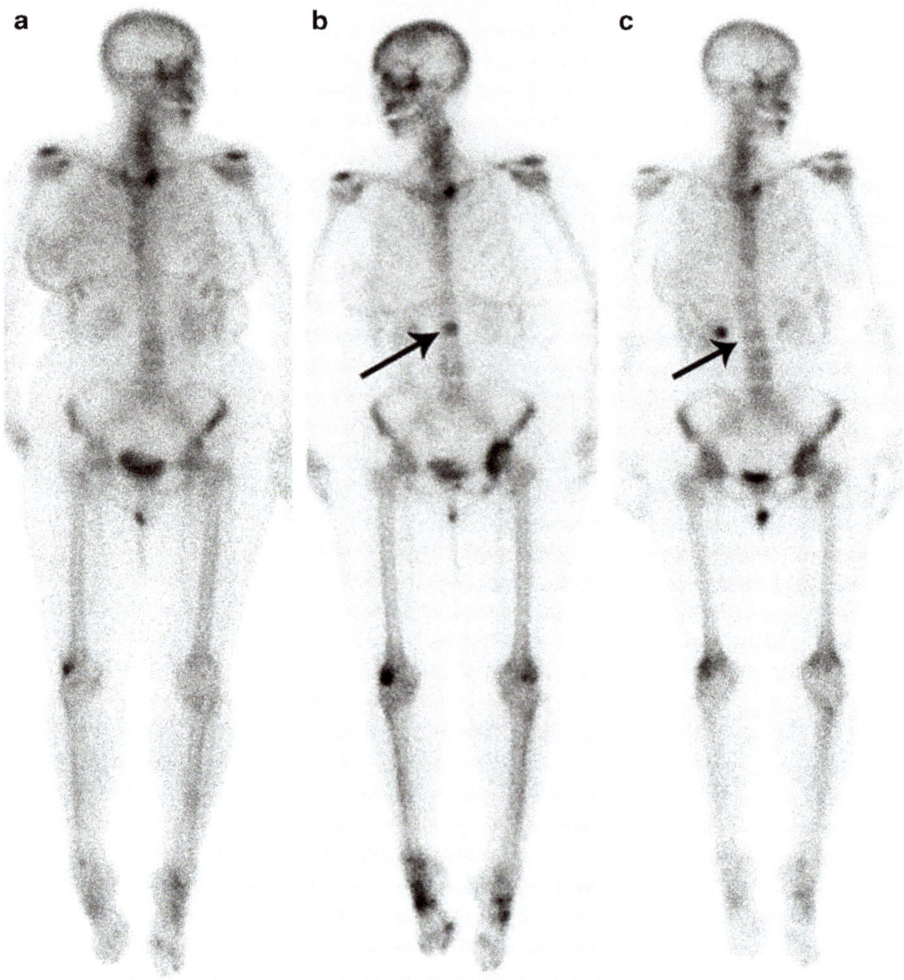

Fig. 3.30 Anterior images from three successive bone scan studies on a patient with breast cancer. The initial staging scan (**a**) is negative, with no areas suspicious for bony metastases. Several areas of activity were consistent with osteoarthritis. Scan performed 3 years (**b**) later shows new focus of activity in the L2 vertebral body (*arrow*) corresponding to a sclerotic metastasis. Following chemotherapy (**c**), activity in the L2 vertebral body (*arrow*) has decreased considerably, indicating response to treatment. Focus in right renal pelvis is an unrelated normal finding due to urine in the collecting system

Positron Emission Tomography Scan

Experience with PET and PET/CT scans for imaging of bone tumors is still relatively limited. However, PET scans can provide information not available from conventional imaging techniques. Available evidence suggests a potential role for PET and, in particular for PET/CT, for the detection, localization, grading, staging, therapeutic monitoring, and follow-up of bone tumors.

PET scans can be performed with various radiotracers. The most common form in current clinical use is based on administration of intravenous FDG, a glucose analog labeled with radioactive positron-emitting fluorine 18, which is used to demonstrate metabolic activity. Lesions with increased levels of metabolic activity accumulate high levels of glucose and show high levels of uptake on FDG-PET scans, whereas lesions with limited metabolic activity do not show significant uptake on FDG-PET scans. In general, PET scanning is well-suited for tumors with high metabolic activity, such as breast, lung, colon carcinoma, and melanoma, but not effective in evaluating low-metabolic lesions, such as prostate, carcinoid, and bronchoalveolar lung cancer. Not all lesions that demonstrate increased uptake are tumors: inflammatory and infectious processes can demonstrate high levels of metabolic activity. Moreover, not all malignant lesions are PET avid.

PET scans allow for evaluation of the entire body, including the skeleton and soft tissues. They can aid in the detection of small hypermetabolic lesions and can demonstrate both intraosseous and extraosseous disease. As a result, they can play a role in either upstaging or downstaging sarcomas, compared with other modalities. When fused with CT scans, PET/CT can improve detection and localization of lesions and improve staging. PET/CT can be used to localize the primary lesion, detect metastatic lesions, and identify a site to biopsy. PET scans may also be used to follow response to treatment: an FDG-avid tumor responding to treatment would be expected to demonstrate decreased PET activity over time (Fig. 3.31). Similarly, PET scans may be used to identify areas of tumor recurrence, in those cases in which the tumor is known to be PET avid.

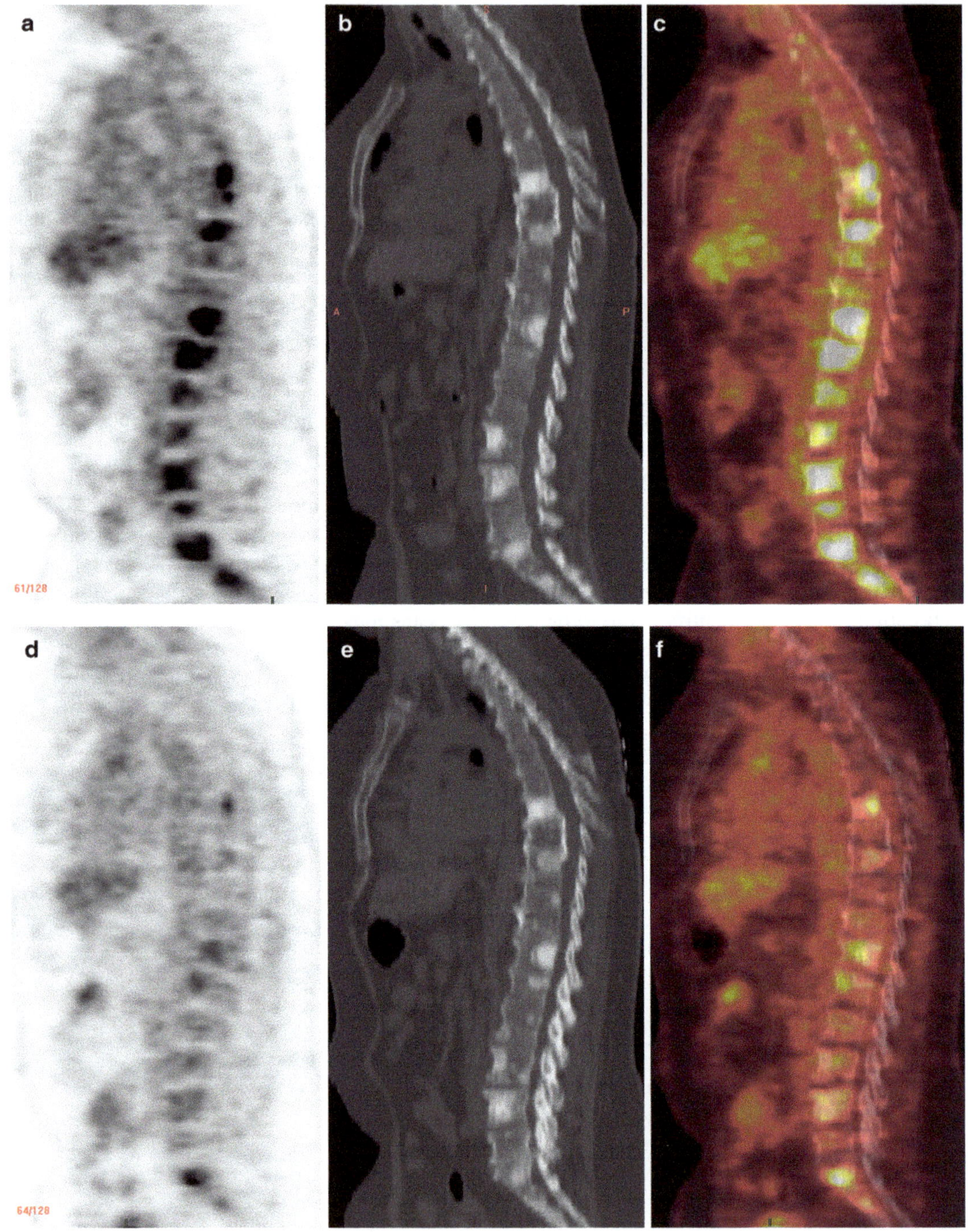

Fig. 3.31 Breast cancer metastases. Sagittal FDG PET (**a**), CT reformat (**b**), and fused PET/CT (**c**) of a patient with breast cancer showing multiple lytic and sclerotic vertebral body metastases with abnormal FDG activity. (**d**–**f**) Analogous images obtained following chemotherapy show a partial response. Abnormal FDG activity remains present, but is less pronounced. Note that the PET scan provides additional information compared to the CT scan, since the sclerotic metastases show no interval change on CT. (Images courtesy of Dr. J. Anthony Parker MD, PhD, Boston, MA.)

Ultrasound

Ultrasound (US) has a limited role in the evaluation of bone tumors, but can be used to guide percutaneous biopsy of bone lesions that have a significant soft tissue component. On ultrasound images, normal bone cortex appears as a uniform, continuous hyperechoic line that creates marked acoustic shadowing, and it often demonstrates reverberation artifact. In most cases, the acoustic shadowing from the cortex completely obscures the bone beneath the cortex. However, when the cortex is markedly thinned or eroded, the underlying medullary cavity may become visible. Normal periosteum is not visible in adults, though it can be seen in certain locations in children as a thin hypoechoic line abutting the cortex, when very-high-frequency probes are used. Areas of irregularity along the cortex, including nutrient foramina and bony exostoses, may be visible. For example, in osteochondromas, US has been shown to provide accurate measurement of cartilage cap thickness and can be used to evaluate overlying soft tissue complications, such as neurovascular impingement and bursa formation. Because of cortical thinning associated with aneurysmal bone cysts, US can demonstrate intralesional fluid–fluid levels, which can be seen to change with patient position. The use of color Doppler imaging for detection and biopsy of the hypervascular nidus of osteoid osteoma has also been described. In bone tumors with significant extraosseous soft tissue extension, US can show the mass and may demonstrate contiguity of the mass with an interruption in the cortex. However, the tumor appearance is variable and nonspecific and does not aid in lesion characterization. When a sizeable extraosseous component has been previously identified on CT or MRI, US can be used to guide percutaneous biopsy (Figs. 3.32 and 3.33). In these cases, US can be helpful in identifying areas of vascularized soft tissue amenable to biopsy, delineating adjacent vessels to be avoided and allowing real-time tracking of the needle. As always, care must be taken regarding sensitive surrounding structures and the biopsy should be performed only after consultation with the orthopedic tumor surgeon who is performing the definitive surgery, in order to avoid seeding a tract that could complicate subsequent surgery.

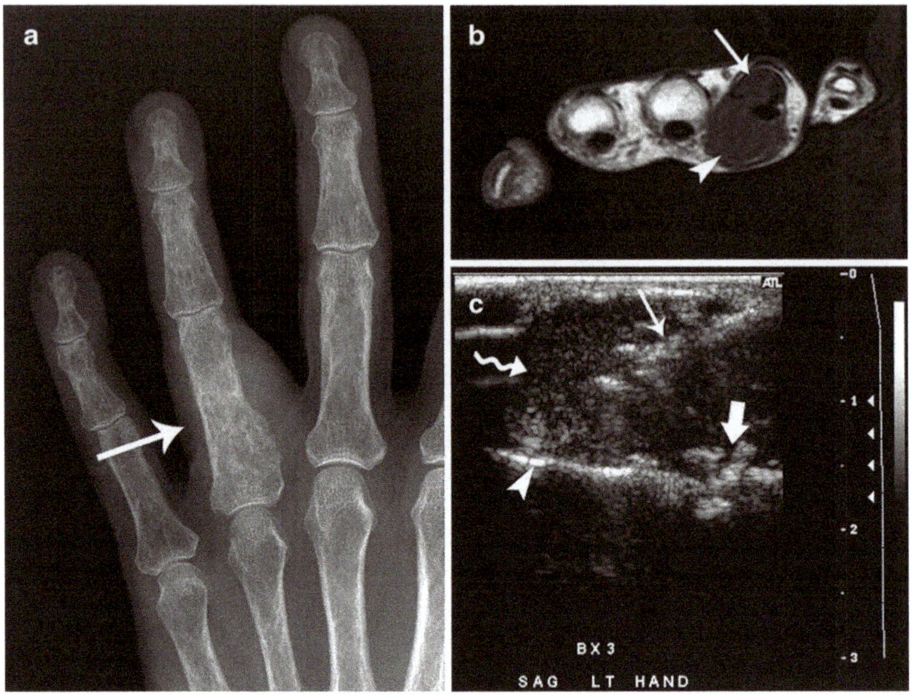

Fig. 3.32 AP radiograph of the hand (**a**) shows a lesion (*arrow*) in the proximal phalanx of the ring finger. Note faint calcifications within the mass. Axial T1-weighted MRI image (**b**) shows abnormal low signal replacing fatty marrow (*arrow*), with soft tissue extension (*arrowhead*). US-guided needle (*arrow*) biopsy (**c**) of the soft tissue component was performed. Bone cortex (*arrowhead*) is seen as a hyperechoic line deep to the soft tissue mass (*wavy arrow*). The medullary cavity of the bone is obscured due to acoustic shadowing from the intact cortex. Note focal cortical interruption (*thick arrow*), where echogenic material is seen deep to the plane of the cortex. Biopsy revealed a chondrosarcoma

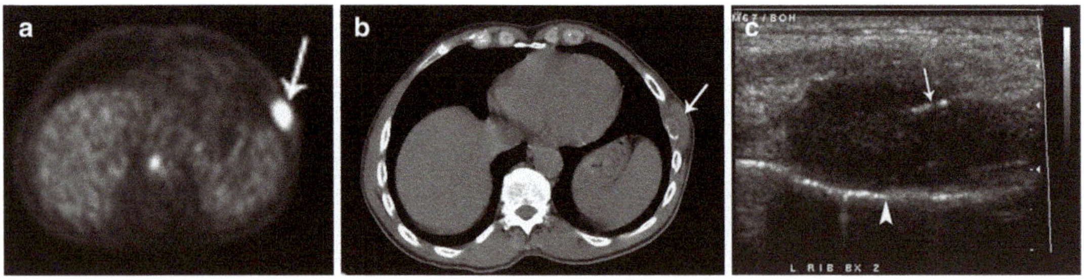

Fig. 3.33 FDG/PET image (**a**) shows abnormal increased activity in the rib (*arrow*) in a patient with both lung and prostate carcinoma. CT image (**b**) from the PET/CT shows a lytic lesion centered in the rib (*arrow*), with a large soft tissue mass expanding out of the rib. US-guided needle (*arrow*) biopsy (**c**) of the soft tissue mass was performed. Bone cortex (*arrowhead*) is seen as a hyperechoic line deep to the soft tissue mass. The medullary cavity of the bone is obscured due to acoustic shadowing by the intact cortex. Biopsy yielded lung metastasis

Staging of Primary Bone Tumors

Most bone tumor staging systems reflect a composite of (1) tumor extent, determined by imaging and (2) grading, determined by histology. Assessment of tumor extent may depend on information gathered from multiple different imaging studies. MRI is often the "workhorse" study for local extent, with some form of whole-body imaging used to determine regional and distant extent. Chest CTs are often obtained to assess for lung metastases in patients with bone sarcomas.

For staging of malignant primary bone tumors, two different systems are in common use: the Musculoskeletal Tumor Society (MSTS)'s Enneking System and the American Joint Committee on Cancer (AJCC) Staging System. The Enneking System, described in 1980, is based on three criteria: (1) tumor extent, (2) nodes, and (3) histologic grade. In the Enneking System, tumors may be intracompartmental (T1—confined within periosteum) or extracompartmental (T2—breach in adjacent joint cartilage, periosteum, fascia lata, quadriceps, joint capsule), without (M0) or with (M1) regional or distant metastases. Histology may be low grade (G1) or high grade (G2). Actual tumor size is not considered. Skip metastases are considered M1. The Enneking System applies only to mesenchymal tumors, not to round cell tumors, such as lymphoma, leukemia, and Ewing sarcoma (Table 3.1).

Table 3.1 Enneking staging system for primary malignant tumors of bone

Stage	Description	Grade	Tumor	Metastases
IA	Low grade, intra compartmental	G1	T1	M0
IB	Low grade, extracompartmental	G1	T2	M0
IIA	High grade, intracompartmental	G2	T1	M0
IIB	High grade, extracompartmental	G2	T2	M0
III	Low or high grade, intracompartmental with metastases	G1 or G2	T1	M1
III	Low or high grade, extracompartmental with metastases	G1 or G2	T2	M1

The AJCC system was revised in 2010 so that tumor extent now refers to tumor size, rather than transcortical extension. In the revised AJCC system, staging is based on four criteria: (1) tumor extent, (2) regional nodes and metastases, (3) distant metastases, and (4) histologic grade. The tumor may be less than (T1) or greater than (T2) 8 cm in greatest dimension or may have skip metastases (T3). Regional lymph nodes or metastases may be absent (N0) or present (N1). Distant metastases may be absent (M0) or present (M1), with a distinction made for lung metastases (M1a) and other distant sites (M1b). Tumors are low grade if well (G1) or moderately (G2) differentiated and high grade if poorly differentiated (G3) or undifferentiated (G4). If the primary tumor, regional lymph node, or histologic grade cannot be assessed, it is designated TX, NX, or GX, respectively. The system applies to primary malignant tumors of bone, including Ewing sarcoma, but does not apply to multiple myeloma or primary lymphoma of bone (Table 3.2).

Table 3.2 American Joint Committee on Cancer Staging System for Primary Malignant Tumors of Bone

Stage	Grade	Tumor	Lymph node	Metastases
IA	G1, G2, or GX	T1	N0	M0
IB	G1, G2, or GX	T2, T3	N0	M0
IIA	G3 or G4	T1	N0	M0
IIB	G3 or G4	T2	N0	M0
III	G3 or G4	T3	N0	M0
IVA	Any G	Any T	N0	M1a
IVB	Any G	Any T	N1	Any M
IVB	Any G	Any T	Any N	M1b

Used with the permission of the American Joint Committee on Cancer (AJCC), Chicago, IL. The original source for this material is the AJCC Cancer Staging Manual, Seventh Edition (2010), published by Springer Science and Business Media LLC, www.springer.com

The key role of the radiologist in tumor staging is to provide the "raw data" for determining tumor extent. The relevant TNM features for making that determination should all be described in the report.

Relevant TNM Features for Staging

- Tumor size (e.g., greatest dimension for AJCC system)
- Extraosseous extension
- Extension into additional other compartments
- Skip metastases (elsewhere in the same bone, but with intervening normal marrow)
- Intra-articular extension
- Encasement or invasion of neurovascular structures
- Regional lymph nodes
- Distant lymph nodes
- Extension to other vital structures

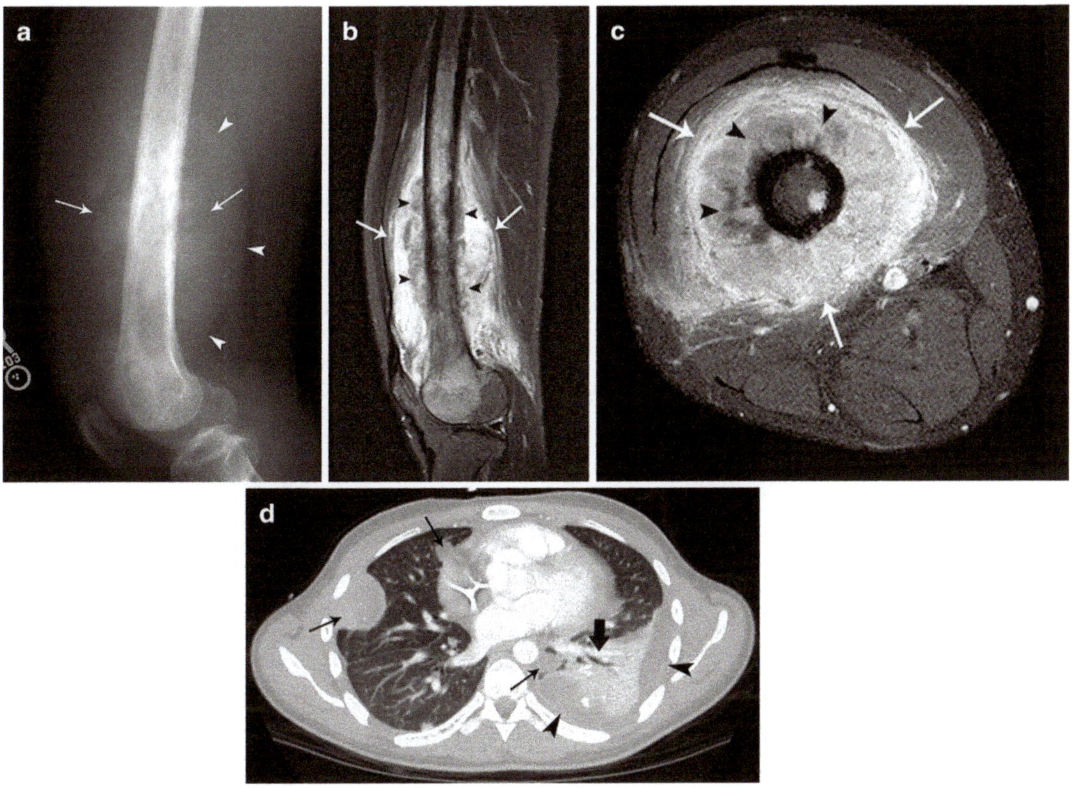

Fig. 3.34 Osteosarcoma. Lateral radiograph of the femur (**a**) shows a lesion centered in the bone with profuse aggressive periosteal reaction (*arrows*). Increased density (*arrowheads*) surrounding the bone is suggestive of a large soft tissue mass. Postcontrast sagittal (**b**) and axial (**c**) fat-saturated T1-weighted MR images confirm the presence of a large soft tissue mass (*arrows*) arising from the femur. Note the low-signal hair-on-end periosteal reaction (*arrowheads*). Chest CT (**d**) revealed lung metastases (*arrows*), left lower lobe collapse (*thick arrow*), and a pleural effusion (*arrowheads*). In the Enneking System, the lesion is considered extracompartmental and would be classified as Stage III, regardless of its histologic grade, because it has distant metastases. In the AJCC system, the lesion would be designated T2 because it is >8 cm in length, N0 for no regional nodes or metastases, and M1a for lung metastases, and would be considered Stage IVa, regardless of histology, based on the presence of lung metastases

Suggested Reading

1. Berquist TH, Dalinka MK, Alazraki N, et al. Bone tumors. American College of Radiology. ACR Appropriateness Criteria. Radiology. 2000;215(Suppl):261–4.
2. Bestic JM, Peterson JJ, Bancroft LW. Use of FDG PET in staging, restaging, and assessment of therapy response in ewing sarcoma. Radiographics. 2009;29:1487–501.
3. Bredella MA, Stoller DW, Johnston JO. Bone and soft tissue tumors. In: Stoller DW, editor. Magnetic resonance imaging in orthopedics and sports medicine, vol. II. 3rd ed. Baltimore: Lippincott Williams & Wilkins; 2007. p. 2045–61.
4. Daldrup-Link HE, Franzius C, Link TM, et al. Whole-body MR imaging for detection of bone metastases in children and young adults: comparison with skeletal scintigraphy and PET. AJR Am J Roentgenol. 2001;177:229–36.
5. Disler DG, McCauley TR, Ratner LM. In-phase and out-of-phase imaging of bone marrow: prediction of neoplasia based on the detection of coexistent fat and water. AJR Am J Roentgenol. 1997;169:1439–47.
6. Edge SB, Byrd DR, Compton CC, editors. AJCC cancer staging manual. 7th ed. New York, NY: Springer; 2010.

7. Espinosa LA, Jamadar DA, Jacobson JA. CT-guided biopsy of bone: a radiologist's perspective. AJR Am J Roentgenol. 2008;190:W283–9.
8. Karcaaltincaba M, Aktas A. Dual-energy CT revisited with multidetector CT: review of principles and clinical applications. Diagn Interv Radiol 2010;17(3):181–194.
9. Landa J, Schwartz LH. Contemporary imaging in sarcoma. Oncologist. 2009;14:1021–38.
10. Lang P, Gramp S, Vahlensieck M, et al. Primary bone tumors: value of MR angiography for preoperative planning and monitoring response to chemotherapy. AJR Am J Roentgenol. 1995;165:135–42.
11. Liu PT, Valadez SD, Chivers S, et al. Anatomically based guidelines for core needle biopsy of bone tumors: implications for limb-sparing surgery. Radiographics. 2007;27:189–206.
12. Robert S. Radionuclide techniques. In: Resnick D, Kransdorf KJ, editors. Bone and joint imaging. 3rd ed. Philadelphia: Elsevier Saunders; 2005. p. 86–118.
13. Stacy GS, Mahal RS, Peabody TD. Staging of bone tumors: a review with illustrative examples. AJR Am J Roentgenol. 2006;186:967–76.
14. Tateishi U, Yamaguchi U, Seki K, et al. Bone and soft tissue sarcoma: preoperative staging with fluorine 18 fluorodeoxyglucose PET/CT and conventional imaging. Radiology. 2007;245(3):839–47.

Cartilage Tumors

4

The neoplasms in this category all produce chondroid matrix, often containing "arcs and rings" of calcifications that can be seen on radiographs and CT. The benign cartilage tumors are typically asymptomatic and represent some of the most commonly encountered incidental bone lesions, with osteochondroma being the most common benign lesion of bone. Osteochondromas demonstrate contiguity of the medullary cavity and cortex with the host bone and pedunculated osteochondromas typically point away from the joint. Enchondromas are very common and are often found in the metaphysis of long bones, hands, and feet. Both enchondromas and osteochondromas can transform into chondrosarcoma and it is important to be familiar with features that suggest malignant transformation. Periosteal chondromas are cartilaginous lesions that arise from the cortical surface and can be difficult to distinguish from periosteal chondrosarcoma or surface osteosarcomas. The smaller size of the periosteal chondroma versus its larger malignant mimickers can be helpful in making the distinction. Chondroblastomas typically occur in skeletally immature patients, arise in the epiphysis, and can have a varied appearance depending on aggressiveness of the lesion. Chondromyxoid fibromas have the least specific imaging features among the benign chondroid lesions. They often do not demonstrate chondroid matrix on imaging, making it difficult to narrow the differential diagnosis. Fortunately, chondromyxoid fibromas are quite rare.

Chondrosarcomas are the third most common primary bone malignancy after multiple myeloma and osteosarcoma and can be divided into primary and secondary chondrosarcomas. Primary chondrosarcomas arise de novo within a bone and account for 80–90% of chondrosarcomas. Secondary chondrosarcomas arise from preexisting cartilage tumors (enchondroma and osteochondroma) or other bony abnormalities (bone infarcts, Paget disease). The majority of chondrosarcomas are the conventional subtype, which are often low grade and most commonly found in the long bones and pelvis. The best feature for distinguishing between enchondroma and low grade chondrosarcoma is endosteal scalloping that involves more than 2/3 of the cortical thickness. Chondrosarcomas tend to occur more frequently in the axial instead of the appendicular skeleton, while enchondromas are more common in the appendicular skeleton. Other primary chondrosarcoma subtypes include clear cell chondrosarcoma and dedifferentiated chondrosarcoma. Clear cell chondrosarcoma occurs in the epiphysis and can be difficult to distinguish from a chondroblastoma. Dedifferentiated chondrosarcoma contains two distinct histologic components, one of which is a high grade noncartilaginous sarcoma. Treatment for chondrosarcoma is highly dependent on achieving adequate surgical resection, as radiation and chemotherapy have limited roles.

J.S. Wu and M.G. Hochman, *Bone Tumors: A Practical Guide to Imaging*,
DOI 10.1007/978-1-4419-0808-7_4, © Springer Science+Business Media, LLC 2012

Benign

Osteochondroma
- Solitary
- Multiple hereditary osteochondromatosis

Chondroma
- Enchondroma
- Periosteal (juxtacortical) chondroma
- Enchondromatosis (Ollier's) and (Maffucci's)

Chondroblastoma

Chondromyxoid fibroma

Malignant

Primary
- Conventional (medullary)
- Clear cell
- Juxtacortical/periosteal
- Mesenchymal
- Dedifferentiated
- Extraosseous

Secondary
- Arises from benign precursor lesions

Osteochondroma

Synonyms: osteocartilaginous exostosis, exostosis

Demographics:
- <30 years at initial diagnosis
- M=F
- Most common benign bone lesion, 3% of population
- 30–50% of benign bone lesions and 10–15% of all bone lesions

Origin:
- Hypothesized to represent growth plate cartilage displaced to the metaphysis

Location:
- Metaphyseal or diametaphyseal
- Femur (distal and proximal), tibia, humerus. Less common in flat bones (ilium and scapula most common)

Clinical symptoms:
- Related to size and mechanical distortion of adjacent tissues
- Neurovascular compression can lead to paresthesias and pseudoaneurysms (especially in popliteal fossa)
- Fracture of lesion (pedunculated types)
- Bursitis from pressure against local soft tissues
- Joint immobility
- Cord compression if near spinal cord

Imaging characteristics:

- Bony exostosis from surface of bone that is contiguous with the marrow/cortex of the host bone and has a cartilaginous cap
- Lesions are (1) sessile or (2) pedunculated and "**cauliflower-like**"
- Often point away from joint, due to local mass effect from surrounding muscles
- Cartilage cap:
  - The cap is thicker in children and thins with age
  - Cartilage cap growth after skeletal maturity is suggestive of malignant transformation
  - Cap greater than 2 cm thick in adults and 3 cm in children is suspicious for malignancy. Average thickness of cap in secondary chondrosarcomas is 5–6 cm
- CT can be unreliable for measuring thickness of cap, as cap cartilage can have similar attenuation to surrounding soft tissue
- US is useful for measuring thickness of cap, but limited for deep lesions
- MRI is most helpful modality to show hyaline cartilage cap (bright T2 due to high water content)

Malignant potential:

- Transformation to conventional chondrosarcoma is <1% with solitary osteochondromas, 3–5% in patients with hereditary multiple exostoses (HME)
- Can also transform to osteosarcoma
- Increase in thickness of cartilage cap or change in the orientation of the calcifications, especially after skeletal maturity, should raise suspicion for malignant transformation

Treatment:

- Depends on symptoms
- Radiographic follow-up recommended for large lesions
- Often not resected until symptomatic or malignant transformation
- Recurrence is 2%

Miscellaneous facts:

- Most common benign tumor associated with radiation—cartilage rests in the epiphyseal plate damaged by radiation can migrate into the medullary cavity

Differential diagnosis:

- Myositis ossificans—is separate from bone
- Parosteal osteosarcoma—medullary and cortical portions are not contiguous with host bone. CT is helpful
- Trevor's disease (dysplasia epiphysealis hemimelica)—developmental disorder in which osteochondromas arise from the epiphyseal articular cartilage, often in lower extremities and associated with limb length discrepancies
- Nora's lesion (bizarre parosteal osteochondromatous proliferation of bone, BPOP)—surface lesion containing bone and cartilage arising from the periosteum. More common in hands and feet and not contiguous with the medullary cavity of the host bone

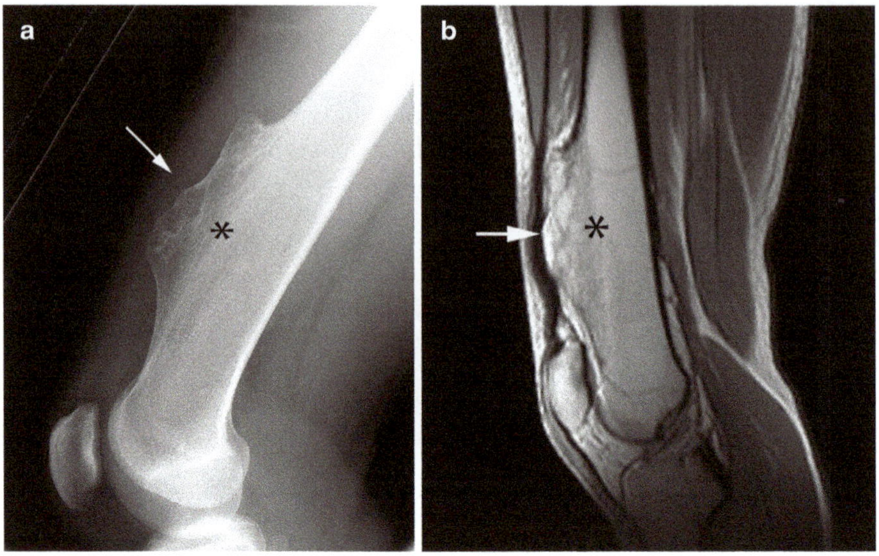

Fig. 4.1 Sessile osteochondroma (*arrows*) with broad-based attachment. Note that the marrow cavity of the lesion is contiguous with that of the host bone (*asterisk*) on both the radiograph (**a**) and T1-weighted MR image (**b**)

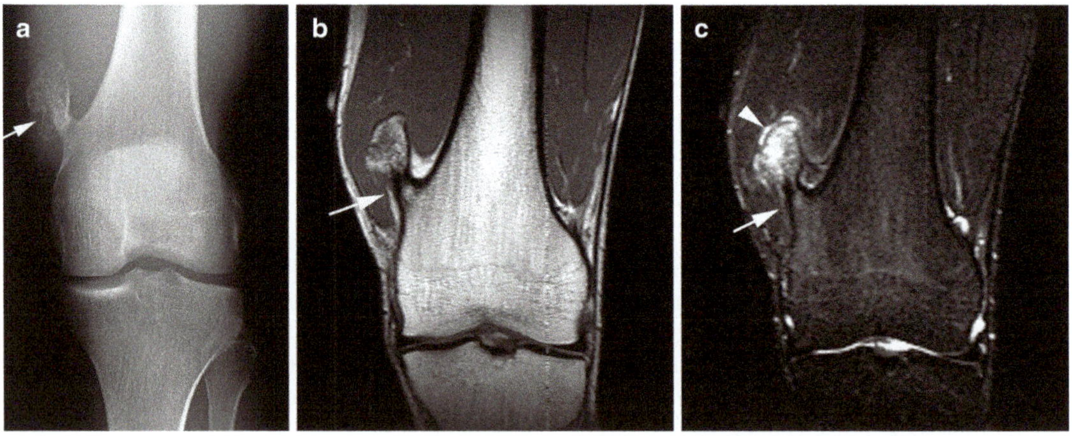

Fig. 4.2 Pedunculated osteochondroma (*arrows*) in the distal femur on radiography (**a**) and MRI (**b**, **c**). Note that the lesion points away from the joint due to mass effect from the adjacent muscles and soft tissues and that the cartilage cap (*arrowhead*) is bright on the T2-weighted MR image (**c**)

Hereditary Multiple Exostoses

- Autosomal dominant disorder characterized by multiple osteochondromas (exostoses). Associated with chromosomes 8, 11, and 19. M>F, 2–1
- Lesions can be sessile or pedunculated
- Patients can have short stature because multiple osteochondromas interfere with longitudinal bone growth and cause limb deformities
- Most lesions in HME are sessile as opposed to pedunculated. However, if >90% are sessile, then higher degree of skeletal deformities
- Sarcomatous transformation (3–5%) is higher than in solitary osteochondromas (<1%), but less than the previously described, 25%
- Transformation occurs at an earlier age than in isolated osteochondromas
- Baseline bone scintigraphy and radiographs of areas difficult to assess at physical exam is recommended
- Lesions should not grow after skeletal maturity
- Although there are no standard guidelines, lesions are typically followed by radiographs every 2–3 years. Symptomatic lesions can be imaged on a more frequent basis

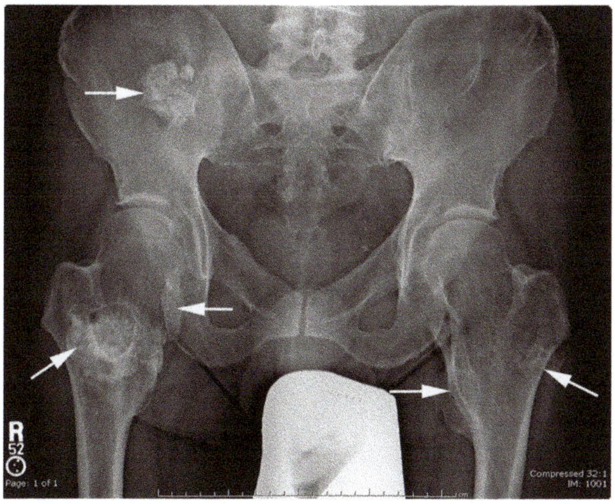

Fig. 4.3 Multiple sessile and pedunculated osteochondromas (*arrows*) in a patient with hereditary multiple exostoses (HME). Lesions which are seen en face can create the appearance of an intramedullary lesion, thus additional views should be interpreted

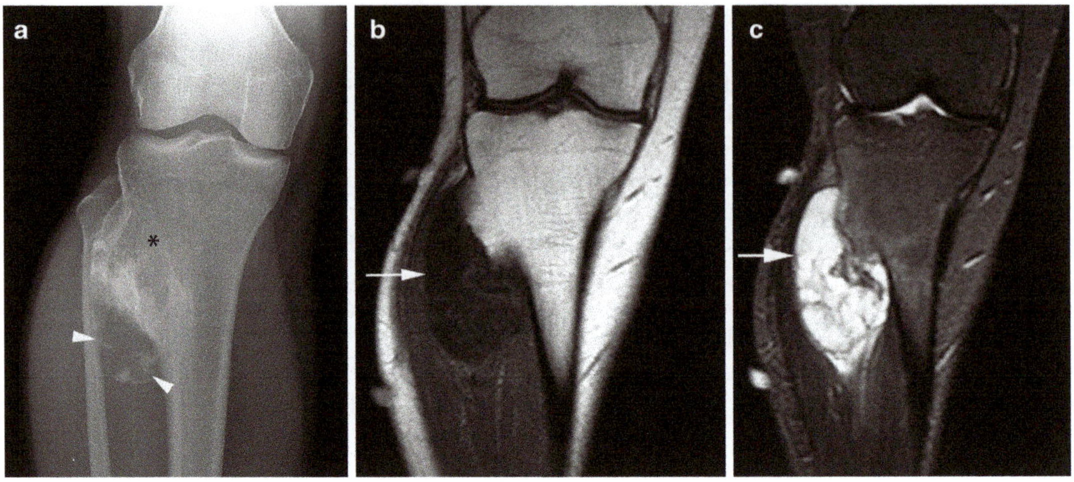

Fig. 4.4 Enlarged cartilaginous cap in malignant transformation of an osteochondroma to a secondary chondrosarcoma. The radiograph (**a**) shows contiguity of the marrow cavities between the tumor and host tibia (*asterisk*) as well as the irregular chondroid calcifications (*arrowheads*) in the periphery. Note the thickened cartilage cap (*arrows*) which is dark on the T1-weighted (**b**) and bright on the T2-weighted (**c**) MR images

Features Suspicious for Malignant Transformation

- Increased size of cartilaginous cap after skeletal maturity
- Cartilaginous cap >2 cm in adults and >3 cm in children
- Areas of lucency within lesion
- Cortical destruction of host bone
- Large soft tissue mass with scattered/irregular calcifications
- Change in orientation of calcifications

Enchondroma

Synonyms: central chondroma, chondroma

Demographics:

- Second to fourth decade at initial diagnosis
- M=F
- Very common. Ten to twenty-five percent of all benign bone tumors. Two to ten percent of all bone tumors.

Origin: benign mature hyaline cartilaginous rests displaced into medullary bone.

Location:

- Most common: proximal humerus, distal femur, tubular bones of hands and feet (50%)
- Uncommon in flat bones

Clinical symptoms:

- Asymptomatic, often discovered incidentally
- Pathologic fractures
- Painful lesions should raise suspicion for degeneration, especially if previously asymptomatic

Imaging characteristics:

- Typically in a central metaphyseal location
- Geographic lesion with stippled "**arcs and rings**" chondroid-type calcified matrix
- Lesions in the small tubular bones of the hands/feet can be expansile and can lack chondroid matrix calcifications
- Some lesions can be entirely calcified
- Mild endosteal scalloping due to the lobular growth pattern (should be less than 2/3 of cortical thickness)
- Can be confused with bone infarcts (no expansion) on radiographs
- CT:
  - Helpful in demonstrating degree of endosteal scalloping, chondroid matrix, and subtle fractures
  - Good for showing areas of nonmineralization for suspected malignant transformation
- MRI:
  - Lobulated low T1 and high T2 signal due to high water content
  - Signal void from calcifications; can obscure the background high T2 signal from the hyaline cartilage content:
  - Chemical shift artifact at periphery of lesion due to the interface of the water content in the hyaline cartilage with the surrounding fat
- Bone scintigraphy:
  - Typically warm or hot
  - Helpful in identifying multiple lesions

Malignant potential:

- Can give rise to chondrosarcoma, especially in axial and large lesions
- Actual rate of transformation of enchondromas to chondrosarcoma is difficult to assess as it is virtually impossible to determine the true incidence of enchondromas, but the rate of transformation is likely <1%

Treatment:

- Followed (especially for large lesions)
- Curettage and bone grafting for large or suspicious lesions. Recurrence is low

Miscellaneous facts:

- Lesions in hands and feet are more likely to be entirely lytic and present with pathologic fracture
- Most common bone tumor in hand

Differential diagnosis:

- Low grade chondrosarcoma—shows more endosteal scalloping, bony destruction and soft tissue component than enchondroma
- Bone infarct—peripheral serpentine calcifications without bony expansion or central cartilaginous matrix

Features to Distinguish Low-Grade Chondrosarcomas from Enchondroma

- Endosteal cortical scalloping >2/3 thickness (best distinguishing feature)
- Pain, especially in a previously asymptomatic lesion
- Growing lesion, especially after skeletal maturity
- Periosteal reaction
- Axial lesions (pelvis, scapula, and sternum) are more likely to be malignant
- Large size (>5 cm)
- Soft tissue component
- Epiphyseal location
- Lucent areas in densely calcified lesions (target these areas for biopsy)
- Uptake of lesion greater than anterior iliac crest on bone scintigraphy
- Older patients

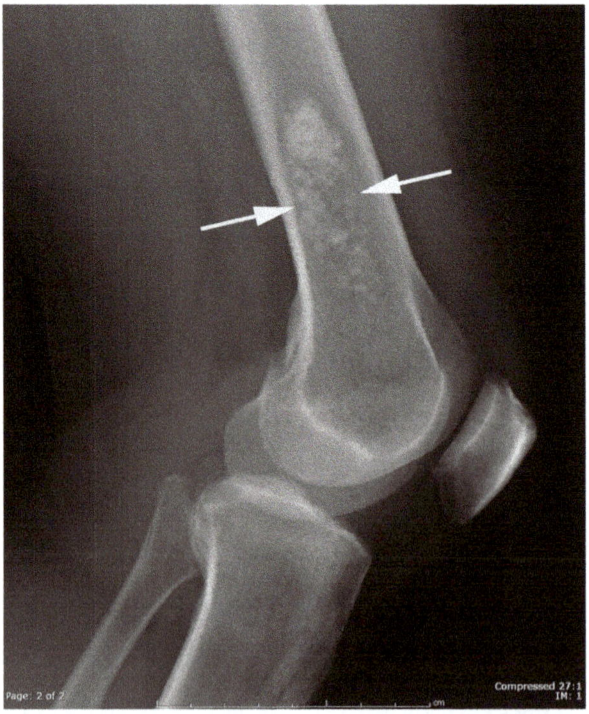

Fig. 4.5 Enchondroma (*arrows*) in the distal femur with "arcs and rings" of chondroid matrix calcification

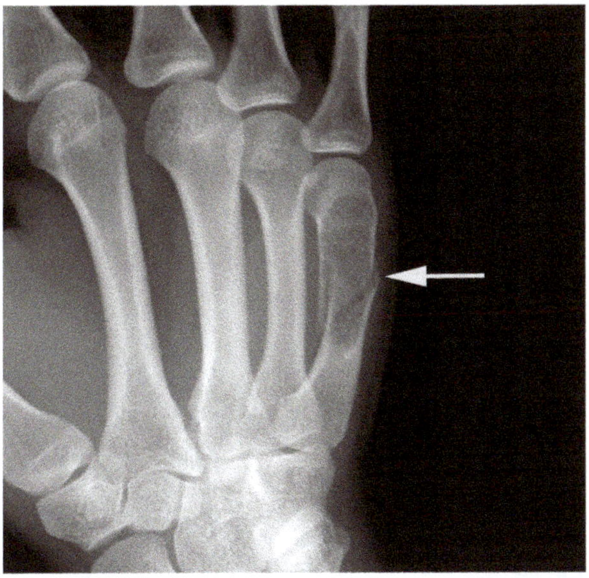

Fig. 4.6 Enchondroma (*arrow*) in fifth metacarpal presenting with pathologic fracture and minimal chondroid matrix

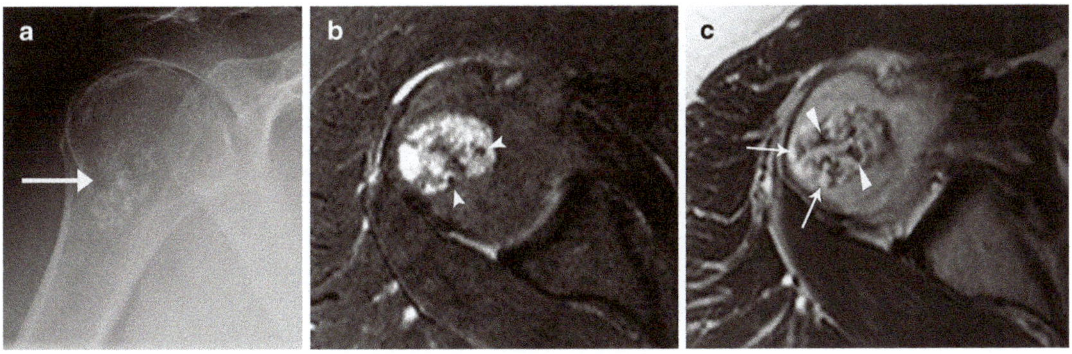

Fig. 4.7 Enchondroma in the proximal humerus. Radiograph (**a**) shows "arcs and rings" chondroid matrix calcifications (*arrow*). The enchondroma is bright on the STIR MR image (**b**) due to the high water content of the hyaline cartilage. The T2-weighted MR image (**c**) shows chemical shift artifact at the periphery of the lesion (*arrows*). The calcifications appear low signal on both MRI images (*arrowheads*)

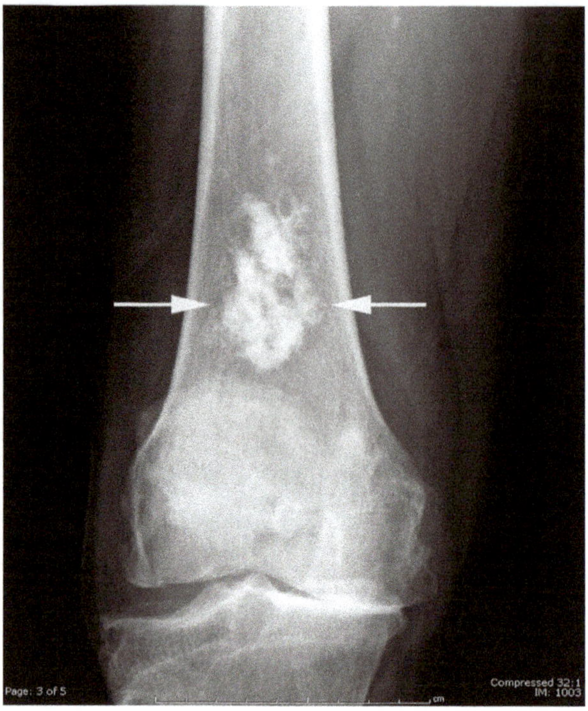

Fig. 4.8 Radiograph of the distal femur shows a densely calcified lobulated enchondroma (*arrows*). The periphery of the lesion shows more typical "arcs and rings" calcification from the chondroid matrix

Multiple Enchondromatosis

- Includes Ollier's disease and Maffucci's syndrome
- Rare congenital disorder with numerous enchondromas
- Not hereditary
- Lesions stop growing at skeletal maturity, but there is usually severe limb deformity and growth disturbance
- Often on one side of the body, with the hands most commonly affected
- "**Columns of cartilage**" with fan-like septations instead of the round or oval forms of cartilage seen in solitary enchondromas
- Increased incidence of malignant transformation to chondrosarcoma (10–25%), even in hands, which is rare for solitary enchondromas
- Maffucci's syndrome versus Ollier's:
  - Maffucci's has multiple cavernous hemangiomas (phleboliths on radiographs)
  - Maffucci's has higher risk of malignant transformation than Ollier's disease

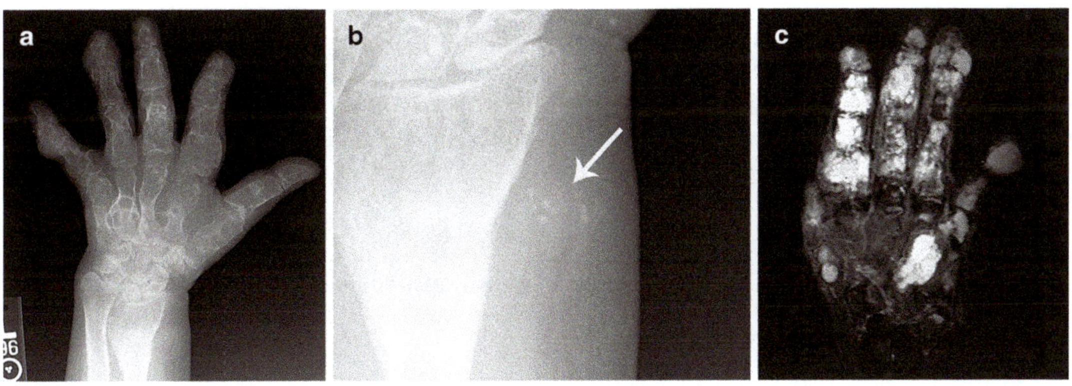

Fig. 4.9 Maffucci's syndrome. Note the multiple enchondromas enlarging the carpal bones leading to severe deformities on the radiograph (**a**). Phleboliths from cavernous hemangiomas (*arrow*) are present in the magnified view (**b**) of the radial soft tissue. The enchondromas (*arrows*) are hyperintense on T2-weighted MR image (**c**) image due to the high water content from the hyaline cartilage

Periosteal Chondroma

Synonyms: juxtacortical chondroma, parosteal chondroma

Demographics:
- <30 years, but has wide age range
- M>F, 2:1
- Rare, 2% of chondromas (enchondroma and multiple enchondromatosis are the others)

Origin:
- Benign cartilage lesion originating at periosteal surface. Slow growing
- Identical histology to enchondroma

Location:
- Long and small tubular bones
- Proximal humerus and hands most common
- Femur and tibia are other sites

Clinical symptoms: pain and swelling. Often palpable due to its periosteal location

Imaging characteristics:
- Small soft tissue mass (2–3 cm) with calcifications (50%), often radiolucent
- Cortical pressure erosion, "**saucerization**", with cortical thickening
- Typically does not extend into the medullary cavity
- Can appear aggressive, mimicking periosteal osteosarcoma/chondrosarcoma or infection
- CT can be helpful to show chondroid matrix
- High T2 signal on MRI
- Can rarely encase the bone, suggesting an intracortical lesion

Malignant potential: benign. Very rare reports of transformation into chondrosarcoma

Treatment: resection (intralesional, marginal, and en bloc)

Miscellaneous facts: associated with tendon and ligament insertions

Differential diagnosis:
- Periosteal osteosarcoma—are more likely to be diaphyseal, and contain sunburst or hair-on-end periosteal reaction, but can be hard to distinguish from a periosteal chondroma
- Juxtacortical (periosteal) chondrosarcoma—occur in older patients, do not have endosteal sclerosis, and are larger (4–5 cm) than periosteal chondromas. In large series, no periosteal chondrosarcomas were <3 cm
- Osteochondroma—contiguous marrow cavity
- Osteomyelitis—signs of infection and lack of large soft tissue component can help distinguish from periosteal chondroma

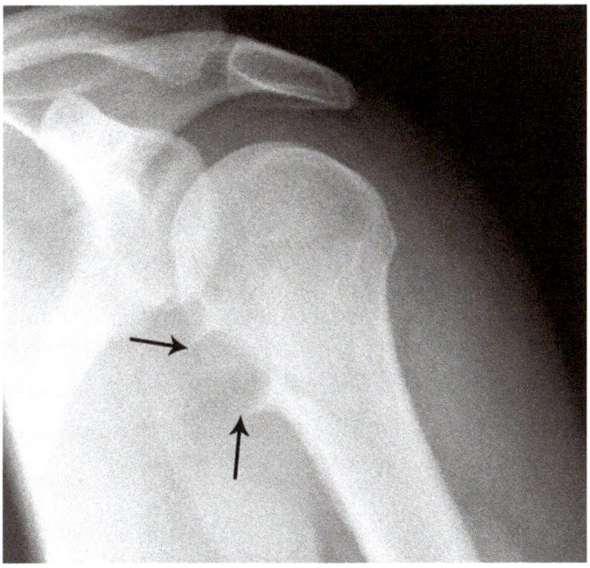

Fig. 4.10 Periosteal chondroma (*arrows*) in the proximal humerus. Note the faint calcifications and cortical erosion "saucerization" on the surface of the bone

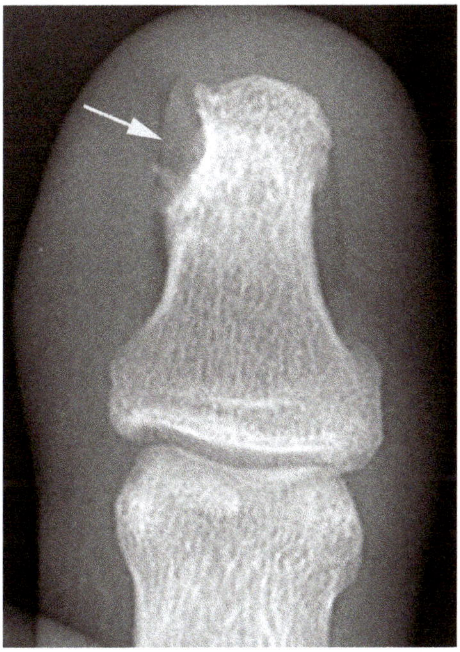

Fig. 4.11 Periosteal chondroma (*arrow*) arising from the distal first phalanx. There is a pressure erosion of the cortical surface and faint calcifications in the lesion. The feet and hands are the most common locations for this tumor

Chondroblastoma

Synonyms: Codman's tumor, calcifying giant cell tumor, epiphyseal chondromatous giant cell tumor

Demographics:
- 10–25 years
- M>F, 2:1
- Rare, <1% of all bone tumors

Origin: benign cartilaginous tumor with abundant chondroblasts and multinucleated giant cells

Location:
- Epiphysis or apophysis
- Long bones (75%): humerus, around the knee (distal femur, proximal tibia) "end of bone" equivalents (pelvic bones, calcaneus, talus, patella, and scapula)

Clinical symptoms:
- Joint pain and stiffness
- Joint effusion (30%)
- Temporal bone lesions can cause deafness, tinnitus, and vertigo

Imaging characteristics:
- Eccentric, well-defined, round or oval lucency centered in the epiphysis, 2–3 cm
- Narrow zone of transition with or without a thin sclerotic margin (60%)
- Chondroid matrix only seen in 1/3 of cases
- Open growth plate in 70%
- Typically nonexpansile. If bone expansion is present, then consider chondroblastoma with associated aneurysmal bone cyst
- Fluid–fluid levels on CT/MRI due to association with ABC
- MRI:
  - Low T1 signal and heterogeneous intermediate signal on T2-weighted images is due to cellular chondroid matrix (unlike the bright T2 hyaline cartilage matrix seen in chondromas)
  - Marrow and soft tissue edema can involve a larger area than expected from the radiographs
- "Aggressive" chondroblastomas may cross growth plate, enter metaphysis or joint space, have thick periosteal reaction, and/or soft tissue component

Malignant potential:
- Very rare risk of transformation to chondrosarcoma
- "Pulmonary metastases" without malignant cells can occur and are associated with prior surgical treatment

Treatment:
- Curettage and packing with bone graft or methylmethacrylate
- Surgical resection
- Local recurrence in 10–15%, typically in first 2 years; higher recurrence if associated with ABC

Miscellaneous facts:
- Also known as Codman's tumor.
- Craniofacial involvement (temporal bone) in older pts (>40 years)
- Metaphyseal based chondroblastomas can be more aggressive
- 15–25% are associated with aneurysmal bone cyst

Differential diagnosis:

- Giant Cell Tumor (GCT)—centered at the physeal scar and extends into epiphysis and metaphysis. Also GCT are seen almost exclusively in skeletally mature patients with closed physes.
- Osteomyelitis—does not have sclerotic rim or chondroid matrix, but can be hard to distinguish from "aggressive chondroblastoma" which can have periosteal reaction, marrow edema, and expansile bony destruction
- Clear cell chondrosarcoma—occurs in older population, larger size, and more likely to extend beyond the epiphysis than chondroblastoma
- Subchondral cyst—usually has signs of osteoarthritis in the joint and do not have chondroid matrix

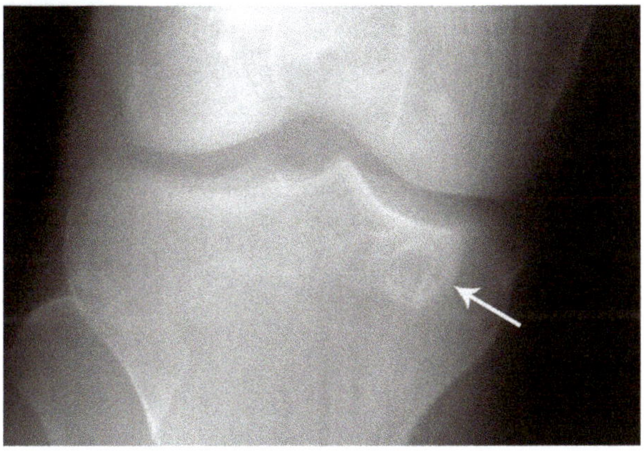

Fig. 4.12 Chondroblastoma (*arrow*) in the proximal tibial epiphysis in a 19-year old male

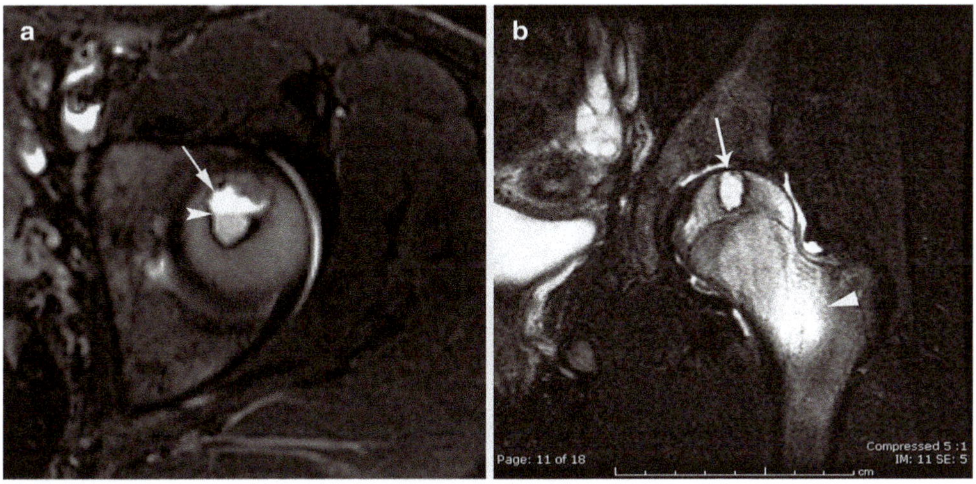

Fig. 4.13 Chondroblastoma (*arrows*) with ABC component in the proximal femoral epiphysis. Note the fluid–fluid level (*arrowhead*) on the axial T2-weighted MR image (**a**) due to the ABC component and the reactive edema in the femoral neck (*arrowhead*) on the coronal T2-weighted MR image (**B**)

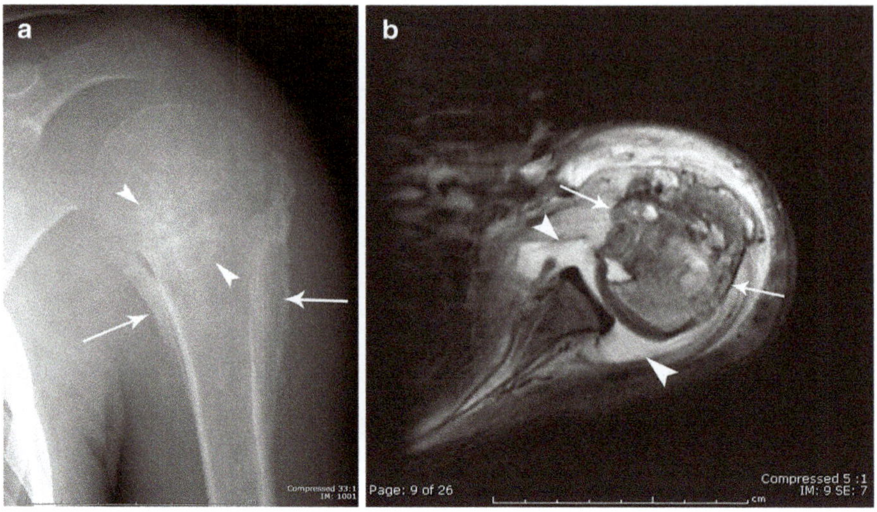

Fig. 4.14 Aggressive chondroblastoma. Radiograph (**a**) shows an epiphyseal lesion in the humeral head with ill-defined margins, cortical destruction, lamellated periosteal reaction (*arrows*), and chondroid matrix (*arrowheads*). Corresponding STIR MR image (**b**) shows extensive marrow edema (*arrows*), adjacent soft tissue edema, and a large joint effusion (*arrowheads*)

Epiphyseal Lesions: Differential diagnosis

- Chondroblastoma
- Subchondral cyst
- Aneurysmal bone cyst
- Langerhans cell histiocytosis
- Osteomyelitis
- Giant cell tumor of bone
- Intraosseous ganglion
- Clear cell chondrosarcoma
- Osteonecrosis

Chondromyxoid Fibroma

Synonyms: fibromyxoid chondroma, myxofibrous chondroma

Demographics:
- Second to third decades
- M>F (slightly)
- Very rare. Two percent of benign tumors

Origin:
- Benign cartilaginous lesion containing fibrous and myxoid tissue
- Can be difficult to distinguish at pathology from chondroblastoma

Location:
- Proximal tibia (most common), pelvic bones, rib, foot, hand
- Differs from chondroblastoma as it has a metaphyseal location
- Rarely crosses growth plate

Clinical symptoms:
- Slowly progressive pain, tenderness, swelling, and loss of mobility
- Occasionally asymptomatic (especially pelvic and rib lesions)

Imaging characteristics:
- Lytic lesion with delicate sclerotic margins (thinner than NOFs)
- Cartilaginous matrix and matrix calcifications are uncommon (7–13%)
- Eccentric, metaphyseal location (chondroblastoma is epiphyseal)
- Often lobulated with cortical expansion "**cortical bubbling sign**", ballooning out from cortex, especially for larger lesions
- Occasionally with septations and periosteal reaction

Malignant potential: rare reports of malignant transformation to chondrosarcoma

Treatment:
- Wide excision, curettage and bone grafting
- High recurrence rate with curettage (15–25%)

Differential diagnosis:
- Chondroblastoma—has epiphyseal location and more likely to have chondroid matrix
- NOF—much more common, have a thicker sclerotic rim, less delicate bubbly appearance, and lack of the "cortical bubbling" that occurs with chondromyxoid fibromas
- Fibrous dysplasia—have ground glass matrix instead of lucent matrix seen in CMFs. Central, instead of eccentric location
- ABC—have fluid–fluid levels and can be difficult to distinguish from CMF
- GCT—usually do not have a sclerotic rim and extend to the articular surface
- Chondrosarcoma—are more likely to have aggressive features, cortical destruction, and soft tissue component. Also much more likely to have chondroid matrix than CMF

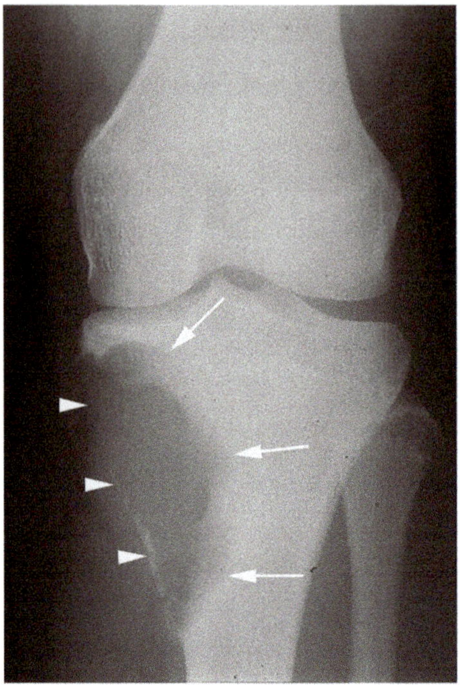

Fig. 4.15 Chondromyxoid fibroma (*arrows*) in the proximal tibia. Note the eccentric location, faint sclerotic margin, lack of intralesional calcifications, and cortical "ballooning" (*arrowheads*). Image courtesy of Dr. Lee Katz, New Haven, CT

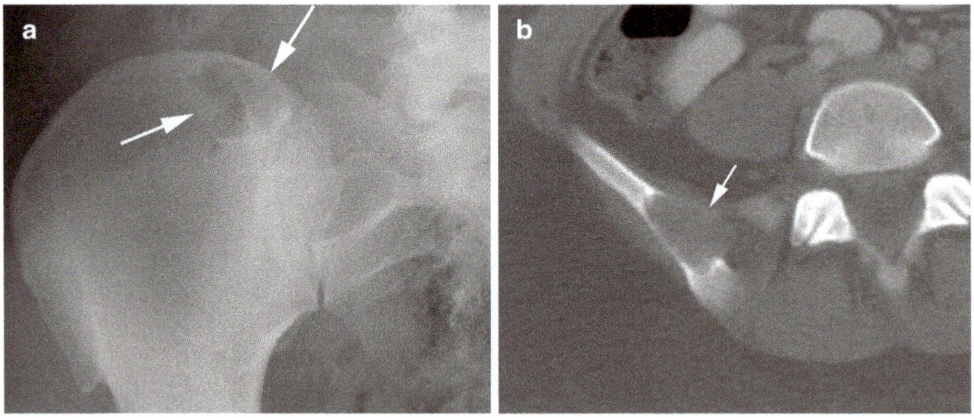

Fig. 4.16 Chondromyxoid fibroma (*arrows*) in the right iliac bone. Note the lucent lesion with narrow zone of transition, faintly sclerotic margin, mild cortical expansion, and lack of internal mineralization on the radiograph (**a**) and CT (**b**) images

Chondrosarcoma (Conventional)

Synonyms: intramedullary chondrosarcoma

Demographics:

- 30–60 years
- M>F (slight)
- 20% of malignant primary bone lesions. 80% of all chondrosarcomas
- Third most common malignant bone (after multiple myeloma and osteosarcoma)

Origin:

- Malignant lesion containing hyaline cartilage
- Typically low grade
- De novo lesions are called primary chondrosarcomas
- Secondary chondrosarcomas arise from preexisting lesions: osteochondroma (most common), enchondroma, periosteal chondroma, Paget disease, irradiated bone

Location:

- Pelvis, long tubular bones (femur, humerus), scapula, sternum, ribs. Rare in hand, feet, and craniofacial bones
- Metadiaphyseal
- If in long bones, usually proximal>>distal
- Axial>appendicular skeleton

Clinical symptoms:

- Slow growing
- Pain and soft tissue swelling (especially in previously asymptomatic lesion)
- Pathologic fracture in 3–17%

Imaging characteristics:

- Mixed lytic and sclerotic lesion arising from medullary cavity with cartilaginous matrix ("arcs and rings" pattern of mineralization)
- Large lesions, usually >4 cm, mean 10 cm
- Variable zone of transition
- Thickened cortex and smooth endosteal scalloping, reflecting slow growth
- Nonaggressive periosteal reaction (if any) due to slow growth
- Aggressive periosteal reaction, cortical breakthrough, permeative pattern are seen in higher grade lesions and other subtypes of primary chondrosarcomas
- CT:
  - More helpful than MRI in showing cartilaginous matrix and subtle endosteal scalloping (best feature to distinguish from enchondroma)
  - Shows entrapment and destruction of surrounding bone by cartilaginous matrix
- MRI:
  - Very bright T2 soft tissue component due to high water content from hyaline cartilage
  - Shows lobulated growth pattern and marrow/soft tissue extension
- Bone scintigraphy:
  - Increased heterogeneous uptake, greater than anterior iliac crest

Malignant potential:

- Dependent on subtype.
- High grade subtypes have a 10% survival at 5 years
- Histologic grade is the most important predictor of local recurrence and metastasis

Treatment:

- Depends on subtype
- Low grade—curettage with thermal/chemical ablation and packing
- Higher grade—adequate wide surgical resection with allograft reconstruction is gold standard
- Adjuvant chemotherapy not very useful
  - Radiation used for lesion not amenable to surgery or when incompletely resected

Differential diagnosis:

- Enchondroma:
  - Lack of aggressive features (i.e., cortical breakthrough, endosteal scalloping, soft tissue component, periosteal reaction)
  - Rare in pelvis, ribs, sternum, and scapula, but chondrosarcoma more common in those sites
  - Very common in hands and feet, but uncommon locations for chondrosarcoma
- Osteosarcoma—osteoid instead of cartilaginous matrix, but can be difficult to distinguish
- Myositis ossificans—not attached to bone and dense mineralization is peripheral
- Osteonecrosis with secondary sarcoma—well-demarcated peripheral, as opposed to central, calcifications

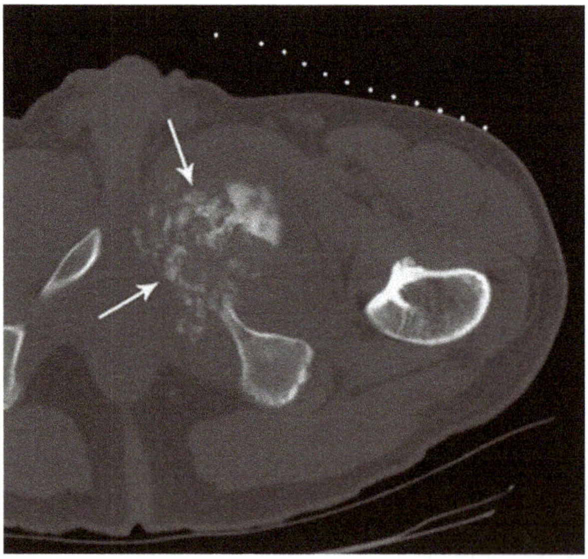

Fig. 4.17 Conventional chondrosarcoma (*arrows*) arising from the left inferior pubic ramus. Note the large size, chondroid matrix, and cortical destruction on the CT image

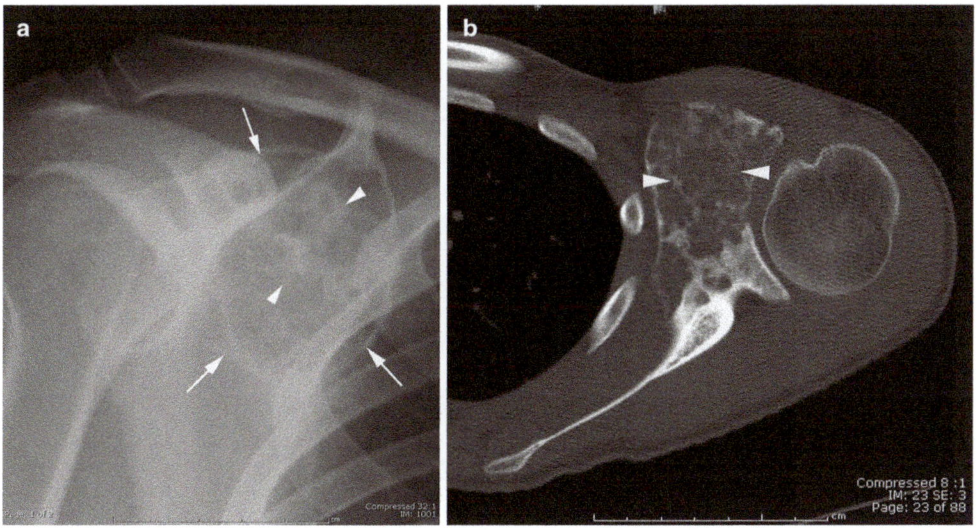

Fig. 4.18 Conventional chondrosarcoma (*arrows*) expanding the scapula. There is chondroid matrix in the lesion (*arrowheads*) which is well seen on the radiograph (**a**) and axial CT (**b**) image

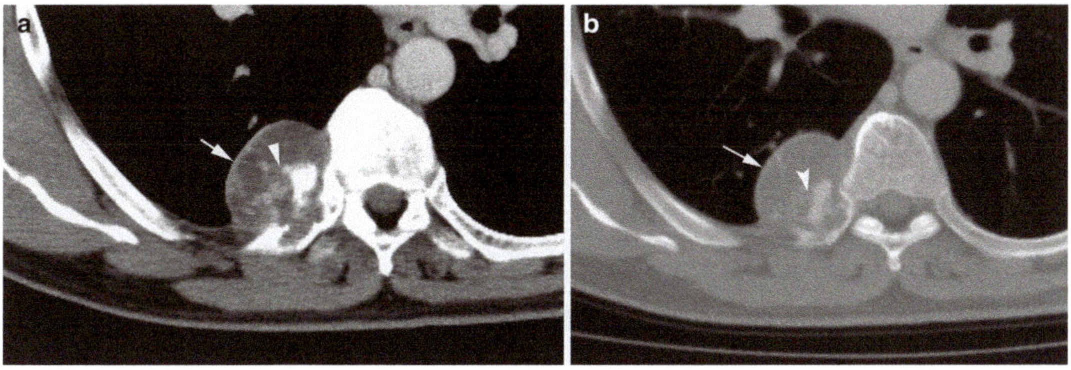

Fig. 4.19 Conventional chondrosarcoma (*arrows*). Soft tissue (**a**) and bone (**b**) window CT images show a lesion arising from the medial portion of a thoracic rib, containing a large soft tissue component and internal chondroid matrix (*arrowheads*)

Chondrosarcoma Subtypes

Primary

- Conventional (intramedullary):
  - Most common
  - Slow growing, well-differentiated
- Clear cell:
  - Very rare. Two percent of chondrosarcomas. M>>F
  - Low grade, nonaggressive appearing
  - "**End of bone**" lucent lesion with sclerotic rim (similar to chondroblastoma).
  - Third to fifth decade
  - Femoral (55%) and humeral heads, followed by pelvis
- Juxtacortical/periosteal:
  - 20–30 years. M>F. Four percent of chondrosarcomas
  - Arises from the periosteal surface of the bone
  - Similar to juxtacortical chondroma and periosteal osteosarcoma in appearance
- Mesenchymal:
  - Very rare. Three percent of chondrosarcomas
  - From primitive mesenchymal cartilaginous rests
  - 20–30 years. M=F
  - Lower limbs and skull (mandible and maxilla)
  - Lytic lesion with soft tissue component
- Dedifferentiated:
  - Occurs in 11% of chondrosarcomas
  - Worst prognosis of all chondrosarcomas
  - Contains at least two distinct components with abrupt transition histologically
    (1) Well differentiated cartilage lesion, such as an enchondroma
    (2) High grade sarcoma component (osteosarcoma, malignant fibrous histiocytoma, fibrosarcoma, and leiomyosarcoma)
  - Pelvis, proximal ends of femur and humerus
  - Look for two distinct radiographic appearances, such as an enchondroma, but with areas of nonmineralized matrix or soft tissue mass
  - Poor prognosis; needs aggressive treatment
- Extraosseous:
  - In soft tissues, especially lower extremities (80%)
  - Very rare. Two percent of soft tissue sarcomas
  - Lobulated pattern of calcification
  - Low grade

Secondary

- Arises from benign precursor lesions:
  - Enchondroma
  - Osteochondroma
  - Irradiated bone
  - Periosteal chondroma
  - Paget disease
  - Synovial chondromatosis

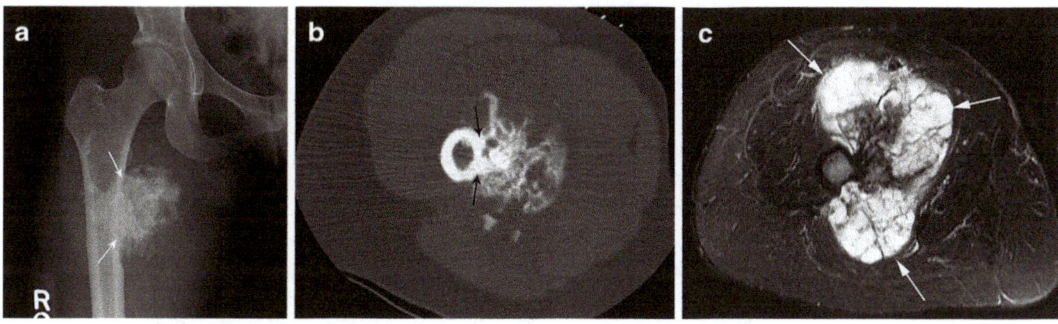

Fig. 4.20 Juxtacortical/periosteal chondrosarcoma. Note the lack of contiguity between the medullary cavities of the lesion and the host bone (*arrows*) on the radiograph (**a**) and CT (**b**) image, distinguishing the lesion from an osteochondroma. The large cartilaginous soft tissue component (*arrows*) is bright on the T2-weighted MR image (**c**)

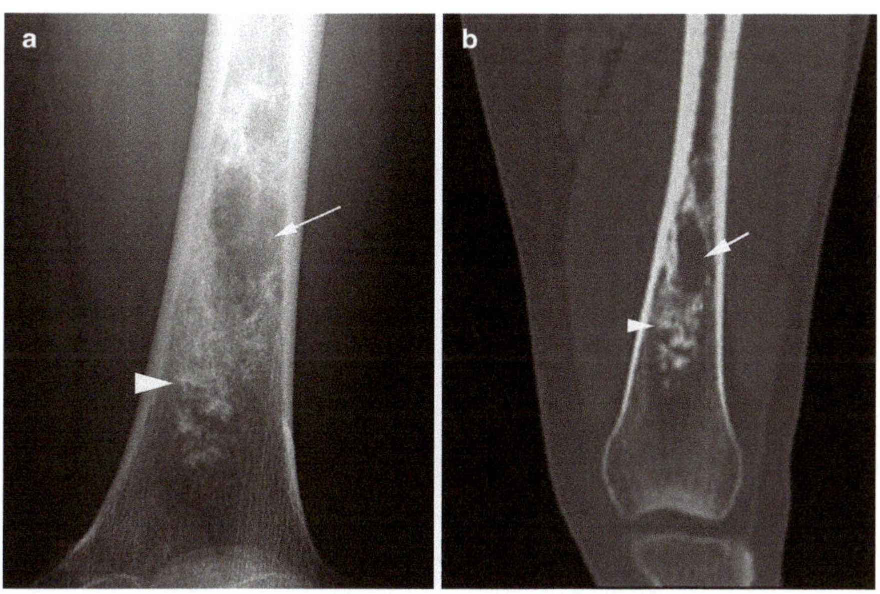

Fig. 4.21 Dedifferentiated chondrosarcoma arising in an enchondroma on radiograph (**a**) and CT (**b**). The non-mineralized matrix (*arrows*) is lucent, better seen on the CT scan, and represents the sarcomatous component. The nonsarcomatous chondroid matrix (*arrowheads*) is best seen at the inferior aspect of the lesion

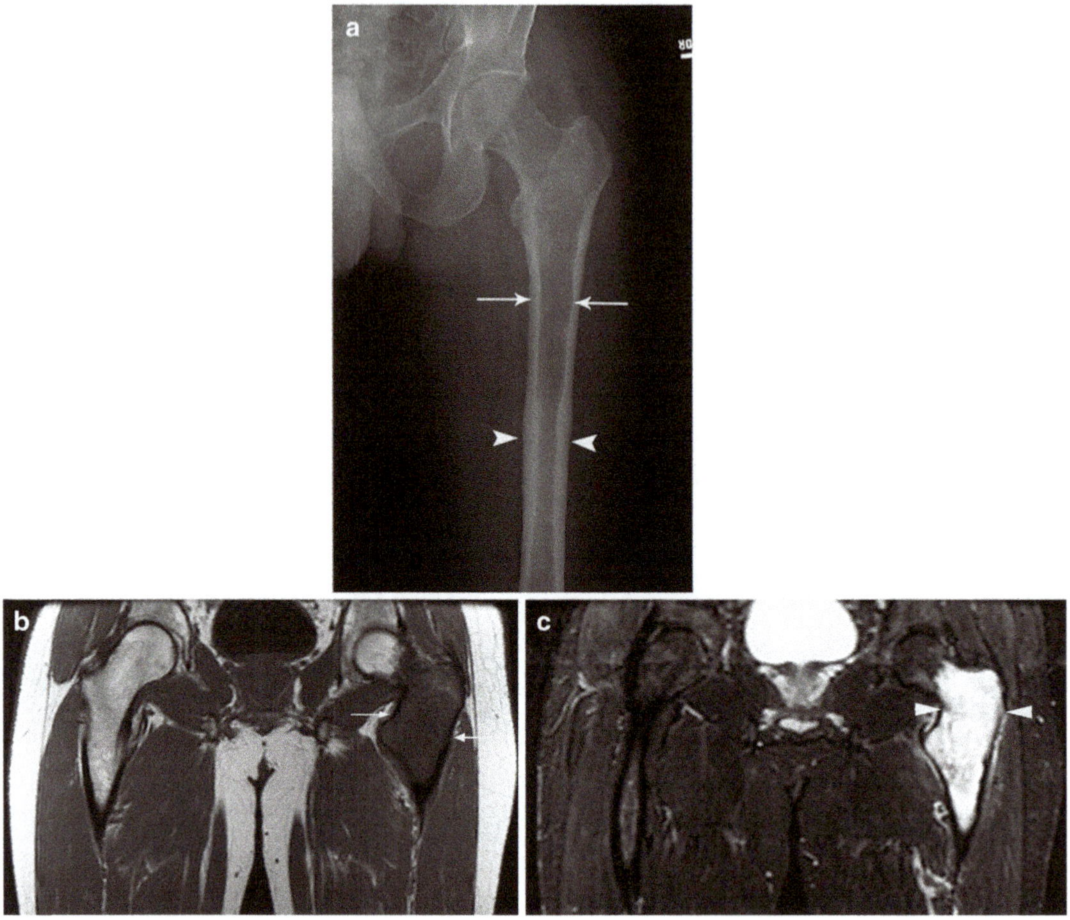

Fig. 4.22 Secondary chondrosarcoma in previously irradiated bone appears as an area of relative lucency (*arrows*) in the proximal femur on the radiograph (**a**). Note the cortical thickening (*arrowheads*) in the mid femoral shaft from prior irradiation. MRI images (**b**, **c**) show an area of marrow abnormality that is slightly darker on T1-weighted (*arrows*) and brighter on T2-weighted images (*arrowheads*) when compared to the adjacent muscle

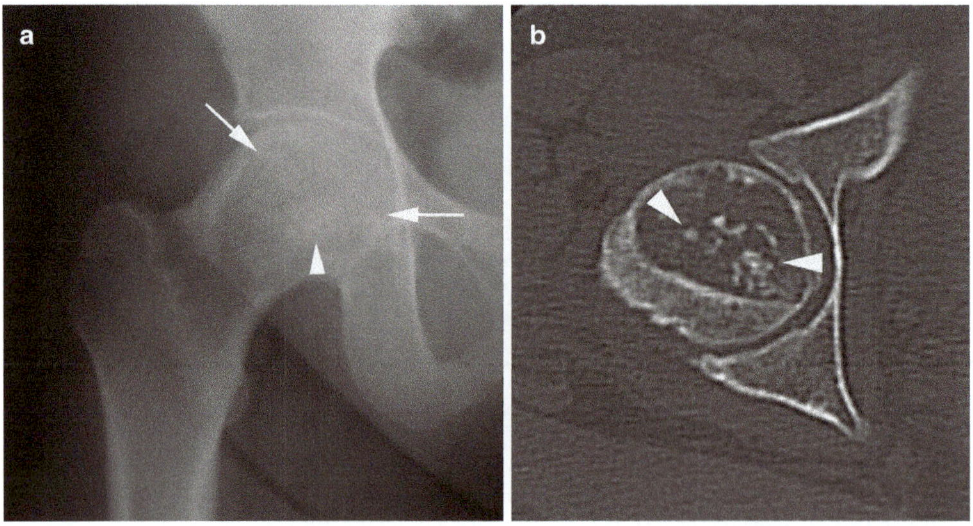

Fig. 4.23 Clear cell chondrosarcoma (*arrows*) in the femoral epiphysis. Note the epiphyseal location of the tumor (*arrows*) and internal chondroid matrix (*arrowheads*) on the radiograph (**a**) and CT (**b**) image. There is an extension of the lesion beyond the epiphysis into the femoral neck, which can help distinguish this epiphyseal lesion from a chondroblastoma. (Images courtesy of Dr. Dieter Lindskog, New Haven, CT)

Suggested Reading

1. Altay M, Bayrakci K, Yildiz Y, Erekul S, Saglik Y. Secondary chondrosarcoma in cartilage bone tumors: report of 32 patients. J Orthop Sci. 2007;12:415–23.
2. Bovee JV. Multiple osteochondromas. Orphanet J Rare Dis. 2008;3:3.
3. Brien EW, Mirra JM, Kerr R. Benign and malignant cartilage tumors of bone and joint: their anatomic and theoretical basis with an emphasis on radiology, pathology and clinical biology. I. The intramedullary cartilage tumors. Skeletal Radiol. 1997;26:325–53.
4. Brien EW, Mirra JM, Luck Jr JV. Benign and malignant cartilage tumors of bone and joint: their anatomic and theoretical basis with an emphasis on radiology, pathology and clinical biology. II. Juxtacortical cartilage tumors. Skeletal Radiol. 1999;28:1–20.
5. Chaabane S, Bouaziz MC, Drissi C, Abid L, Ladeb MF. Periosteal chondrosarcoma. AJR Am J Roentgenol. 2009;192:W1–6.
6. Fletcher CD, Unni KK, Mertens F, editors. WHO classification of tumours: pathology and genetics of tumours of soft tissue and bone. Lyon, France: IARC; 2002.
7. Greenspan A, Jundt G, Remagen W. Differential diagnosis in orthopaedic oncology. 2nd ed. Philadelphia, PA: Lippincott Williams & Wilkins; 2007.
8. Lee KC, Davies AM, Cassar-Pullicino VN. Imaging the complications of osteochondromas. Clin Radiol. 2002;57:18–28.
9. Littrell LA, Wenger DE, Wold LE, et al. Radiographic, CT, and MR imaging features of dedifferentiated chondrosarcomas: a retrospective review of 174 de novo cases. Radiographics. 2004;24:1397–409.
10. Miller TT, Schweitzer ME. Diagnostic musculoskeletal imaging. New York, NY: McGraw-Hill; 2005.
11. Murphey MD, Choi JJ, Kransdorf MJ, Flemming DJ, Gannon FH. Imaging of osteochondroma: variants and complications with radiologic–pathologic correlation. Radiographics. 2000;20:1407–34.
12. Murphey MD, Walker EA, Wilson AJ, Kransdorf MJ, Temple HT, Gannon FH. From the archives of the AFIP: imaging of primary chondrosarcoma: radiologic–pathologic correlation. Radiographics. 2003;23:1245–78.
13. Pannier S, Legeai-Mallet L. Hereditary multiple exostoses and enchondromatosis. Best Pract Res Clin Rheumatol. 2008;22:45–54.
14. Resnick D, editor. Diagnosis of bone and joint disorders. 4th ed. Philadelphia, PA: W.B. Saunders; 2002.
15. Robinson P, White LM, Sundaram M, et al. Periosteal chondroid tumors: radiologic evaluation with pathologic correlation. AJR Am J Roentgenol. 2001;177:1183–8.

5 Osseous Tumors

The neoplasms in this category all form osseous matrix and are divided into benign and malignant tumors. Although bone islands and osteomas are not classified by the World Health Organization (WHO) as true tumors, they are included here under benign osteogenic tumors for simplicity and due to their common occurrence. Bone islands and osteomas appear as dense lesions within and on the surface of bone, respectively, and the major concern is distinguishing them from sclerotic metastases. Osteoid osteomas and osteoblastomas are bone-forming tumors with a highly vascular central nidus and are often surrounded by dense reactive sclerosis. They are nearly identical histologically, and the distinction is made based on imaging. Osteoid osteomas have a nidus smaller than 2 cm and are more common in the appendicular skeleton. Osteoblastomas have a nidus greater than 2 cm, and have a more varied appearance, ranging from a dense lesion with a poorly visualized nidus to an expansile lytic lesion. Osteoblastomas also have a more varied clinical presentation than osteoid osteomas and may not respond to aspirin.

The osteogenic malignant tumors include conventional osteosarcomas, surface-based osteosarcomas, and secondary osteosarcomas. These tumors all form osseous matrix, with the conventional subtype accounting for 80% of osteosarcomas. The surface-based osteosarcomas typically occur in a slightly older age group, characterized by bone formation arising from the cortical surface, and can have a cartilage cap. Secondary osteosarcomas arise from bone with a preexisting condition such as Paget disease, osteonecrosis, or prior radiation.

J.S. Wu and M.G. Hochman, *Bone Tumors: A Practical Guide to Imaging*,
DOI 10.1007/978-1-4419-0808-7_5, © Springer Science+Business Media, LLC 2012

Benign

Bone island
Osteoma
Osteoid osteoma
Osteoblastoma

Malignant

- Osteosarcoma
  - Conventional
  - Telangiectatic
  - Parosteal
  - Periosteal
  - High grade surface
  - Low grade intramedullary
  - Small cell
  - Secondary
    - Paget disease
    - Osteonecrosis
    - Irradiated bone

Bone Island

Synonyms: enostoses, bone nucleus, calcific island in bone focal sclerosis

Demographics:
- Very common. Incidental finding
- M=F

Origin:
- Normal compact bone arising in the medullary cavity
- Not classified as a neoplasm by the WHO
- Considered a hamartoma (normal tissue in abnormal location)

Location:
- Periarticular
- Can occur anywhere, most common in pelvis, proximal femurs, and ribs
- Rare in spine, especially uncommon in cervical spine

Clinical symptoms: none

Imaging characteristics:
- Well-defined oval lesion
- Typically < 1 cm, giant bone islands >2 cm
- Parallel to the long axis of host bone
- Radiographs and CT:
  - "**Brush border**" margin with radiating spicules
  - Uniformly dense lesion

- MRI:
  - Uniformly low signal on all pulse sequences
  - Absence of surrounding edema to distinguish from sclerotic metastases
- Bone scintigraphy:
  - Usually normal (no uptake)
  - Large or metabolically active lesions may have mild uptake

Malignant potential:

- None
- Can grow, shrink, or disappear
- Actively growing lesion can have uptake on bone scintigraphy

Treatment:

- None
- Need to distinguish from osteoblastic metastasis
- Consider biopsy if lesion grows >25% in 6 months or >50% in 1 year

Miscellaneous facts:

- Higher incidence in people with leprosy

Differential diagnosis:

- Sclerotic metastasis—do not have radiating spicules, PSA >10 ng/mL
- Low grade osteosarcoma—usually larger than bone island
- Melorheostosis—thickened cortical bone with "**candle-wax dripping**" appearance in a sclerotome distribution and often extending from the cortical surface
- Osteopoikilosis—multiple bone islands, often in pelvis or shoulder girdle
- Osteopathia striata—autosomal dominant disorder with linear or fan-like areas of sclerosis in the long bones and pelvis
- Osteoid osteoma—typically cortically based

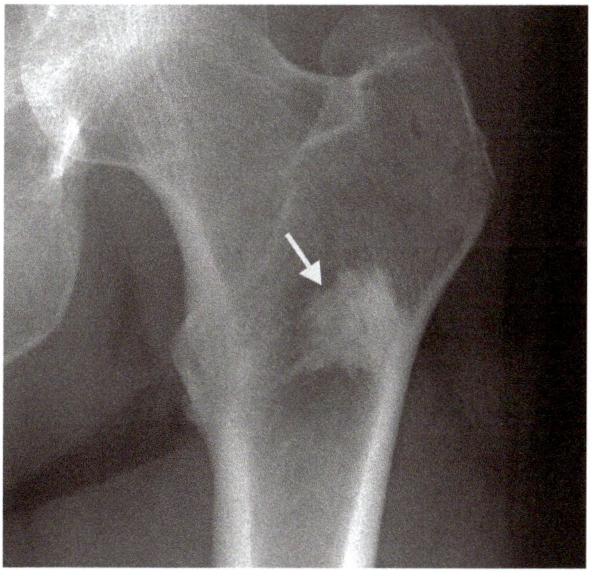

Fig. 5.1 Large bone island in the proximal femur (*arrow*). Note the spiculated "brush border" margin

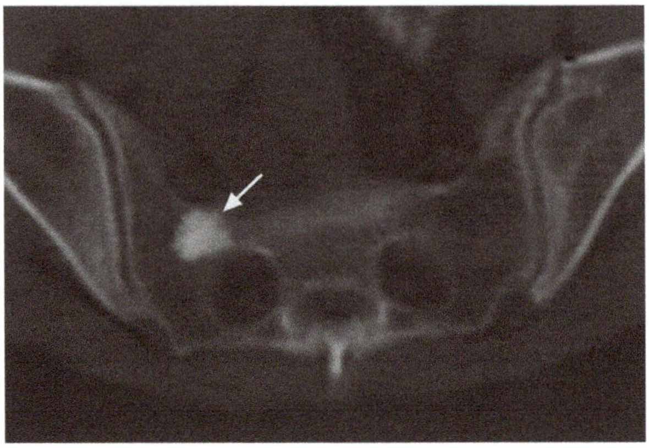

Fig. 5.2 Bone island (*arrow*) in the right sacral ala on CT

Osteoma

Synonyms: ivory exostoses

Demographics:

- Fourth to fifth decade
- M>F

Origin:

- Normal cortical bone, but abnormally thickened and arising from the periosteum
- Not classified as a neoplasm by the WHO
- Considered a hamartoma (normal tissue in abnormal location)

Location:

- Skull and sinuses. Frontal sinus (70%)
- Sphenoid lesions have high association with Gardner's syndrome
- Very rare in flat bones

Clinical symptoms:

- Typically asymptomatic
- Cosmetic issues
- Inner table skull lesions (rare) can cause neurologic symptoms
- Infection from obstruction of the frontonasal sinus
- Vision problems can occur from orbital osteomas

Imaging characteristics:

- Very dense bony lesion on surface of bone
- Well-circumscribed with smooth borders
- No appreciable medullary cavity
- MRI: uniformly low signal on all sequences and no enhancement or surrounding edema
- Bone scintigraphy: usually no uptake, mild uptake for metabolically active lesions

Malignant potential: none

Treatment: surgical excision if symptomatic

Miscellaneous facts:

- Associated with Gardner's syndrome: GI polyps, skin disorders (desmoids), osteomas. Autosomal dominant
- Associated with tuberous sclerosis

Differential diagnosis:

- Parosteal osteosarcoma—often has cortical invasion, which is rare with osteomas, and a less dense periphery than osteomas due to a soft tissue component
- Osteochondroma—has contiguity between host bone marrow cavity and lesion
- Melorheostosis—is more longitudinal and may involve multiple bones (sclerotome)
- Bone island—occurs in the medullary cavity, not the surface
- Parosteal lipoma—has a fatty component which is best seen on MRI
- Myositis ossificans—is not as uniformly dense as osteoma and not attached to bone surface

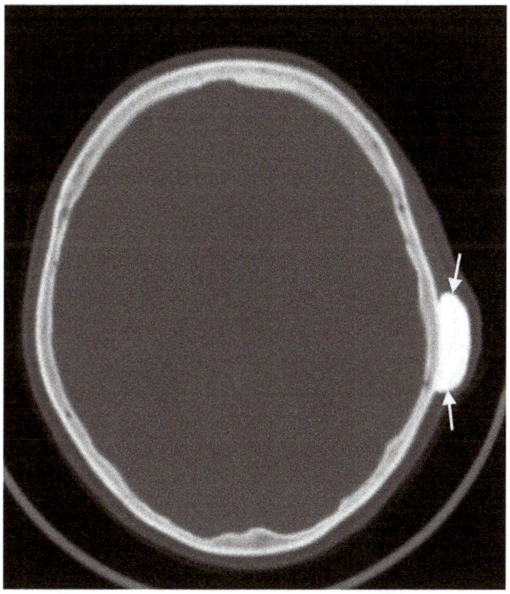

Fig. 5.3 Dense osteoma (*arrows*) arising from the outer table of the skull

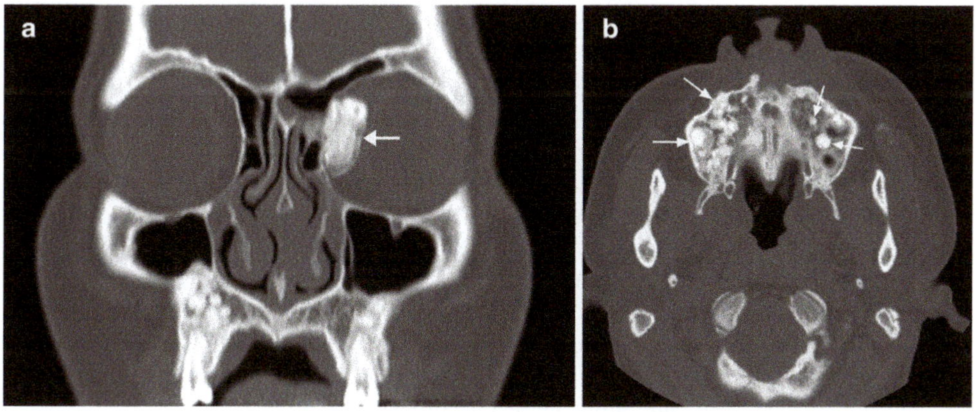

Fig. 5.4 Multiple osteomas in a patient with Gardner's syndrome. There is a large osteoma (*arrow*) arising from the medial wall of the left orbit on the coronal CT image (**a**) which is causing proptosis and visual impairment. Multiple small osteomas (*arrows*) are seen in the maxilla on the axial CT image (**b**). (Images courtesy of Dr. Gul Moonis, Boston, MA)

Osteoid Osteoma

Demographics:

- 7–25 years. Rare cases in very young, elderly, blacks
- M>F, 3:1
- 12% of benign bone tumors and 3% of primary bone tumors
- Classified based on location: cortical, medullary (cancellous), and subperiosteal

Origin: osteoblastic neoplasm with central core of highly vascularized connective tissue

Location:

- Femur and tibia are most common locations (60%)
- Spine (posterior elements in 90%), long bones, talus, and hand (proximal phalanx and metacarpal)
- Very rare in skull, clavicle, and sternum (no reported cases)

Clinical symptoms:

- Almost always painful, consider a different diagnosis if pain is not present
- Pain worse at night and relieved by aspirin quickly (interferes with prostaglandin release by tumor)
- Painful scoliosis or torticollis for spinal lesions (usually on concave aspect of the scoliotic curve near the apex)
- Lesions are rarely painless, but if asymptomatic, many occur in the hand
- Epiphyseal lesions are rare, but can lead to growth disturbances, inflammatory synovitis, joint effusion, and swelling

Imaging characteristics:

- Usually cortically based (80%), but can be medullary (cancellous), or subperiosteal
- Typically in diaphysis of long bones
- The tumor is the round lucency (nidus) and the surrounding sclerosis represents the reaction by the surrounding bone
- Majority of niduses are <1 cm
- Amount of sclerosis depends on location; intra-articular lesions can have minimal sclerosis due to absence of overlying periosteum
- Radiographs:
  - Cortical thickening
  - Nidus often not visible due to the dense reactive sclerosis
  - Poor for identifying lesions in the spine and pelvis
- CT:
  - Best modality for demonstrating the lucent nidus (based on ACR appropriateness guidelines)
  - The lucent nidus can contain variable amounts of central mineralization (punctate, amorphous, ring-like, and dense) which represents mineralized osteoid
  - Mineralization within the nidus is seen in 50% of cases using CT
  - Use bone windows with thin slices (1 mm)
- MRI:
  - Can be hard to assess with MRI alone
  - Nidus not as well seen as compared with CT
  - Nidus is low signal on T1-weighted and high on T2-weighted images, but often obscured by adjacent marrow edema
  - Edema and enhancement can mimic aggressive processes

- Bone scintigraphy:
  - Uptake on all three phases (vascular, blood pool, and delayed)
  - "**Double density**" sign: central focus of intense uptake surrounded by area of less intense uptake

Malignant potential:

- None
- Slow growing

Treatment:

- Can resolve spontaneously, possibly due to infarction of the nidus
- Treat with NSAIDS
- Painful lesions can be (1) excised or (2) treated with radiofrequency ablation
- Presurgical localization can be performed under CT guidance
- Incomplete removal of nidus can lead to recurrence

Differential diagnosis:

- Stress fracture—has a lucency that is linear and perpendicular to cortical surface
- Brodie's abscess—is an intramedullary lesion and may have a sinus tract
- Osteoblastoma—has nidus >2 cm, more common in spine
- Osteosarcoma—is more aggressive, look for soft tissue mass in osteosarcoma
- Osteoma—does not have nidus, cold on bone scintigraphy and no edema on MRI
- Bone island—does not have nidus, cold on bone scintigraphy and no edema on MRI
- Chondroblastoma—can have reactive sclerosis and marrow edema; intramedullary and epiphyseal location can help distinguish from osteoid osteoma, which is usually cortical and diaphyseal

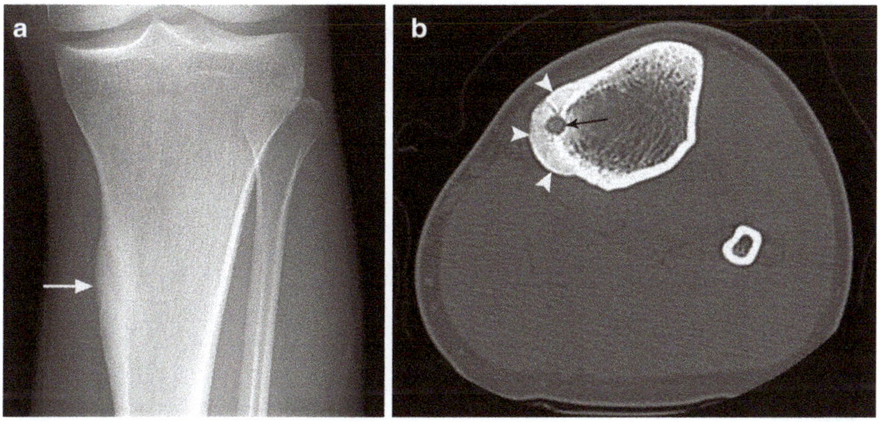

Fig. 5.5 Osteoid osteoma (*arrow*) causes smooth nonaggressive periosteal reaction in the tibial cortex (**a**). The lucent nidus (*black arrow*) with surrounding cortical thickening (*arrowheads*) and sclerosis is better appreciated on the CT (**b**) than on the radiograph

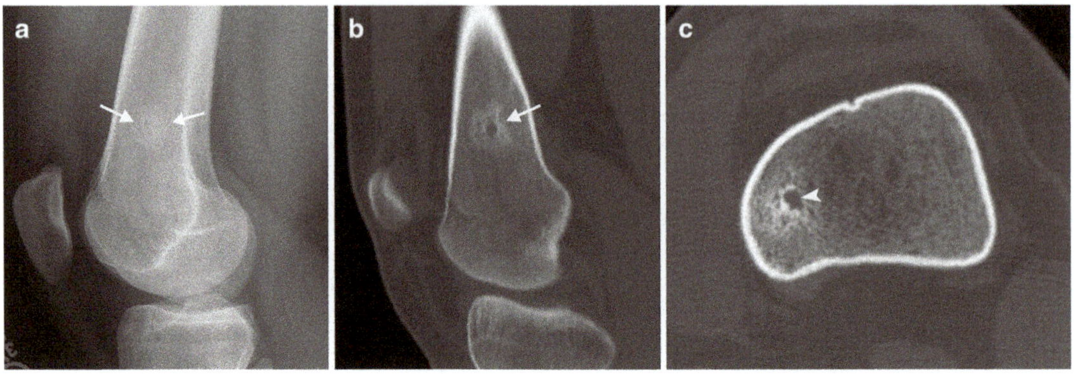

Fig. 5.6 Intramedullary osteoid osteoma (*arrows*) has minimal sclerosis on the radiograph (**a**) and is better seen on the sagittal CT image (**b**). The axial CT image (**c**) shows that the lucent nidus (*arrowhead*) is in a medullary, not cortical, location

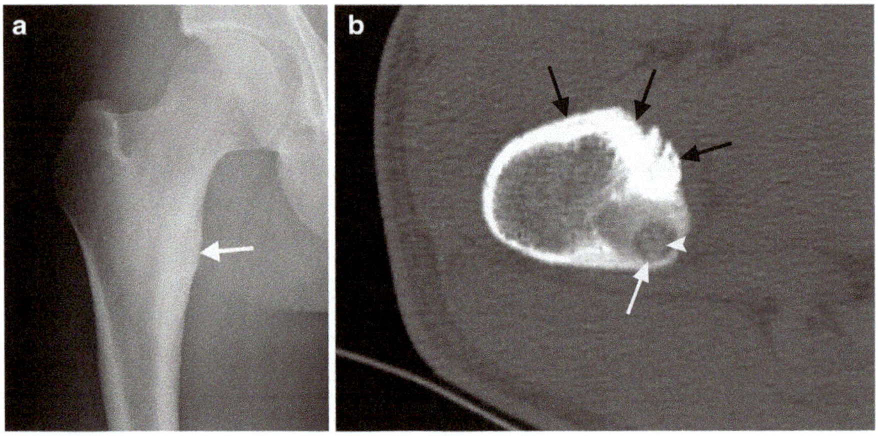

Fig. 5.7 Osteoid osteoma in the medial femoral cortex. Note the dense cortical thickening (*arrow*) obscuring the nidus on the radiograph (**a**). The lucent nidus (*white arrow*) is well seen on the axial CT image [**b**, contains amorphous central mineralization (*arrowhead*), and has adjacent cortical thickening (*black arrows*)]

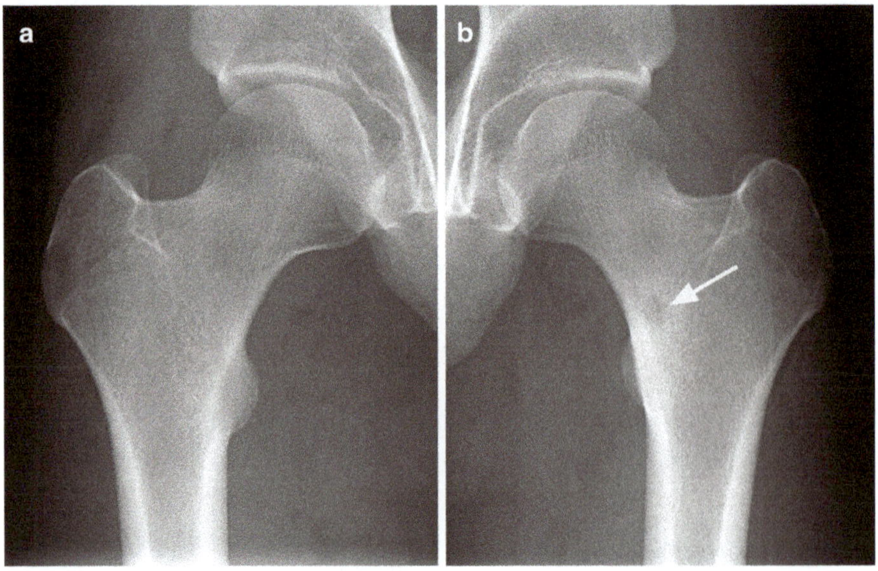

Fig. 5.8 Intra-articular osteoid osteoma (*arrow*) in the left femoral neck (**a**). There is minimal sclerosis surrounding the lucent nidus characteristic of intra-articular osteoid osteomas. The normal right femur is provided for comparison (**b**)

Osteoblastoma

Synonyms: giant osteoid osteoma, osteogenic fibroma, ossifying giant cell tumor

Demographics:
- 10–35 years
- M>F, 2:1
- 1% all bone tumors and 3% of benign bone tumors

Origin:
- Benign bone forming neoplasm with numerous osteoblasts and vascular osteoid matrix
- Same appearance histologically as osteoid osteoma

Location:
- Half are seen in the spine (posterior elements) and sacrum
- Femur, jaw and tibia are the next most common sites
- Most are in a medullary location, occasionally cortically based

Clinical symptoms:
- Pain and tenderness, but less severe than osteoid osteoma
- Scoliosis, back spasms, and neurologic symptoms from spine lesions
- Tooth pain if in jaw
- Not as responsive to aspirin as osteoid osteomas
- Can cause systemic osteomalacia, potentially due to release of humoral factors that impair proximal tubular renal function

Imaging characteristics:
- Varied appearance depending on location (four types)
  (1) Identical to osteoid osteoma, slightly expansile, well-defined lytic lesion which is enclosed by a periosteal shell of reactive bone. Nidus >2 cm
  (2) ABC-like lytic, expansile lesion with central radiodensities (common in the spine)
  (3) Aggressive lesion with periosteal reaction, often seen in the "aggressive osteoblastoma"
  (4) Very rare juxtacortical (periosteal) mass with thin shell of periosteal bone
- Lytic lesion with lucent nidus >2 cm (in osteoid osteoma, nidus is <2 cm)
- Most are 2–3 cm, however giant osteoblastomas can be >15 cm
- Can have focal internal calcification (30%)
- May have soft tissue component, unlike osteoid osteoma
- CT:
  - Best imaging modality
  - Very helpful for identifying lesions in spine
  - Also useful for showing nidus and central calcifications
- MRI:
  - Useful to evaluate for spinal compromise
  - Can have ABC-like features with fluid–fluid levels
  - Shows extent of marrow and soft tissue involvement
- Bone scintigraphy:
  - Intense uptake on all three phases

Malignant potential:
- "Aggressive osteoblastomas" have a more concerning histologic appearance and there are rare case reports of recurrent lesions causing death

Treatment:

- Curettage or excision
- Recurrence in 10–15%
- Aggressive osteoblastomas have recurrence of 50%
- Do not regress and disappear like osteoid osteomas

Miscellaneous facts:

- Some authors believe osteoid osteoma and osteoblastomas are the same pathologic process
- Osteoblastoma can be associated with secondary ABC

Differential diagnosis:

- ABC—have fluid—fluid levels without internal mineralization
- Osteoid osteoma—has nidus <2 cm
- Osteosarcoma—may have soft tissue component
- Brodie's abscess—may have sinus tract or adjacent abscess

Conventional Versus Aggressive (Malignant) Osteoblastoma

- No well-established distinction between the two lesions
- Death of a few patients with "aggressive" osteoblastomas has led to controversy
- Mostly a pathologic distinction
- See atypical cells, frequent mitoses, and multinucleated giant cells
- Similar to conventional osteosarcoma

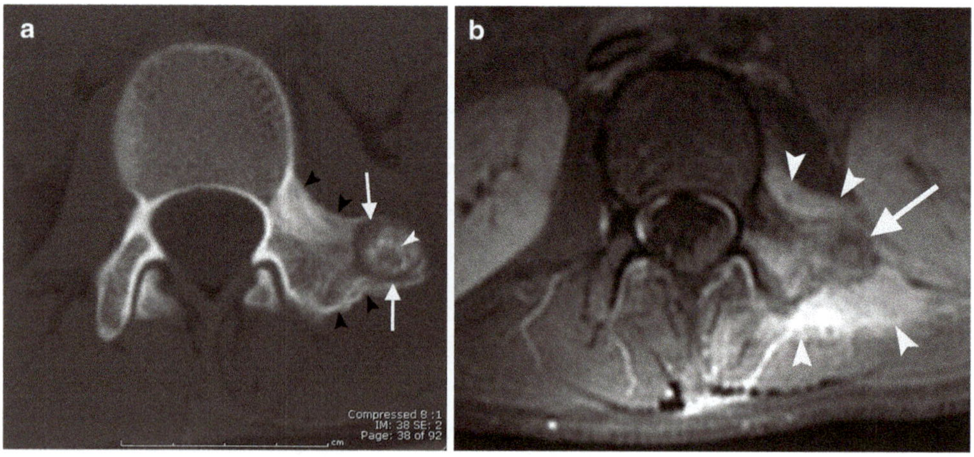

Fig. 5.9 A 22-year-old male with an osteoblastoma in the left transverse process. Note the large lucent central nidus (*arrows*), prominent internal calcifications (*white arrowhead*), and thick surrounding reactive sclerotic bone (*black arrowheads*) in the pedicle and transverse process on the CT image (**a**). There is enhancement of the nidus (*arrow*) and adjacent soft tissues (*arrowheads*) on the post contrast T1-weighted MR image (**b**)

Conventional Osteosarcoma

Synonyms: intramedullary osteosarcoma, classical osteosarcoma, osteogenic sarcoma, central osteosarcoma, primary osteosarcoma

Demographics:
- 10–25 years
- M>F, 3:2
- Second most common primary tumor of bone (#1 is myeloma), 20% of all bone malignancies, and 75% of osteosarcomas
- 30% of osteosarcomas occur in patients over age 40 (often with predisposing conditions such as Paget disease or irradiated bone)

Origin: intramedullary malignant neoplasm that produces osteoid matrix

Location:
- Distal femur (40%), proximal tibia, proximal humerus most common
- Usually metaphyseal (90%)
- Very rare in the hands and feet

Clinical symptoms:
- Dull aching pain, especially at night
- Limited range of motion
- Palpable mass
- Not associated with significant lymphadenopathy (if present, think osteomyelitis)
- Elevated alkaline phosphatase and lactic acid dehydrogenase

Imaging characteristics:
- Variable appearance on radiographs depending on the amount of osseous matrix (amorphous or cloud-like) and aggressiveness
- Typically a focal lesion with mixed lucency and sclerosis
- Wide zone of transition with aggressive features (cortical breakthrough, soft tissue mass)
- Aggressive periosteal reaction (disorganized, sunburst, and Codman's triangle)
- Staging workup:
  - CT and MRI useful for preoperative planning
  - Bone scintigraphy to assess for skip lesions (i.e., metastases in the same bone) and distant metastases
  - Chest CT for pulmonary metastases

Malignant potential:
- Metastases to lung (80%) and bone associated with very poor prognosis

Treatment:
- Preoperative chemotherapy to reduce vascularity, followed by surgical resection
- Seek >90% tumor necrosis prior to surgery
- Preservation of knee joint is of high priority
- Allografts (longer rehab, late complications)
- Endoprosthesis (long-term complication is loosening)

Miscellaneous facts:

- Osteosarcoma metastases to lung associated with pneumothorax from tumor necrosis at pleural surface
- Pulmonary metastases with osteoid matrix have poorer prognosis than those without
- May contain chondroblastic or fibroblastic elements (i.e., chondroblastic osteosarcoma). Even if only 1% osseous component, is still classified as an osteosarcoma

Differential diagnosis:

- Osteosarcoma with lytic appearance
  - Infection—can have infection history, sinus tracts, soft tissue ulcers, and less mass-like appearance
  - Fracture—can have trauma history, no soft tissue mass, and heals
- Osteosarcoma with dense appearance
  - Chondrosarcoma—has higher occurrence in axial skeleton and contains cartilaginous matrix
  - Myositis ossificans—does not arise from bone and has more mature calcifications peripherally
  - Avulsive cortical irregularity (cortical desmoid)–occurs in the posterior distal femoral metaphysis

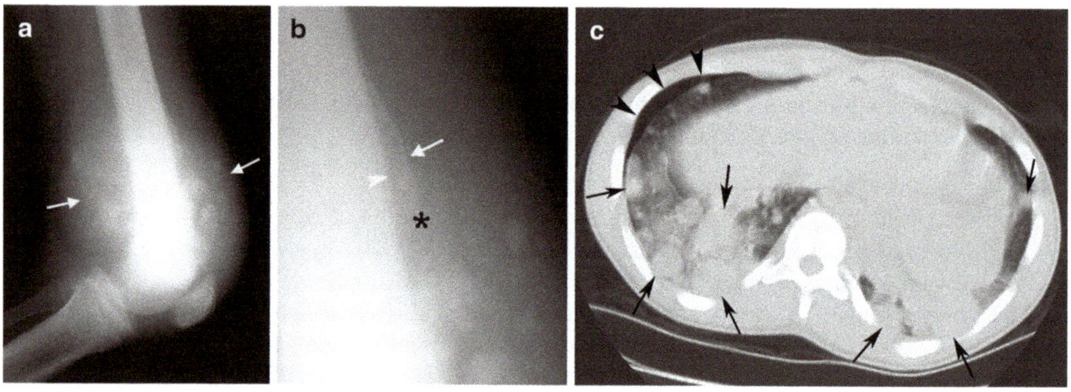

Fig. 5.10 Conventional osteosarcoma of the distal femur. Note the large soft tissue mass with osseous matrix (*arrows*) centered in the meduallary cavity of the distal femur on the radiograph (**a**). Magnified view (**b**) demonstrates a Codman's triangle at the anterior femoral cortex with three components: (1) lifted periosteum (*arrow*), (2) femoral cortex (*arrowhead*), and (3) soft tissue tumor mass (*asterisk*). Chest CT image (**c**) shows multiple pulmonary metastases (*arrows*) at the time of presentation which is associated with very poor prognosis. Right sided pneumothorax (*arrowheads*) is due to pleural based tumor necrosis

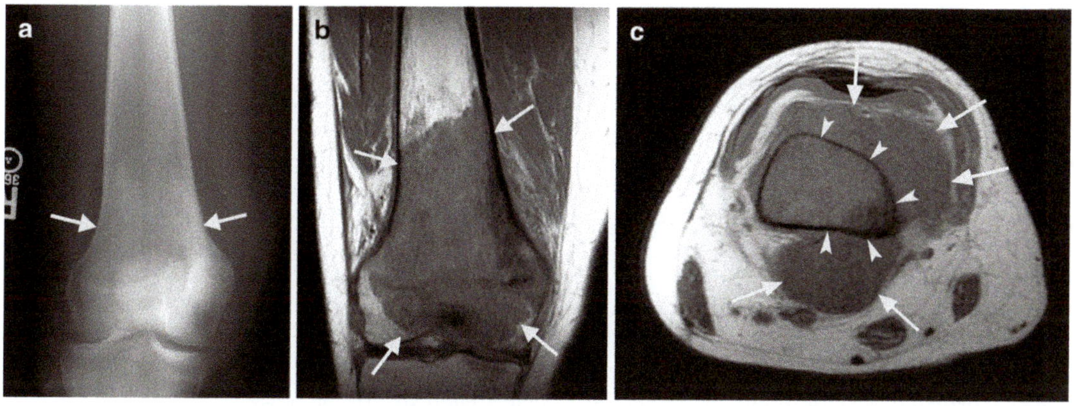

Fig. 5.11 Conventional osteosarcoma with minimal osteoid matrix. The AP radigraph of the distal femur (**a**) shows only mild subtle sclerosis (*arrows*). The tumor (*arrows*) is dark on the T1-weighted MR image (**b**). On the axial MR image (**c**), the large soft tissue component (*arrows*) extends outside the cortical margin of the femur (*arrowheads*) without cortical destruction as if "oozing from the bone"

Telangiectatic Osteosarcoma

Synonyms: malignant bone aneurysm, hemorrhagic osteosarcoma, aneurysmal bone cyst-like osteosarcoma

Demographics:
- Similar to conventional. 10–25 years
- M>F, 2:1
- <5% of osteosarcomas

Origin: malignant bone forming neoplasm containing necrosis and large cystic cavities containing hemorrhage

Location:
- Similar to conventional: distal femur, proximal tibia, and proximal humerus

Clinical symptoms:
- Pain
- Pathologic fracture in 25% of cases at presentation

Imaging characteristics:
- Radiographs show a lytic and expansile geographic lesion
- Little or no mineralization or sclerosis
- Cortical breakthrough with soft tissue component seen in 89% cases by MRI
- MRI and CT may show multiple blood-filled cystic spaces, "**fluid–fluid**" levels, "**bag of blood**"
- Bone scintigraphy shows a rim of peripheral uptake with central photopenic area, "**donut sign**"

Malignant potential:
- Most aggressive appearing osteosarcoma subtype
- Similar prognosis to conventional osteosarcoma, 68% 5-year survival

Treatment:

- Tumor removal with limb salvage
- Chemotherapy (pre- and postoperative)

Miscellaneous facts:

- Can be mistaken for aneurysmal bone cyst (look for nodular tumor components in telangiectatic osteosarcomas)
- Has been associated with Paget disease and retinoblastoma

Differential diagnosis:

- ABC—unlike ABCs, telangiectatic osteosarcomas have:
  (1) Thick, solid nodular tissue surrounding the cystic spaces
  (2) Matrix mineralization in the periphery, best seen on CT (but can be subtle)
  (3) Cortical destruction with associated nonencapsulated soft tissue mass
- GCT—has epiphyseal location and no osseous matrix
- Conventional osteosarcoma—typically has more osseous matrix, no fluid–fluid levels
- Osteomyelitis—fluid—fluid levels and hemorrhage less likely
- Fibrous dysplasia—ground glass appearance without cortical breakthrough or hemorrhage

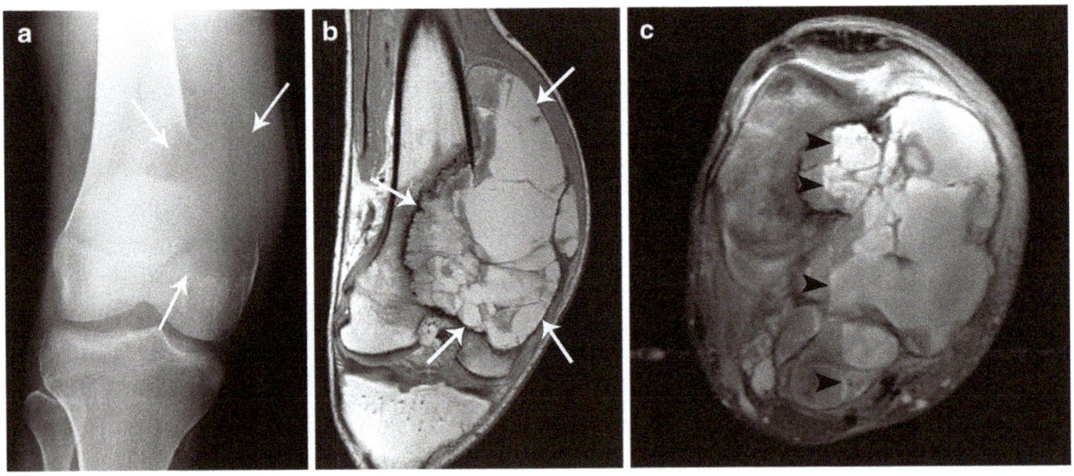

Fig. 5.12 Telangiectatic osteosarcoma in the distal femur. Note the aggressive lytic lesion with cortical breakthrough (*arrows*) on the radiograph (**a**). On the coronal (**b**) and axial (**c**) T1-weighted MR images, there is a large cystic soft tissue component tumor (*arrows*). Several internal fluid–fluid levels are seen the axial MR image (*arrowheads*). The patient was scanned on his side. (Images courtesy of Dr. Daniel Siegal, Detroit, MI)

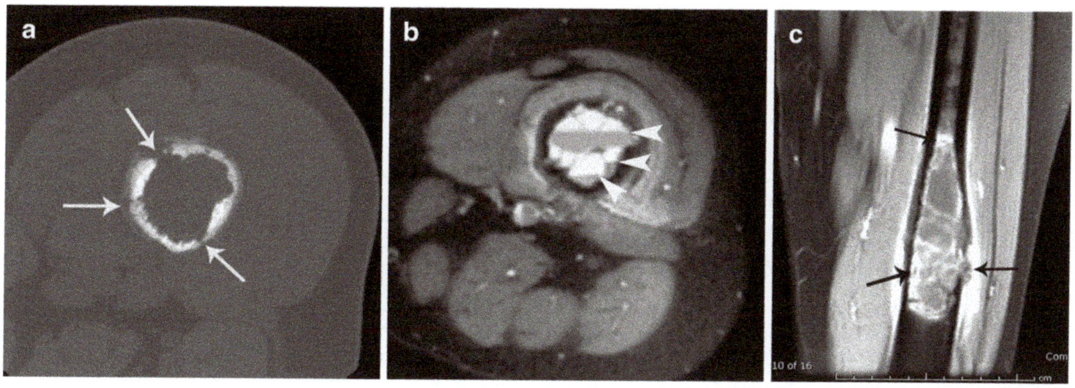

Fig. 5.13 Telangiectatic osteosarcoma of distal femoral shaft. Note the aggressive cortical breakthrough (*arrows*) on the CT image (**a**), fluid–fluid levels (*arrowheads*) on the axial STIR MR image (**b**), and enhancing peripheral nodular components (*black arrows*) on the coronal postcontrast fat-saturated T1-weighted MR image (**c**)

Parosteal Osteosarcoma

Synonyms: juxtacortical osteosarcoma

Demographics:
- 50% after age 30 (older than conventional)
- F>M
- 4% of osteosarcomas

Origin: bone forming tumor that arises from outer layer of periosteum

Location:
- Similar to conventional osteosarcoma
- Posterior aspect of distal femur (70%), proximal humerus, and proximal tibia
- Uncommon in flat bones (ilium and scapula)

Clinical symptoms:
- Painless or painful swelling
- Difficult to flex leg if in distal femur posteriorly

Imaging characteristics:
- "**Cleavage plane**" between lesion and host bone
- "**Stuck on**" cauliflower appearance to the surface of bone
- Occasionally wraps around the bone
- CT and MRI useful in delineating extent of mass and proximity to neurovascular structures and joint space
- Can have cap-like area containing cartilage similar to periosteal osteosarcomas and osteochondromas
- Marrow and soft tissue invasion occasionally (25%)

Malignant potential:
- Better prognosis than conventional, as lesions are typically low grade (91% survival at 5 years)
- Dedifferentiated lesions following recurrence have worse outcome
- Metastatic spread to lung

Treatment:

- Tumor removal with limb salvage
- Chemotherapy

Differential diagnosis:

- Myositis ossificans—will be separate from bone
- Osteochondroma—has contiguous marrow cavity with host lesion
- Periosteal osteosarcoma—is difficult to distinguish, but periosteal osteosarcomas are rarer than parosteal osteosarcomas. Also periosteal osteosarcomas are more likely to have sunburst periosteal reaction
- Parosteal lipoma—has fatty component and are more rare
- Nora's lesion (also known as bizarre parosteal osteochondromatous proliferation or BPOP)—typically occurs in hands and feet

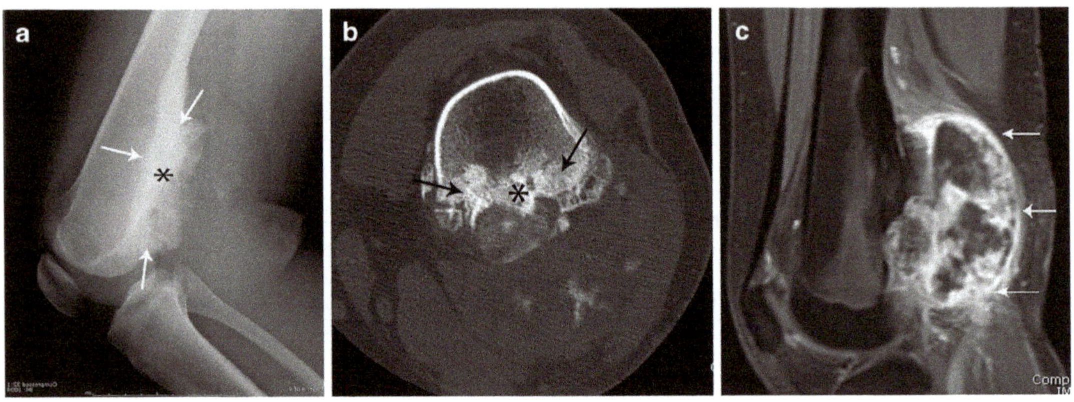

Fig. 5.14 A 16-year-old female with parosteal osteosarcoma of the distal femur. On the radiograph (**a**) and axial CT image (**b**), there is extensive thickening of the cortical surface (*arrows*) where the tumor arises. Note the lack of medullary and cortical contiguity between the lesion and the host bone (*asterisk*) which help distinguish the tumor from an osteochondroma. The large soft tissue component (*arrows*) has heterogeneous signal intensity on the sagittal fat-saturated T1 postcontrast MR image (**c**)

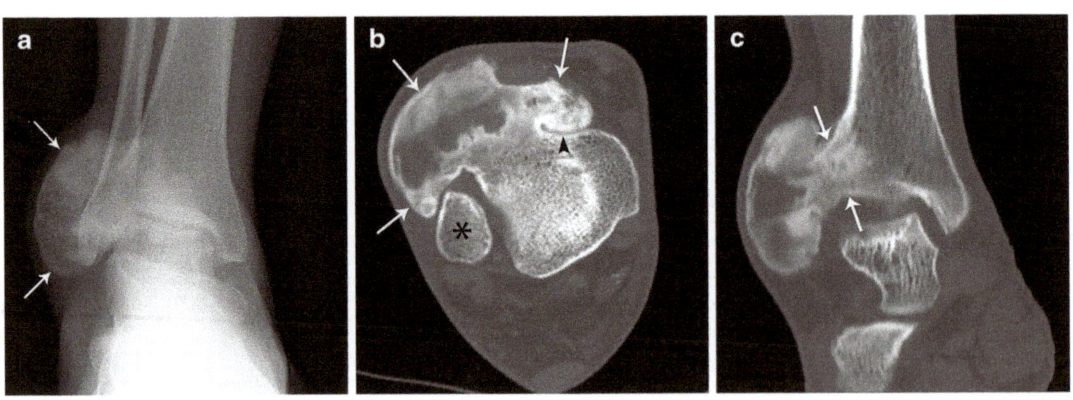

Fig. 5.15 Parosteal osteosarcoma of the distal tibia. Whether the lesion (*arrows*) arises from bone or is entirely in the soft tissues is difficult to assess on the radiograph (**a**) alone. The axial CT image (**b**) shows that the lesion (*arrows*) is arising from the tibia, wrapping around distal fibula (*asterisk*). Note the "cleavage plane" that the lesion forms with the tibia (*black arrowhead*). Also note the lack of contiguous medullary extension (*arrows*) on the coronal CT reformatted image (**c**) which helps distinguish this "cauliflower-like" parosteal osteosarcoma from an osteochondroma

Periosteal Osteosarcoma

Synonyms: juxtacortical osteosarcoma, juxtacortical chondroblastic osteosarcoma

Demographics:
- Second to third decade (slightly older than conventional)
- Very rare

Origin:
- Osseous neoplasm that arises from the inner layer of periosteum (parosteal arises from outer layer)
- Often contains large amount of cartilaginous matrix

Location:
- Lower extremities (femur, tibia, and humerus), and other long bones
- More diaphyseal than metaphyseal, as seen in many other osteosarcoma subtypes

Clinical symptoms:
- Painless mass with swelling
- Gradual progression to pain and tenderness

Imaging characteristics:
- Variable appearance on radiographs ranging from spiculated periosteal reaction perpendicular to cortex (sunburst) to a smooth dense mass arising from the surface of the bone
- Scalloping of outer cortex with cartilaginous soft tissue mass
- Typically does not enter medullary cavity
- Markedly thickened and dense cortex due to osteoid material
- CT and MRI important for staging and surgical planning

Malignant potential:
- Worse than parosteal osteosarcoma but better than conventional osteosarcoma

Treatment:
- Tumor removal with limb salvage
- Chemotherapy

Differential diagnosis:
- Juxtacortical (periosteal) chondroma/chondrosarcoma—can have pressure erosions and cartilaginous matrix, however, can be difficult to distinguish from a periosteal osteosarcoma
- High grade surface osteosarcoma—is difficult to distinguish by imaging
- Parosteal osteosarcoma—is difficult to distinguish by imaging
- Osteochondroma—has contiguous medullary component with host bone
- Osteoid osteoma—has nidus and lacks soft tissue component
- Osteomyelitis—often has circumferential periosteal involvement instead of a focal mass on the cortical surface

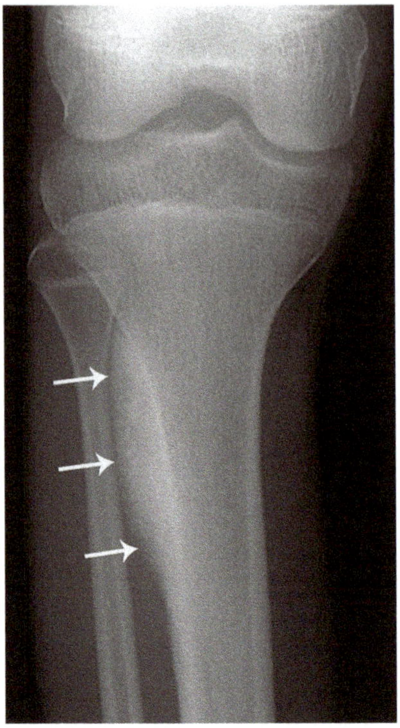

Fig. 5.16 Periosteal osteosarcoma of the proximal tibial metaphysis. Note the dense periosteal bone formation (*arrows*) arising from the lateral cortex without extension into the medullary cavity. (Image courtesy of Dr. Andrew Haims, New Haven, CT)

Additional Osteosarcoma Subtypes

- High grade surface
  - Very rare, <1% of osteosarcomas
  - Same histology as conventional but arising from surface of the bone
  - Long bones (femur, tibia, humerus, and fibula)
  - Can be difficult to distinguish from periosteal osteosarcoma
- Low grade intramedullary
  - Similar to conventional but low grade
  - Older population than conventional. M=F
  - Difficult to diagnose histologically
  - Appearance is less aggressive: more sclerosis but can have areas of cortical breakthrough
  - Better prognosis than conventional subtype but can recur as a high grade lesion if inadequately resected
- Small cell osteosarcoma
  - 1.5% of osteosarcomas
  - Composed of small cells on histology
  - Similar to Ewing sarcoma
  - Slight F>M
  - Predominantly lytic and permeative but can contain small areas of osteoid
  - Likes to extend along shaft of bone
  - Slightly worse prognosis than conventional

- Secondary osteosarcoma
  - Arises in older patients with long-standing preexisting conditions in bone
    Paget disease
    - Occurs in <1% of cases of Paget disease
    - Accounts for 50–60% of sarcomas in Paget disease
    - More likely to occur in polyostotic than monostotic Paget disease
    Prior radiation
    - Account for 50–60% of radiation-induced sarcomas
    - Especially in children
    - Median latent period following radiation is 11 years
    - Higher dose associated with higher risk (typically >55 Gy)
    Osteonecrosis
    - Fibrous dysplasia
    - Osteogenesis imperfecta
    - Hardware
    - Osteomyelitis

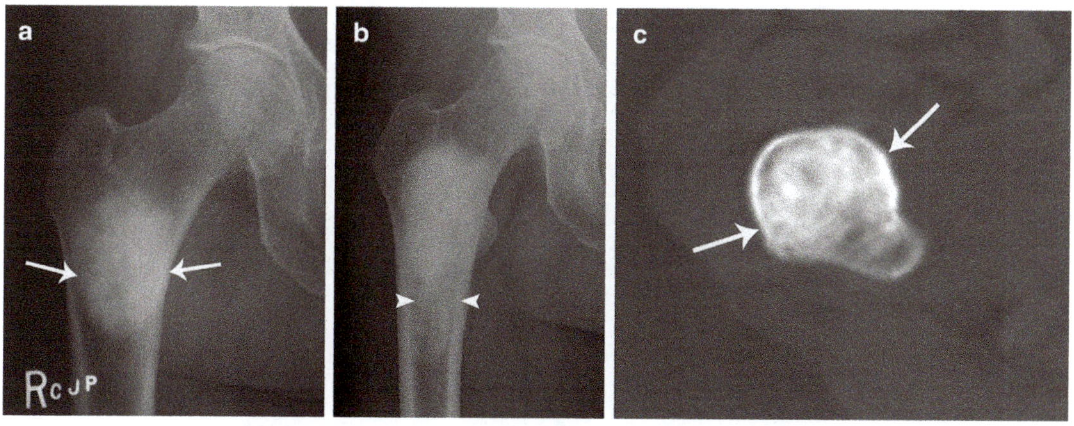

Fig. 5.17 A 77-year-old woman with large sclerotic lesion in the proximal femur. On the initial radiograph (**a**) the lesion (*arrows*) has nonaggressive features (no cortical breakthrough or periosteal reaction, and a narrow zone of transition). Follow-up radiograph (**b**) in 3 months shows growth of the tumor at the inferior aspect (*arrowheads*) which would be atypical for a giant bone island. The axial CT image (**c**) shows a very dense lesion (*arrows*) filling the majority of the medullary cavity. Biopsy revealed a low-grade osteosarcoma

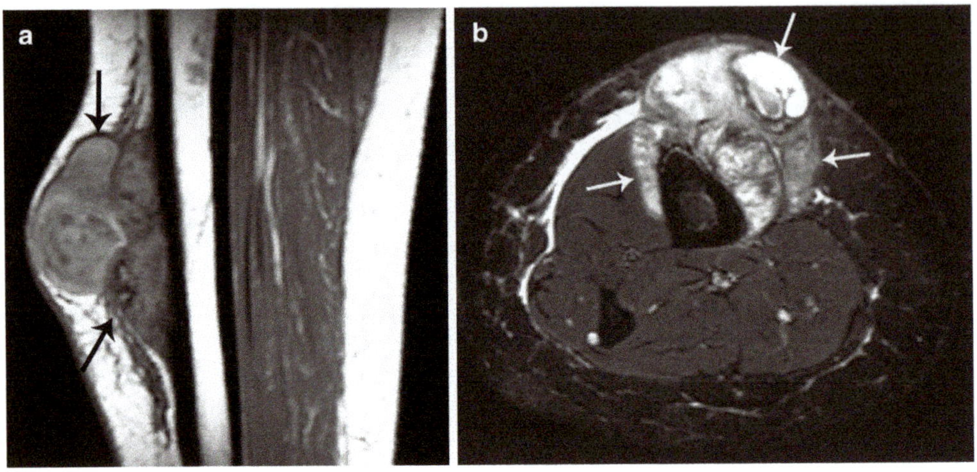

Fig. 5.18 T1-weighted (**a**) and STIR (**b**) MR images show a high grade surface osteosarcoma (*arrows*) arising from the anteromedial tibial cortex. The lesion contains a large soft tissue component without medullary involvement

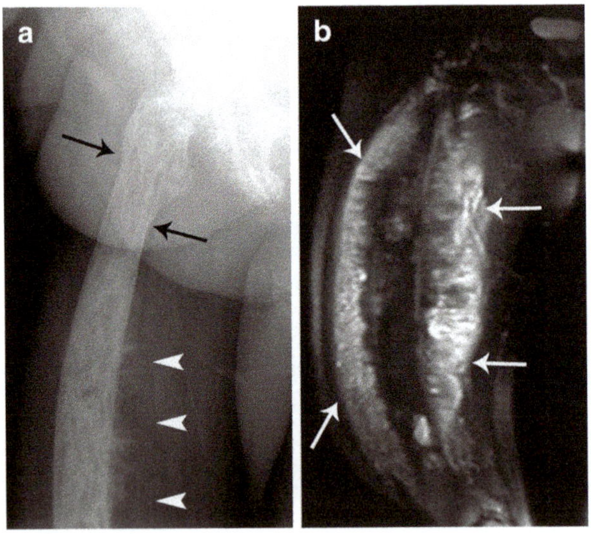

Fig. 5.19 Secondary osteosarcoma in the femoral shaft of a patient with longstanding Paget disease. On the radiograph (**a**), there is poor corticomedullary differentiation and trabecular thickening in the femur (*black arrows*) consistent with baseline Paget disease. The secondary osteosarcoma causes aggressive sunburst periosteal reaction (*arrowheads*) along the medial femoral cortical surface. The coronal STIR MR image (**b**) shows the large soft tissue component (*arrows*) of the tumor

Suggested Reading

1. Chai JW, Hong SH, Choi JY, et al. Radiologic diagnosis of osteoid osteoma: from simple to challenging findings. Radiographics. 2010;30:737–49.
2. Deyrup AT, Montag AG, Inwards CY, Xu Z, Swee RG, Unni KK. Sarcomas arising in Paget disease of bone: a clinicopathologic analysis of 70 cases. Arch Pathol Lab Med. 2007;131:942–6.
3. Fletcher CD, Unni KK, Mertens F, editors. WHO classification of tumours: pathology and genetics of tumours of soft tissue and bone. Lyon, France: IARC; 2002.
4. Greenspan A. Benign bone-forming lesions: osteoma, osteoid osteoma, and osteoblastoma. Clinical, imaging, pathologic, and differential considerations. Skeletal Radiol. 1993;22:485–500.
5. Greenspan A, Jundt G, Remagen W. Differential diagnosis in orthopaedic oncology. 2nd ed. Philadelphia, PA: Lippincott Williams & Wilkins; 2007.
6. Greenspan A, Steiner G, Knutzon R. Bone island (enostosis): clinical significance and radiologic and pathologic correlations. Skeletal Radiol. 1991;20:85–90.
7. Jelinek JS, Murphey MD, Kransdorf MJ, Shmookler BM, Malawer MM, Hur RC. Parosteal osteosarcoma: value of MR imaging and CT in the prediction of histologic grade. Radiology. 1996;201:837–42.
8. Kransdorf MJ, Stull MA, Gilkey FW, Moser Jr RP. Osteoid osteoma. Radiographics. 1991;11:671–96.
9. Kroon HM, Schurmans J. Osteoblastoma: clinical and radiologic findings in 98 new cases. Radiology. 1990;175:783–90.
10. Moore TE, King AR, Kathol MH, el-Khoury GY, Palmer R, Downey PR. Sarcoma in Paget disease of bone: clinical, radiologic, and pathologic features in 22 cases. AJR Am J Roentgenol. 1991;156:1199–203.
11. Murphey MD, Robbin MR, McRae GA, Flemming DJ, Temple HT, Kransdorf MJ. The many faces of osteosarcoma. Radiographics. 1997;17:1205–31.
12. Murphey MD, Jelinek JS, Temple HT, Flemming DJ, Gannon FH. Imaging of periosteal osteosarcoma: radiologic–pathologic comparison. Radiology. 2004;233:129–38.
13. Murphey MD, wan Jaovisidha S, Temple HT, Gannon FH, Jelinek JS, Malawer MM. Telangiectatic osteosarcoma: radiologic–pathologic comparison. Radiology. 2003;229:545–53.
14. Resnick D, editor. Diagnosis of bone and joint disorders. 4th ed. Philadelphia, PA: W.B. Saunders; 2002.
15. Suresh S, Saifuddin A. Radiological appearances of appendicular osteosarcoma: a comprehensive pictorial review. Clin Radiol. 2007;62:314–23.

6 Fibrous Tumors

The lesions in this category include both neoplastic and nonneoplastic lesions that contain fibrous constituents (i.e., collagen). The World Health Organization (WHO) groups fibrous bone lesions into two main categories: (1) fibrogenic and (2) fibrohistiocytic tumors. However, unlike the WHO classification, this chapter also includes fibrous dysplasia (FD) and fibrous xanthomas [fibrous cortical defects (FCD) and non-ossifying fibromas (NOFs)]. The WHO actually classifies FD as a miscellaneous lesion with "undefined neoplastic nature" and excludes fibrous xanthomas, even though they have fibrohistiocytic constituents, probably because they are considered developmental defects that often heal, rather than true bone tumors. Nonetheless, these lesions are commonly encountered and we include them here for completeness. In fact, aside from fibrous xanthomas and FD, most of these lesions are quite rare. In general, fibrous lesions appear as lucent areas on radiographs due to the absence of mature bony matrix.

Fibroxanthomas include FCD and NOF, which are benign developmental defects with fibrohistiocytic components. The two lesions are identical histologically, but vary in size and appearance. FCD is smaller and is centered in the cortex, whereas NOF tends to be larger and is centered in the medullary cavity. In fact, there is no agreed upon cutoff size, though an upper limit of 3 cm is often cited for FCD. These lesions are extremely common, particularly in the first two decades, and often present as an asymptomatic incidental finding. The majority occur about the knee, in the posteromedial metaphysis of the distal femur or proximal tibia.

According to the WHO, fibrous dysplasia (FD) and osteofibrous dysplasia (OFD) are "tumors of undefined neoplastic nature." They may have cytogenetic features of neoplasms, but behave more like nonneoplastic lesions. FD is a benign nonhereditary developmental anomaly that is relatively common, particularly in its monostotic form. It can occur as an incidental finding and can be associated with prominent increased activity on bone scintigraphy. FD classically appears as a long lesion in a long bone, with ground glass density. It can occur in flat bones and can have variable appearances, including a cystic or chondroid appearance. Polyostotic forms of FD can be associated with McCune–Albright and Mazabraud syndromes. OFD is a rare benign fibroosseous lesion, usually arising in the anterior cortex of the tibia during infancy and childhood. It can be mistaken for adamantinoma, which is malignant, but OFD tends to occur in younger patients and tends to be less extensive and aggressive. OFD is distinct in histopathology and appearance from FD. Its relationship to adamantinoma is controversial.

J.S. Wu and M.G. Hochman, *Bone Tumors: A Practical Guide to Imaging*,
DOI 10.1007/978-1-4419-0808-7_6, © Springer Science+Business Media, LLC 2012

The WHO category of fibrogenic tumors includes desmoplastic fibroma (DF) and fibrosarcomas, both of which are rare. Desmoplastic fibroma represents the intraosseous version of the much more common soft tissue desmoid tumor. However, DF can be locally aggressive, with cortical breakthrough and soft tissue extension, and can be mistaken for a malignant lesion. Fibrosarcomas are rare malignant neoplasms, with a nonspecific aggressive imaging appearance. However, some fibrosarcomas can contain a bony sequestrum.

The WHO category of fibrohistiocytic tumors, although long accepted, is currently being challenged on the basis of its histogenic accuracy. This category includes benign fibrous histiocytoma and malignant fibrous histiocytoma (MFH) of bone, both of which are rare. Benign fibrous histiocytoma is histologically similar to FCD and NOFs, but it occurs in adults and is seen in different locations from NOFs. MFH is a highly malignant intraosseous counterpart of soft tissue MFH. Approximately one quarter of both MFH and fibrosarcoma bone tumors occur as secondary lesions in a preexisting bony abnormality, such as Paget disease, bone infarct, or prior irradiation.

Fibrogenic

Desmoplastic Fibroma (DF)
Fibrosarcoma

Fibrohistiocytic

Benign Fibrous Histiocytoma
Malignant Fibrous Histiocytoma (MFH)

Fibrous Xanthoma (not in WHO classification)

Fibrous Cortical Defect (FCD)
Non-ossifying Fibroma (NOF)

Fibrous Dysplasia (FD)

Monostotic Fibrous Dysplasia
Polyostotic Fibrous Dysplasia
- McCune–Albright syndrome
- Mazabraud Syndrome

Osteofibrous Dysplasia (OFD)

Desmoplastic Fibroma

Synonyms: desmoid tumor of bone

Demographics:
- Rare, approximately 0.1% of all primary bone tumors
- 5–10 × less common than soft tissue desmoids
- Most common in adolescent and young adults
- M=F

Origin:
- Intraosseous form of soft tissue desmoid tumor, abundant collagen and fibroblasts

Location:
- Femur, tibia, humerus, radius, mandible, and pelvis are the most common locations

Clinical symptoms:
- Asymptomatic until large
- Chronic pain or swelling
- Pathologic fracture in 15%

Imaging characteristics:
- Lobulated geographic lucent lesion with narrow zone of transition, often expansile with cortical thinning, and occasionally with cortical destruction and soft tissue extension
- Internal trabeculation common, results in "**soap bubble**" or "**honeycomb**" pattern
- Periosteal reaction rare
- MRI:
  - Low-intermediate T1 and variable T2; low T2 signal reflects collagen and/or sclerosis
  - Variable pattern and intensity of contrast enhancement, usually in cellular portions
- Bone scintigraphy:
  - Increased activity

Malignant potential:
- Benign; locally aggressive and slowly progressive
- Local recurrence: 72% following curettage and 17% following resection
- Local recurrence reported as late as 8 years following primary surgery

Treatment:
- En bloc resection or definitive curettage and bone graft

Miscellaneous facts:
- Cortical breakthrough (seen in 29% of cases) should not be mistaken for malignancy

Differential diagnosis:
- GCT—both can extend into epiphysis, but GCT is rounder and DF is more oval
- Fibrous dysplasia—involves longer segment of bone, typically has "ground glass" matrix, often has sclerotic rim
- ABC—have more eccentric and "blown out" expansion than fusiform DF
- NOF—has eccentric, scalloped margin, and sclerotic rim; NOF pseudotrabeculation tends to be more curvilinear
- Simple bone cyst (SBC)—can be indistinguishable on radiographs, but has fluid content on CT and MRI
- Low grade fibrosarcoma—fibrosarcoma has a permeative pattern and wider zone of transition compared with geographic DF; distinction can be difficult histologically
- Fibroblast-predominant low-grade osteosarcoma—also similar histologically, but has mineralized tumor matrix

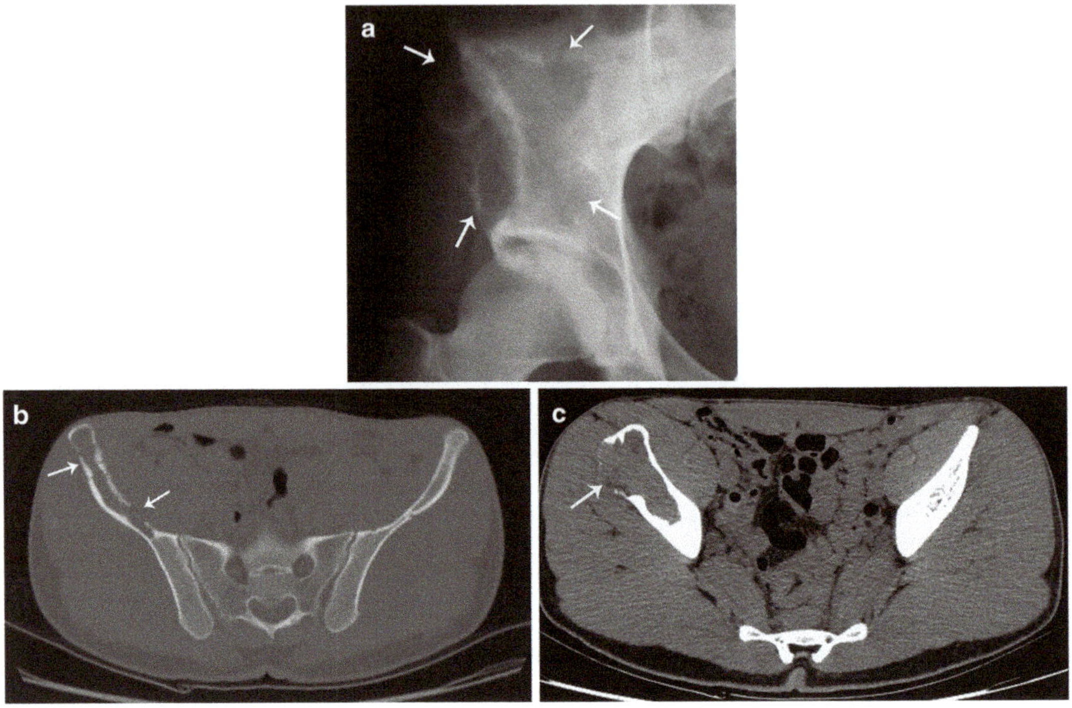

Fig. 6.1 Hip radiograph (**a**) shows a desmoplastic fibroma (DF) in the right iliac bone, seen as a bubbly, expansile, lytic lesion (*arrows*). (**b**) CT better demonstrates lesion borders. Note expansion and cortical penetration and absence of periosteal new bone formation (*arrows*). (**c**) Soft tissue windows show soft tissue expansion beyond confines of bone (*arrow*)

Fibrosarcoma

Demographics:

- Uncommon, ≤5% of all primary malignant bone tumors
- Precise incidence difficult because of inconsistent terminology for fibrosarcoma versus MFH of bone
- Relatively uniform incidence from second to sixth decades
- M=F

Origin:

- Malignant spindle cell neoplasm with variable amounts of collagen, in "**herringbone**" pattern, and no other differentiating features, such as osteoid or cartilage
- Most are primary; approximately 25% occur secondary to another process, such as prior radiation, Paget disease, bone infarct, chronic osteomyelitis

Location:

- Metaphysis or metadiaphysis of long bones, can extend to epiphysis
- 40–80% occur around knee (distal femur, proximal tibia), also humerus, iliac, sacrum

Clinical symptoms:

- Local pain and swelling
- Pathologic fracture in 19%

Imaging characteristics:

- Lucent, predominantly permeative or moth-eaten lesion, without sclerotic margin, often with cortical destruction and soft tissue extension
- Can have bony sequestrum
- CT:
  - Isodense to muscle ± areas of hypodensity secondary to necrosis
- MRI:
  - Nonspecific; low-intermediate T1; heterogeneously intermediate-to-high T2; often hemorrhage and necrosis
  - Prominent heterogeneous gadolinium contrast enhancement
- Bone scintigraphy:
  - Nonspecific; peripheral increased activity
  - Shows additional sites

Malignant potential:

- Tends to recur and metastasize
- Favorable imaging findings: eccentric location, geographic pattern, involving less than two quadrants of bone circumference
- Poor prognosis: over 40 years old, axial skeleton, high grade tumor
- Metastases common, seen in 45% or more, to lungs and other bones
- 10-year survival 83% low grade, 34% high grade

Treatment:

- Surgical resection with wide margins; amputation when necessary
- High grade: adjuvant chemotherapy for better survival
- Usually resistant to radiation

Miscellaneous facts:

- Include fibrosarcoma in differential for aggressive lesion with a "sequestrum" (small fragment of cortical and/or trabecular bone within an aggressive lytic lesion)—the differential diagnosis for sequestra includes osteomyelitis, MFH, lymphoma, and LCH
- Calcifications within or at the periphery of a fibrosarcoma suggests secondary fibrosarcoma arising in bone infarct

Differential diagnosis: fibrosarcoma has a nonspecific aggressive appearance, leading to a wide differential

- Chondrosarcoma—has chondroid matrix
- Osteosarcoma—has osteoid matrix
- GCT—extends to subchondral bone
- Desmoplastic fibroma—is more geographic
- MFH—little to differentiate, both can have sequestra
- Ewing sarcoma—can have a larger soft tissue mass, more likely to have sclerotic component, saucerization of cortex may be present, periosteal new bone more likely
- Langerhans cell histocytosis (LCH)—lamellated periosteal new bone formation more likely

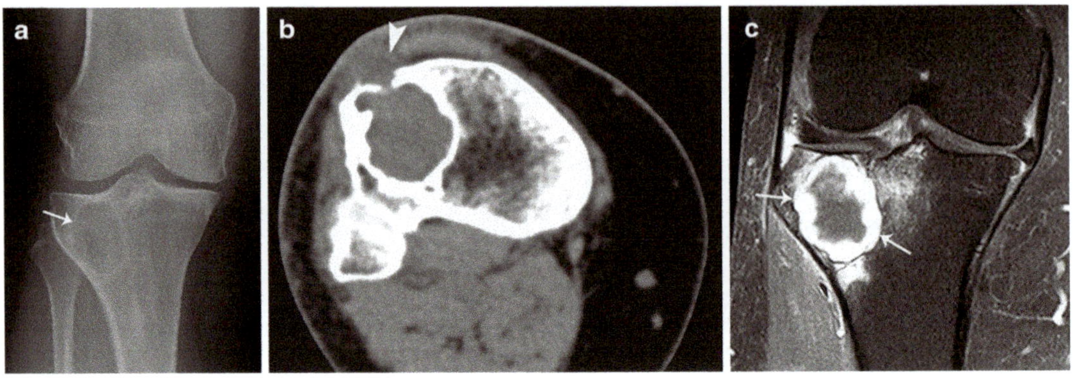

Fig. 6.2 Radiograph (**a**) shows a lytic fibrosarcoma in the lateral proximal tibia (*arrow*). The lesion commonly occurs about the knee, is often centered in the metaphysis, and can extend into the epiphysis. The geographic pattern of bone destruction is somewhat unusual for this entity, which is often moth-eaten or permeative, with a wide zone of transition. However, the axial CT image (**b**) demonstrates aggressive features, including cortical penetration and a soft tissue component extending outside the bone anteriorly (*arrowhead*). Coronal postcontrast MR image (**c**) shows a thick rind of peripheral enhancement (*arrows*)

Malignant Fibrous Histiocytoma

Synonyms: malignant histiocytoma, xanthosarcoma, malignant fibrous xanthoma, fibroxanthosarcoma

Demographics:

- Rare, <2% of all primary malignant bone lesions
- Second and eighth decades; higher incidence >40 years old
- M>F (slight)

Origin:

- Malignant neoplasm composed of fibroblasts, histiocytes, and pleomorphic cells, with a storiform (whorled) pattern
- Approximately 28% occur as secondary tumors and arise in Paget disease, bone infarct, prior site of irradiation, chronic osteomyelitis

Location:

- 90% arise in central metaphysis of long bones, with frequent epiphyseal extension
- Lesions originating in diaphysis are uncommon and tend to be eccentric
- Majority occur about the knee
- Femur (30–45%), tibia, humerus, iliac bone

Clinical symptoms:

- Pain and, less often, swelling (average 7–9 months)
- Pathologic fractures in approximately 20%

Imaging characteristics:

- Moth-eaten, permeative and/or partially geographic lytic lesion, often with cortical destruction and soft tissue extension
- Can have partial sclerotic margin, especially when metaepiphyseal
- Periosteal reaction is uncommon, but typically aggressive
- May see mineralization at periphery of soft tissue component, due to periosteal reaction; matrix calcification is otherwise rare
- In secondary MFH, may see evidence of underlying primary process
- CT:
  - Useful for cortical destruction, but MRI is superior for intra- and extraosseous extent
- MRI:
  - Nonspecific aggressive lesion; low-intermediate T1; heterogeneous intermediate-high T2 and fat-saturated T2; can have hemorrhagic foci and peritumoral edema; gadolinium contrast enhancement is heterogeneous and nodular, often intense, and often more pronounced at periphery
  - Findings s/p treatment can mimic tumor growth—enlargement due to nonenhancing necrotic foci, hemorrhage; calcification in areas of necrosis
- Bone scintigraphy:
  - Helps identify metastatic disease
  - Tc-99m MDP—nonspecific increased activity throughout intraosseous portion of tumor (mechanism uncertain)
  - Ga-67—higher sensitivity for both primary and (extraosseous) metastatic lesions than Tc-99m MDP

Malignant potential:

- Highly malignant, with propensity to metastasize and recur

Treatment:

- Preoperative chemotherapy and wide en bloc excision ± radiation therapy for residual tumor
- Metastases—to lungs in up to 50% of patients, to regional lymph nodes in 4%
- Ten-year survival: low grade 60%; high grade 46%; secondary MFH 36%
- Extent of necrosis in resected specimen has prognostic significance

Miscellaneous facts:

- In secondary MFH arising in osteonecrosis, bone destruction begins at edge of infarct
- MRI shows joint invasion in ~30%

Differential diagnosis: nonspecific aggressive appearance

- Differential is similar to fibrosarcoma
- Look for underlying process indicative of secondary MFH

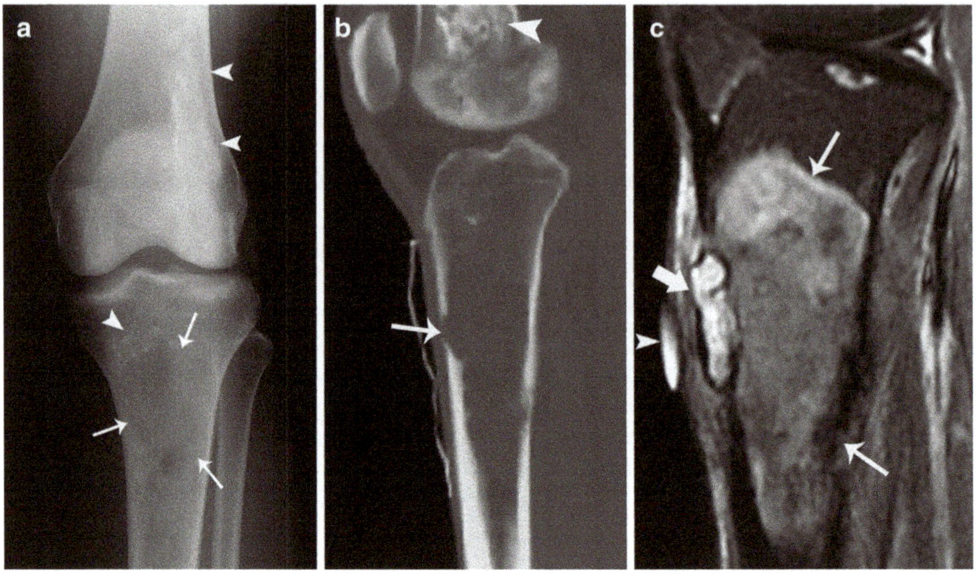

Fig. 6.3 AP radiograph of the knee (**a**) shows a large lytic lesion (*arrows*) in the proximal tibia caused by a secondary MFH arising in a bone infarct. The patient developed bone infarcts during CHOP therapy for lymphoma 15 years earlier. Bone infarcts (*arrowheads*) are visible in the distal femur and the proximal tibia. Sagittal CT image (**b**) better demonstrates the cortical erosion by the MFH (*arrow*) and the bone infarct in the distal femur (*arrowhead*). On the sagittal fat-saturated T1-weighted MR image (**c**) the MFH has heterogeneous high signal (*arrows*) with extra-osseous soft tissue extension (*thick arrow*), accounting for the cortical defect. Oval skin marker (*arrowhead*) is seen on the anterior skin surface

Fibrous Xanthoma: Fibrous Cortical Defect and Non-ossifying Fibroma

Synonyms: fibroxanthoma, fibrous metaphyseal defect, nonosteogenic fibroma, xanthogranuloma

Demographics:
- Common, FCD seen in 30% of normal population during first two decades
- Peak age second decade; rarely seen on radiographs after age 20
- M:F=2:1

Origin:
- FCD and NOF—essentially the same lesion, but different in size and primary location
- Benign developmental defects comprised of fibroblastic spindle cells, collagen, giant cells, and hemorrhage
- Lesions themselves do not make bone, but reactive bone forms at periphery, resulting in healing
- May occur due to traumatic injury to the physeal plate at the site of tendon or ligament insertion, resulting in focal hemorrhage; muscle pull during weight-bearing may contribute

Location:
- Metaphysis of long bone; usually posterior and medial (rather than lateral)
- Migrates from metaphysis into diaphysis as patient ages and bone lengthens
- 55% around knee (distal femur, proximal tibia); distal tibia; occasionally fibula
- Occurs, but rarely, in upper extremity (proximal humerus, distal radius)

Clinical symptoms:

- FD asymptomatic
- NOF asymptomatic, except for large lesions
  - Pain, focal bony enlargement, pathologic fracture in up to 20%
  - Greater likelihood of fracture in lesions >3 cm, >50% of diameter, and in weight-bearing bones
  - Stress fractures can also occur

Imaging characteristics:

- Imaging usually diagnostic—classic "**don't touch**" lesion
- The terms FCD and NOF are often used interchangeably. However, FCD is smaller and is centered in the cortex; NOF tends to be larger and extends into the medullary cavity. In fact, there is no agreed upon cut-off size between FCD and NOF, though an upper limit of 3 cm has been suggested for FCD
- FCD—1–3 cm well-circumscribed, oval or rounded lucent lesion with thin sclerotic rim, centered in cortex of long bone metaphysis; length>width; negligible involvement of medullary bone
- NOF—0.5–7 cm well-circumscribed, elliptical lucent lesion with thin sclerotic rim, positioned eccentrically in medullary cavity of long bone metaphysis; usually involves but does not breach cortex (e.g., endosteal scalloping, cortical thinning, and slight cortical expansion), often lobulated like a "**bunch of grapes**"; bubbly due to ridging of inner surface of cortex
- No intralesional matrix mineralization
- Most undergo partial or complete spontaneous regression (healing), usually beginning at the end of adolescence, taking up to 1 year (FCD) or longer (NOF); see gradual centripetal filling-in of trabecular bone from periphery
- CT:
  - Well-depicted; Hounsfield units may be higher than normal bone marrow
- MRI:
  - Isointense to muscle on T1, variable on T2 due to heterogeneous histology (can have hyperintense components)
  - Peripheral rim of low T2 sclerosis
  - Variable enhancement in FCD; peripheral contrast enhancement in NOF
  - Surrounding bone is normal, unless fracture
- Bone scintigraphy:
  - Not part of routine workup
  - Three-phase bone scintigraphy activity varies with maturity of lesion
  - Healing: mild hyperemia and moderate bone uptake
  - Healed: no activity or slightly increased
  - Superimposed fracture or other lesion—intense hyperemia and markedly positive scan

Malignant potential:

- None

Treatment:

- No treatment necessary unless atypical clinical or radiologic features or large enough to be at risk for pathologic fracture, in which case treat with biopsy, curettage, and bone graft packing
- Small asymptomatic lesions can be followed with serial radiographs; if unchanged at 3 months, then every 6–12 months, until regress or become symptomatic

Miscellaneous facts:

- Should not appear for first time in adults
- Presence of soft tissue mass precludes diagnosis of FCD or NOF
- If in fibula or ulna, can occupy entire diameter and be mistaken for simple bone cyst, ABC, or Langerhans cell histiocytosis
- Has been associated with vitamin-D-resistant rickets and osteomalacia, which disappears after removal of tumor, though the cause for this in these lesions is unknown
- 8% of NOFs are multiple—when multiple, can be familial or seen in neurofibromatosis (von Recklinghausen's disease) or Jaffe–Campanacci syndrome
- Benign fibrous histiocytoma is a rare lesion whose existence is controversial: identical to fibroxanthoma (NOF) on pathology, but patients are older and is often symptomatic; radiologically appears as larger lesion, more expansion, more medullary involvement

Differential diagnosis:

- Avulsive cortical irregularity (cortical desmoid)—occurs in the posteromedial distal femur, but saucer-like concavity of the outer cortex, as opposed to convexity with NOFs; margins are less well defined; has adjacent sclerosis, periostitis, and soft tissue swelling
- Fibrous dysplasia—tends to be central, diaphyseal or metadiaphyseal
- Abscess—has associated marrow and soft tissue edema; larger high T2 component
- Osteoid osteoma—has more prominent sclerosis, surrounding marrow and soft tissue edema, characteristic clinical symptoms
- ABC—is more expansile, fluid levels on MRI
- Simple bone cyst—is central, unilocular, cystic

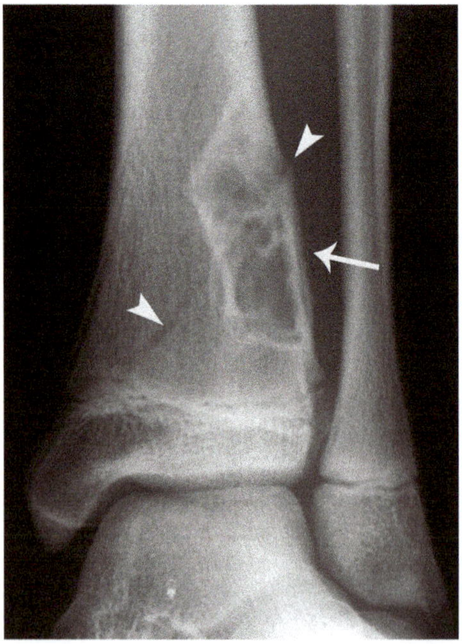

Fig. 6.4 NOF in distal tibia (*arrow*). Note eccentric positioning in the metaphysis, "bunch of grapes" morphology, sclerotic rim, and mild bone expansion in a skeletally immature individual, with unfused physes. The patient presented with a pathologic fracture through the lesion (*arrowheads*)

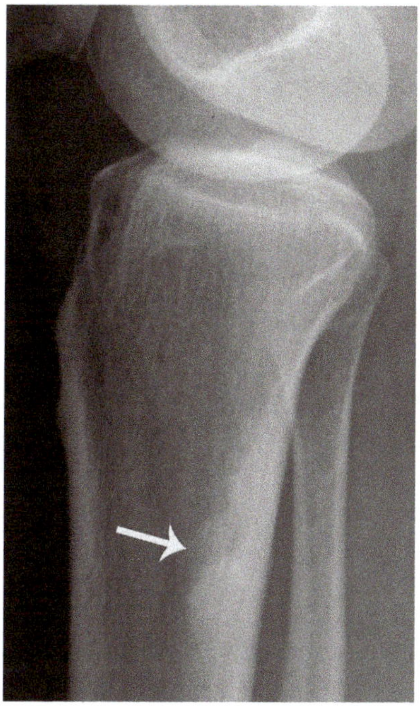

Fig. 6.5 Healed NOF in proximal tibia (*arrow*). Residual sclerosis is present

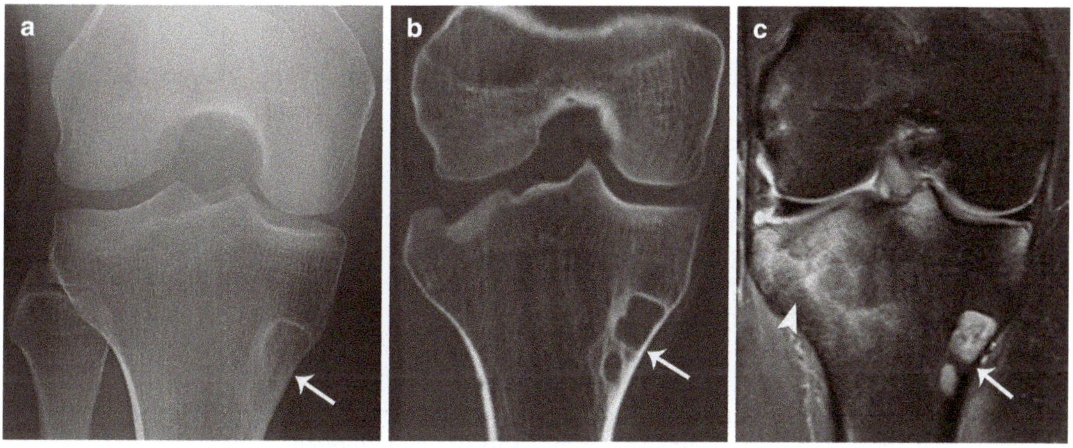

Fig. 6.6 Radiograph (**a**) shows a NOF (*arrow*) in the proximal tibia, abutting the cortex. Coronal reformat CT image (**b**) shows full extent of the lesion (*arrow*), including its multi-locular appearance and sclerosis in the surrounding bone. On the coronal fat-saturated PD-weighted MR image (**c**), the lesion (*arrow*) is lobulated, but well-demarcated, and has heterogeneously high signal, without surrounding edema. Edema elsewhere in the proximal tibia (*arrowhead*) is due to a nondisplaced fracture. As here, NOFs are often an asymptomatic, incidental finding

Fibrous Dysplasia

Synonyms: fibrocartilaginous dysplasia, generalized fibrocystic disease of bone, fibroosseous dysplasia, Lichtenstein–Jaffe disease

Demographics:

- Approximately 5% of benign bone tumors
- Monostotic form 6× more common than polyostotic
- Any age, but majority detected under 30 years old, younger in polyostotic
- M=F

Origin:

- Benign nonhereditary developmental anomaly linked to mutation in GNAS1 gene
- Abnormal remodeling of immature woven to mature lamellar bone, resulting in dysplastic fibrous tissue and immature trabeculae, with variable cystic, chondroid, and osteoid components

Location:

- Intramedullary; diaphysis and metadiaphysis
- Monostotic: femur (35–40%), tibia (20%), skull and facial bones (10–25%), ribs (10%); uncommonly in hands, feet, spine, and clavicle
- Polyostotic:
  - Extent varies from two bones to >75% of skeleton
  - Majority involve predominantly one side of body
  - Craniofacial (50%), femur (91%), tibia (81%), pelvis (78%), and foot (73%)

Clinical symptoms:

- Monostotic disease is often an asymptomatic, incidental finding on radiographs
- In general, age of onset, lesion size, extent and severity of skeletal involvement, and frequency of clinical symptoms is increased in polyostotic disease
- Pain, tenderness, swelling, and limp
- Bowing, leg-length discrepancy, craniofacial deformity (hypertelorism, exophthalmos, cranial neuropathies, and sinus disorders), scoliosis
- Pathologic and stress fractures

Syndromes and associations:

- **McCune–Albright syndrome**—a triad of (1) polyostotic FD, (2) cafe au lait spots (irregular borders, "coast of Maine"), (3) precocious puberty and/or other endocrine abnormalities, e.g., acromegaly, Cushing syndrome, hyperparathyroidism, hyperthyroidism, and diabetes. Complete triad is uncommon. Need to have two of three in the triad to make the diagnosis. F>M
- **Leontiasis ossea (lion face)**—rare, polyostotic FD involving craniofacial bones, causing facial deformity and enlargement
- **Cherubism**—autosomal dominant, fibroosseous enlargement of mandible, maxilla and other gnathic structures; although originally attributed to FD, now thought to be variant of giant cell granuloma
- **Mazabraud syndrome**—extremely rare syndrome consisting of FD (predominantly polyostotic) and intramuscular myxomas
- Hypophosphatemic rickets and osteomalacia—reported with mono- and polyostotic dysplasia; may respond to resection of the FD bone lesion

Imaging characteristics:

- Well-circumscribed lucent (ground glass) or mixed lucent and dense lesion in diaphysis of long bones or in skull, rib, or pelvis, with peripheral sclerotic rind of variable thickness, and occasionally with endosteal scalloping and mild bone expansion
- Variable density—depends on composition:
  - Woven bone ~ hazy ground glass
  - More fibrous or cystic ~ more radiolucent
  - More ossified ~ denser
  - Some have large percentage of cartilage, with chondroid calcifications (fibrocartilaginous dysplasia)
- No periosteal reaction unless fracture or malignant transformation
- "**Long lesion in a long bone**"—tends to extend along longitudinal axis of long bone
- "**Shepherd's crook**" deformity—varus bowing of femoral neck and proximal shaft
- "**Parrot beak**" deformity—stress fracture along medial femoral neck, radiolucent line perpendicular to cortex, surrounded by reactive bone
- Bowing—coxa vara, tibia, and protrusio acetabuli
- Rib—fusiform enlargement of one or more ribs
- Skull—widening of diploic space, outer table convexity; deformity of orbits, sella, paranasal sinuses, and foramina
- Spine—well-defined expansile lucent lesion with multiple septations; usually in vertebral body, occasionally pedicles and arch; ± neural foraminal narrowing; rare paraspinal soft tissue extension and vertebral collapse with angulation and spinal cord compression
- Rare exophytic variant of FD may be mistaken for osteochondroma or parosteal lesion
- CT:
  - Good for demonstrating fibrous dysplasia in skull, pelvis, and spine
  - Good for showing well-circumscribed geographic borders and lack of periosteal reaction
- MRI:
  - Appearance depends on composition
  - Well-circumscribed low to low-intermediate T1; variable (low to high) T2
  - Low signal rim of variable thickness
  - Occasional septations, cystic changes
  - Variable gadolinium contrast enhancement
  - If recent fracture, see periosteal and juxtacortical contrast enhancement
- Bone scintigraphy:
  - Helpful for demonstrating polyostotic disease
  - Normal to marked activity
  - Not all ground glass or cystic lesions show increased activity

Malignant potential:

- Malignant transformation very rare, seen in 0.4–4%, occurs in both mono- and polyostotic FD, with and without history of prior radiation
- Rapid onset pain and swelling, lesion enlargement, cortical destruction, soft tissue mass
- Can transform to osteosarcoma, fibrosarcoma, chondrosarcoma, or MFH

Treatment:

- Usually conservative
- Both monostotic and polyostotic forms cease or slow growth at puberty, but deformities in polyostotic disease can continue after puberty
- Early experience with bisphosphonates for relief of symptoms
- Surgery for fracture, deformity, symptomatic lesions, and nerve compression

Miscellaneous facts:

- Most common benign lesion of rib
- Can be painful during menstruation or pregnancy, due to estrogen receptors within lesion
- Lesion enlargement can occur due to malignant transformation, cystic degeneration, or secondary aneurysmal bone cyst formation

Differential diagnosis:

- **Monostotic**
  - Simple bone cyst—more radiolucent, more expansile, moves away from growth plate with skeletal growth
  - Aneurysmal bone cyst—more eccentric and aneurysmal, with marked thinning of cortex; fluid levels more typical in ABC
  - Giant cell tumor—eccentric, centered in metaphysis, much more likely to extend into epiphysis and subchondral bone
  - Non-ossifying fibroma—centered eccentrically in metaphysis, lacks intralesional ossification, "heals" from periphery inward
  - Osteofibrous dysplasia—rare, almost always in tibia or fibula, centered in anterior cortex
  - Low grade central (intramedullary) osteosarcoma—rare variant of OS, lack of reactive shell, permeative borders, denser mineralization, more aggressive, appearance changes over time
  - Paget disease (lytic phase)—older individuals, thickened cortex and trabeculae, marked elevation in serum alkaline phosphatase
  - Liposclerosing myxofibrous tumor of bone (LSMFT)—few distinguishing imaging features; tends to have higher T2 signal intensity and may contain minute speckles of fat. LSMFT occurs almost exclusively in the intertrochanteric region of the femur
- **Polyostotic**
  - Multiple enchondromas—enchondromas may extend into epiphysis, radiolucent streaks extending from growth plate into metaphysis
  - Neurofibromatosis—long bone deformity without intramedullary bone density changes typical of fibrous dysplasia
  - Jaffe–Campanacci syndrome (multiple NOFs)—NOFs as above, with additional nonskeletal features

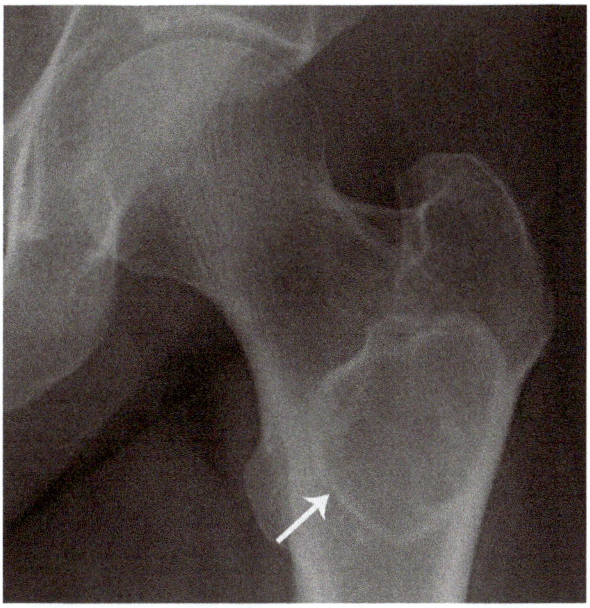

Fig. 6.7 AP view of the proximal femur shows a common location and appearance of fibrous dysplasia (FD) (*arrow*). The lesion lies in the proximal femur, has hazy, ground glass density and a sclerotic rim. This appearance is essentially pathognomic for FD. However, the differential includes liposclerosing myxofibrous tumor of bone

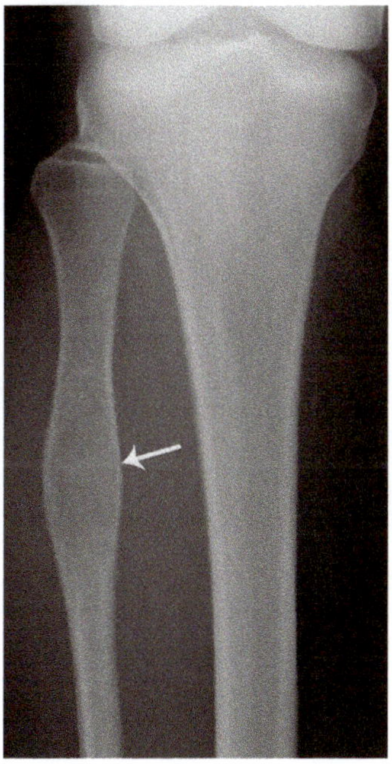

Fig. 6.8 FD seen as a typical "long lesion in a long bone." AP view of the knee shows an elongated focal lucent lesion in the proximal fibula (*arrows*), with subtle endosteal scalloping and cortical thinning and slight expansion of this small-diameter bone. The lesion's ground glass density is similar to surrounding bone, but is slightly heterogeneous and it lacks the normal trabecular pattern

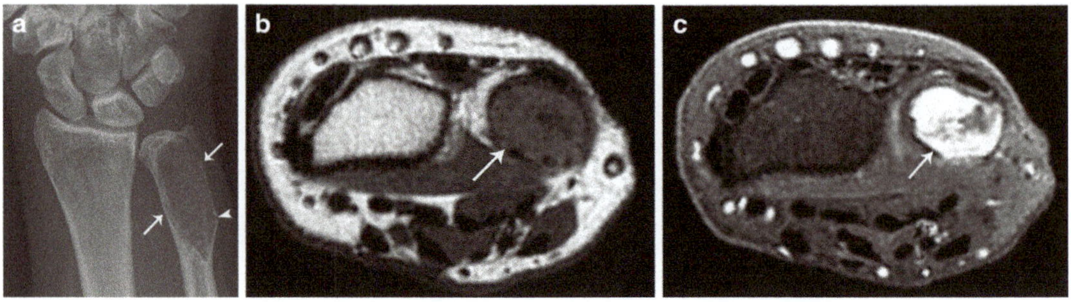

Fig. 6.9 Fibrous dysplasia. AP radiograph of the wrist (**a**) shows a geographic lytic lesion in the distal ulna (*arrows*), with thinning of the cortex and aneurysmal expansion of the bone. Buckling of the cortex (*arrowhead*) indicates subtle pathologic fracture. Axial T1-weighted MR image (**b**) in the same patient shows that the lesion (*arrows*) is isointense to muscle and high signal on the corresponding fat-saturated T2-weighted MR image (**c**)

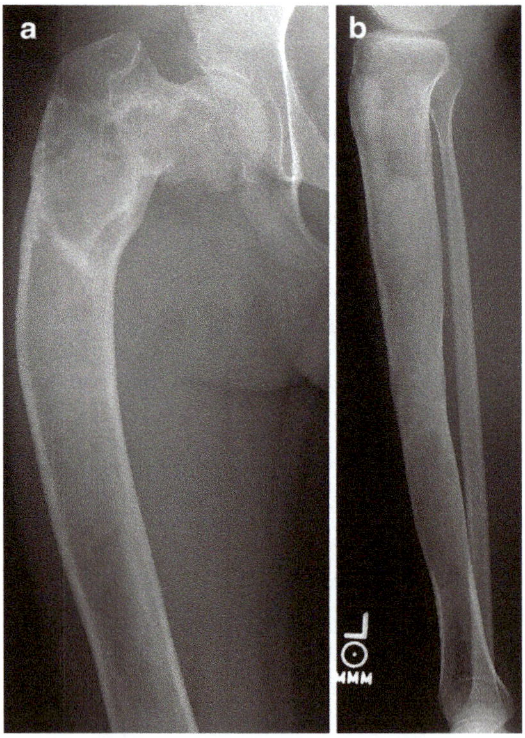

Fig. 6.10 Fibrous dysplasia. AP view of the femur (**a**) shows a long lesion in a long bone, with classic ground glass matrix and "shepherd's crook" deformity (varus bowing). Lateral view of the tibia (**b**) in the same patient shows an ipsilateral focus of fibrous dysplasia, with denser, more sclerotic matrix. Cortical thinning and mild bone expansion are seen distally

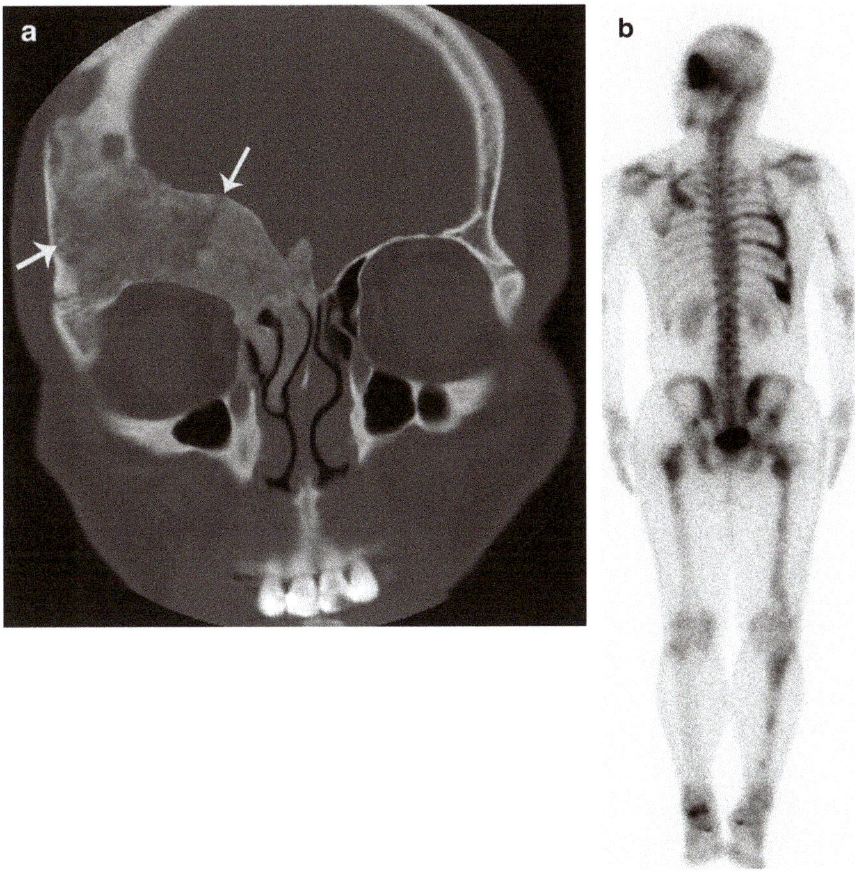

Fig. 6.11 Coronal reformatted CT image (**a**) demonstrates fibrous dysplasia (*arrows*) with ground glass matrix, expansion of the diploic space, and deformity of the orbit and ethmoid sinuses. Bone scintigraphy (**b**) helps depict extent and distribution of the polyostotic FD. Note lesions in the skull, mandible, ribs, pelvis, and extremities

Osteofibrous Dysplasia

Synonyms: ossifying fibroma of the tibia and/or fibula, intracortical or cortical fibrous dysplasia, Kempson–Campanacci lesion, congenital fibrous defect of the tibia, congenital osteitis fibrosa, congenital pseudoarthrosis, and juvenile adamantinoma

Demographics:

- Rare, 0.2% of biopsied primary bone tumors
- Usually <10 years old, rare after 16 years old
- M>F (slight)

Origin:

- Benign self-limited fibroosseous lesion, usually arising in the anterior cortex of the mid-shaft of the tibia during infancy and childhood
- Fibrous connective tissue and immature nonlamellar bone

Location:

- Tibia (75–80%); proximal or middle third most common
- Usually centered in anterior cortex of tibia; medullary extension in ~10%
- Can be bilateral, can involve ipislateral or contralateral fibula; rarely in radius or ulna

Clinical symptoms:

- Can be asymptomatic
- Localized pain and/or swelling; anterior tibial bowing or protuberance; pathologic fracture

Imaging characteristics:

- Multiloculated lucent lesion with well-circumscribed sclerotic margins, centered in anterior cortex of midtibial diaphysis, that may extend inward to involve medullary canal
- Individual lucent foci have hazy, ground glass density; the grouping of contiguous lucent lesions creates an overall lobulated contour with a scalloped, sawtoothed, or bubbly appearance; can be multifocal; ranges from ~3 cm long to entire length of bone
- Anterior bowing (in >80%), fracture (13%), and pseudoarthrosis
- CT:
  - Show features well—intracortical centering, sclerotic rim, absence of breakthrough into soft tissues
- MRI:
  - Multiple low-intermediate T1/high T2 signal intracortical foci, separated by low T1/lowT2 signal cortical bone and sclerotic reaction, with prominent enhancement
- Bone scintigraphy:
  - Increased activity

Malignant potential:

- Controversial—probably not, but some believe it is a precursor of (malignant) adamantinoma; others describe an OFD-subtype of adamantinoma that is distinct from conventional OFD
- Gradual slow growth in kids, until 15 years old, then heals or spontaneously regresses
- Can be locally aggressive; frequently recurs after excision

Treatment:

- In kids <15 years old, surgery for pseudoarthroses, marked bowing, and/or large lesions that have fractured or are at risk for fracture
- Curettage with cryosurgery and bone grafting, or excision with wide margins and bone grafting

Miscellaneous facts:

- Some suggest OFD is a form of fibrous dysplasia, but this concept is not widely accepted
- Relationship to adamantinoma is controversial, possibly two separate lesions that can coexist or two related lesions on a continuum from benign to malignant. According to WHO, there is an OFD-subtype of adamantinoma—distinct from conventional de novo OFD—that has been reported to rarely progress to adamantinoma; distinction of OFD-like adamantinoma from actual OFD is radiographically and histologically difficult
- In fibula, OFD can extend across entire diameter of bone

Differential diagnosis:

- Adamantinoma—patients tend to be older, usually more extensive and aggressive
- FD—centered in medullary canal with cortical thinning (rather than bubbly appearance)
- Osteomyelitis—clinical presentation differs, has marrow and soft tissue edema, not ground glass

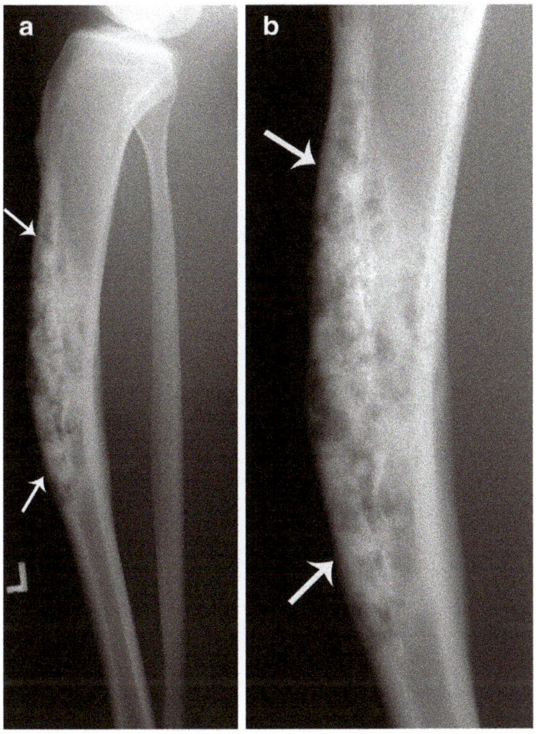

Fig. 6.12 Lateral radiograph of the tibia (**a**) shows osteofibrous dysplasia (OFD) (*arrows*). Note the tibial bowing. The lesion is centered in the anterior cortex, but extends into the medullary cavity. The magnified view (**b**) of the lesion shows confluent rounded, bubby, lucent lesions (*arrows*), creating an overall lobulated contour. The individual lucent lesions usually have ground glass density

Suggested Reading

1. Betsy M, Kupersmith LM, Springfield DS. Metaphyseal fibrous defects. J Am Acad Orthop Surg. 2004;12:89–95.
2. DiCaprio MR, Enneking WF. Fibrous dysplasia. Pathophysiology, evaluation, and treatment. J Bone Joint Surg Am. 2005;87:1848–64.
3. Fitzpatrick KA, Taljanovic MS, Speer DP, et al. Imaging findings of fibrous dysplasia with histopathologic and intraoperative correlation. AJR Am J Roentgenol. 2004;182:1389–98.
4. Frick MA, Sundaram M, Unni KK, et al. Imaging findings in desmoplastic fibroma of bone: distinctive T2 characteristics. AJR Am J Roentgenol. 2005;184:1762–7.
5. Kahn LB. Adamantinoma, osteofibrous dysplasia and differentiated adamantinoma. Skeletal Radiol. 2003;32:245–58.
6. Link TM, Haeussler MD, Poppek S. Malignant fibrous histiocytoma of bone: conventional x-ray and MR imaging features. Skeletal Radiol. 1998;27:552–8.
7. Ritschl P, Hajek PC, Pechmann U. Fibrous metaphyseal defects: magnetic resonance imaging appearances. Skeletal Radiol. 1989;18:251–9.
8. Taconis WK, Mulder JD. Fibrosarcoma and malignant fibrous histiocytoma of long bones: radiographic features and grading. Skeletal Radiol. 1984;11:237–45.
9. Weidner N. Review and update: oncogenic osteomalacia-rickets. Ultrastruct Pathol. 1991;15:317–33.

Miscellaneous Tumors

7

Several chapters in this book are based on lesions that resemble specific cell types, depending on their pattern of differentiation—osseous, cartilaginous, and fibrous lesions. In this chapter, we describe lesions that arise from more diverse origins: marrow elements (lymphoma/leukemia, myeloma, Ewing sarcoma, Langerhans cell histiocytosis, giant cell tumor, and intraosseous lipoma), vascular structures (hemangioma and angiosarcoma), smooth muscle (leiomyoma and leiomyosarcoma), and notochord (chordoma). Also included are lesions for which the origin remains speculative (solitary or unicameral bone cyst, aneurysmal bone cyst, and adamantinoma). The WHO, in total, divides bone tumors into ten different categories, with separate categories for Ewing sarcoma/primitive neuroectodermal tumors; hematopoietic tumors; giant cell tumors; notochordal tumors; vascular tumors; myogenic, lipogenic, neural, and epithelial tumors; and tumors of undefined neoplastic nature, as well as the previously reviewed cartilage, osteogenic, fibrous, and fibrohistocytic tumors. For the purpose of this book, we have chosen to group the former lesion categories together into a single very heterogeneous "miscellaneous" grouping because, on radiographs, most of these entities appear as nonspecific lucent lesions. In practice, age, location, and clinical presentation prove to be the most helpful factors for discriminating these lesions. This is in contrast to osteogenic, chondroid, and fibrous lesions, where lesion matrix also plays an important role in lesion characterization. The miscellaneous tumors presented in this chapter have been further divided into benign and malignant miscellaneous lesions.

Benign	Malignant
Langerhans cell histiocytosis (LCH)	Ewing sarcoma
Intraosseous hemangioma	Adamantinoma
Giant cell tumor (GCT)	Chordoma
Simple bone cyst (SBC)	Lymphoma
Aneurysmal bone cyst (ABC)	Non-Hodgkin lymphoma
Lipoma of bone	Hodgkin lymphoma
	Leukemia
	Angiosarcoma
	Multiple myeloma
	Plasmacytoma
	POEMS

J.S. Wu and M.G. Hochman, *Bone Tumors: A Practical Guide to Imaging*,
DOI 10.1007/978-1-4419-0808-7_7, © Springer Science+Business Media, LLC 2012

Langerhans Cell Histiocytosis

Synonyms: eosinophilic granuloma, histiocytosis X, Langerhans cell granulomatosis

Demographics:
- Relatively rare, <1% of all bone lesions
- 80–85% under 30 years old
- M:F = 2:1, >95% Caucasian

Origin:
- Proliferation of Langerhans cells, from bone marrow precursors
- Likely neoplastic (in past, thought to be a disorder of immune regulation)

Location:
- Solitary form is twice as common as diffuse
- 70% involve flat bones, most commonly skull (25%) and pelvis (20%)

Clinical symptoms:
- The WHO currently refers to this disease as Langerhans cell histocytosis, with four subcategories: (1) NOS, (2) unifocal, (3) multifocal, and (4) disseminated. Knowledgeable authors advise that the historical terms eosinophilic granuloma, Letterer–Siwe disease, Hand–Schüller–Christian disease, and diffuse reticuloendotheliosis should be abandoned. The preferred means of defining LCH is in terms of whether it involves a single site (organ) or is a diffuse disease
- Historically, LCH was thought of as three clinical syndromes that tended to be more severe in younger patients:
  - *Letterer–Siwe disease*—rapidly progressive syndrome most frequent in children <3 years old; involvement of multiple visceral organs; any bone may be involved, including hands and feet; most die from sepsis within 1–2 years
  - *Hand–Schüller–Christian*—triad of bone lesions, diabetes insipidus, exophthalmos; skull involved in >90%; skeletal lesions may be widespread; prognosis varies; usually protracted course; fatal in 10–30%
  - *Eosinophilic Granuloma of Bone (EGB)*—adults with lesions in one or just a few bones; can be incidental finding; may have local pain, tenderness, swelling, fever, ↑ESR; neurologic symptoms (vertebral body collapse); otitis media or mastoiditis (temporal bone); and loosening of teeth (mandible)

Imaging characteristics:
- *Early phase*—aggressive, permeative lucency with laminated periosteal reaction
- *Mid-phase*—well-demarcated lucent lesion that can enlarge; may have endosteal scalloping, sclerotic rim, thick periosteal new bone formation, and soft tissue mass (in 5–10%)
- *Late-phase*—peripheral or patchy diffuse sclerosis (indicating healing) and maturation of periosteal new bone
- Radiographs:
  - Long bones—radiolucent lesion in diaphysis (79%)
  - Skull—lytic lesion 1–4 cm, tends to be "**punched out**," characteristic beveled edge (due to unequal involvement of deep and superficial edges); may have button sequestrum composed of residual bone within center of lytic lesion
  - "**Hole within hole**"—multiple small lesions coalesce and overlap, resulting in one rounded lucency superimposed over another

  - Spine—severe compression known as "**vertebra plana**" or "**silver-coin**" appearance (can regain partial height when healed)
  - Mandible/maxilla—"**floating teeth**"—tooth surrounded by lytic lesion
- CT: good for areas of bony overlap, e.g., spine and pelvis
- MRI:
  - Can show radiographically or scintigraphically occult lesions
  - Low-intermediate T1, heterogeneously high T2
  - Focal lesion surrounded by extensive, ill-defined bone marrow and soft tissue edema
  - Can appear aggressive: cortical interruption, soft tissue extension, and linear periosteal high T2 signal
  - Marked gadolinium enhancement, including perilesional enhancement
- Bone scintigraphy:
  - Shows distribution of unknown lesions
  - Variable activity (55% increased, 35% normal, and 10% decreased)

Malignant potential:

- Evidence of clonal origin (i.e., derived from common originating cell, also a feature in neoplasms), but solitary bone lesions do not metastasize

Treatment:

- Prognosis and treatment depends on the extent of disease at presentation and whether "risk" organs (i.e., liver, spleen, lung, and bone marrow) are involved
- Solitary lesions—can treat conservatively and follow; may regress
- If symptomatic or unstable—curettage or excise; can recur
- Radiation for large, enlarging, or vertebral lesions

Miscellaneous facts:

- Consider LCH in infant or child with lytic lesions in the pelvis or skull
- Rapid progression and disappearance of lytic lesions is characteristic
- Bone scan helps distinguish from Ewing sarcoma, which is rarely multifocal

Differential diagnosis:

- Solitary, Aggressive
  - Ewing sarcoma—occurs in younger patients, has larger soft tissue mass
  - Osteomyelitis—may be indistinguishable
  - Telangiectatic osteosarcoma—has large expansile lesion with fluid levels
- Solitary, Well-Defined
  - GCT—is expansile, extension into subchondral epiphysis
  - SBC—is a unilocular cystic lesion, no bone or soft tissue edema unless fractured
  - Brown tumor—has other findings of hyperparathyroidism
  - ABC—is expansile, multilocular cystic lesion with multiple fluid levels
  - Fibrous dysplasia—is a long lesion, with ground glass density and possible bone expansion
- Solitary, Healing Phase
  - Non-ossifying fibroma—is lobulated, usually abutting posterior cortex
- Multifocal
  - Can be difficult to differentiate from hematogenous osteomyelitis, but multifocal forms of LCH have additional signs and symptoms and systemic findings

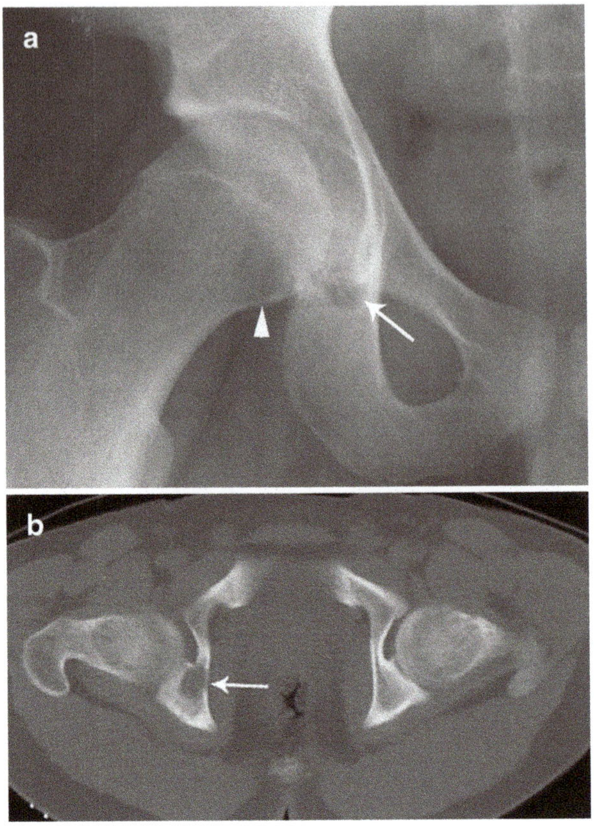

Fig. 7.1 Langerhans cell histiocytosis. The focal lucent lesion in the posterior column (*arrow*) is difficult to discern on the hip radiograph (**a**), due to overlying bone. Lucency in inferomedial femoral head (*arrowhead*) represents normal stress shielding. Axial CT (**b**) readily depicts the focal lytic lesion (*arrow*), absence of matrix mineralization, very faint sclerotic rim, and cortical interruption

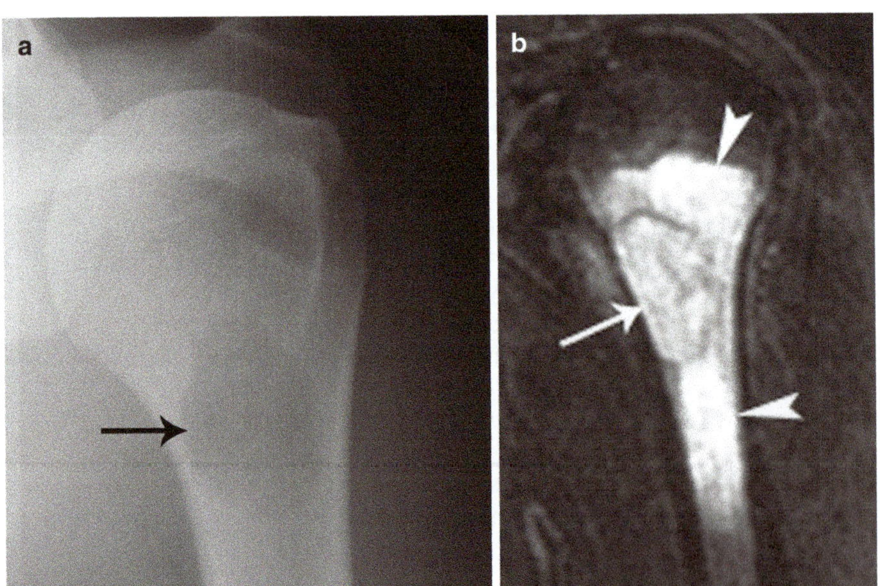

Fig. 7.2 Langerhans cell histiocytosis. Radiograph (**a**) shows a well-demarcated lucent lesion in the metadiaphysis (*arrow*) without sclerotic rim. Fat-saturated T2-weighted MR image (**b**) shows a large area of marrow edema (*arrowheads*) surrounding the focal lesion (*arrow*). A small area of soft tissue edema is also visible medially

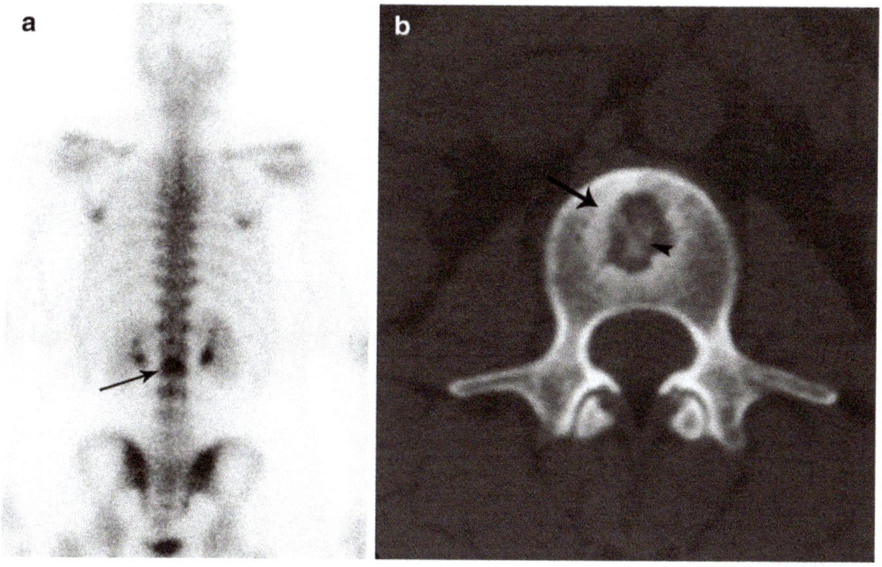

Fig. 7.3 Langerhans cell histiocytosis. Bone scintigraphy (**a**) demonstrates a focus of increased activity in the L2 vertebral body (*arrow*), corresponding to the site of symptoms in a young adult. Axial CT image (**b**) shows a well-circumscribed lytic lesion (*arrow*), with surrounding reactive sclerosis and a central sequestrum (*arrowhead*), compatible with Langerhans cell histiocytosis

Intraosseous Hemangioma

Synonyms: capillary cavernous, venous or histiocytoid hemangioma, angioma

Demographics:
- Found on 10% of spine autopsies
- Incidence increases with age, most present after fourth decade
- M:F = 2:3

Origin:
- Benign hamartoma comprised of endothelial-lined spaces, most are capillary or cavernous, rare arteriovenous shunting

Location:
- Vertebral bodies, calvarium (especially frontal and parietal)

Clinical:
- Vast majority are asymptomatic, incidental finding
- Vertebral posterior element lesion more likely symptomatic
- Can expand or fracture (with hematoma) and compress cord and/or nerves
- May enlarge during pregnancy and cause cord compression

Imaging:

- Vertebrae—focal lucent lesion with coarse vertical striations representing thickened vertical trabeculae (“**corduroy**,” “**honeycomb**,” or “**polka dot**” appearance)
- Flat bones—lucent lesion, with characteristic radiating trabecular pattern, causing “**spokewheel**,” “**web-like**,” or “**sunburst**” appearance; may cause slight expansion of skull (outer>inner table)
- Small tubular bones—can be expansile, mimicking ABC
- Periosteal or cortical lesion—cortical erosion and periosteal reaction
- CT:
  - Fat density, cross-sectional “polka dot” appearance of thickened trabeculae can be diagnostic
- MRI:
  - Classically, high T1 due to fat components and high T2 due to slow-flowing blood; presence of high T1 signal in spinal lesion is highly suggestive of hemangioma
  - Mild to marked gadolinium contrast enhancement
  - A subset of atypical hemangiomas does not demonstrate high T1 signal and cannot be distinguished from other lesions, including metastases
  - Rarely, see atypical hemangiomas with extension through cortex into surrounding soft tissues, with potential for cord and root compression
- Bone scintigraphy:
  - Often normal; may range from photopenic to moderately increased activity

Malignant potential:

- Malignant degeneration to angiosarcoma is very rare

Treatment:

- Most are incidental findings; no treatment
- For spinal compression, surgery; may get pre-operative arteriography and/or embolization
- For painful or recurrent vertebral lesions, radiation and/or embolization
- Vertebroplasty can treat pain, but may not be effective for long-term relief

Miscellaneous facts:

- Angiomatosis—multiple hemangiomas or large regional hemangioma

Differential diagnosis:

- Angiosarcoma—are more likely to be infiltrative, and do not have fat
- Paget disease (vertebra)—bone is enlarged, endplates are thickened, and striations are less regular
- Metastasis—does not have thickened intralesional trabeculae or fat
- Langerhans cell histiocytosis—is more likely to present with vertebral compression fracture (which is rare for hemangiomas) and does not have fat
- Intraosseous lipoma—many have characteristic central or ring-like calcification or ossification

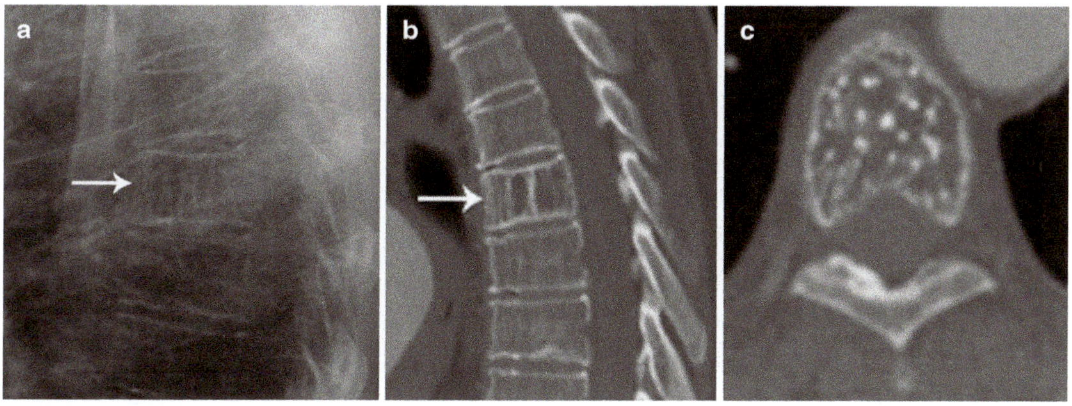

Fig. 7.4 Radiograph (**a**) and sagittal CT image (**b**) show thickened vertical trabeculae associated with an intravertebral hemangioma (*arrows*), known as the "corduroy" sign. On the axial CT image (**c**), these thickened trabeculae have a characteristic "polka dot" appearance. Together with surrounding fat density, this appearance is pathognomonic for a hemangioma

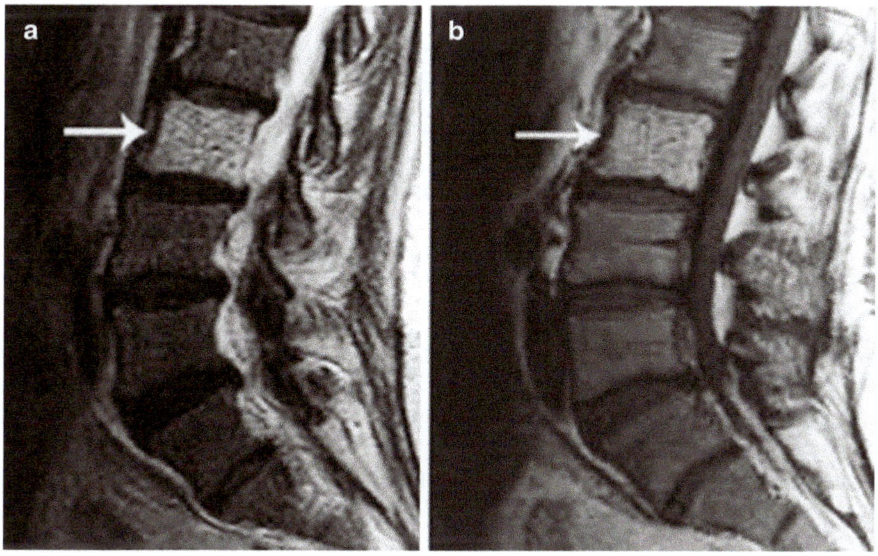

Fig. 7.5 Fat-saturated T2-weighted MR image (**a**) shows nonspecific high signal diffusely within the L3 vertebral body. On the T1-weighted MR image (**b**) there is high signal (from fat) in the L3 vertebral body, confirming an intraosseous hemangioma. Note faint low signal vertical striations, reflecting thickened trabeculae. Intravertebral hemangioma may also occur as a smaller, focal, rounded lesion

Giant Cell Tumor

Synonyms: osteoclastoma

Demographics:

- Relatively common, 4–5% of all primary bone tumors
- Peak incidence 20–45 years old, in the skeletally mature
- Benign F:M = 1.5:1; aggressive M:F = 3:1

Origin:

- Composed of osteoclast-like giant cells and neoplastic mononuclear cells; may contain hemorrhage, necrosis, and ABC-like areas
- Can be primary or secondary

Location:

- Originate in metaphysis and extend into subarticular epiphysis or epiphyseal equivalent
- Majority in long bones (75–90%), most surrounding knee (distal femur, proximal tibia)
- Also distal radius, proximal humerus, sacrum, and spine (vertebral body)
- Rarely hands and feet, ischium, scapula, ribs, and patella

Clinical symptoms:

- Pain, swelling, tenderness; may have decreased range of motion of adjacent joint
- Pathologic fracture in 5–10%

Imaging characteristics:

- Eccentric, well-defined geographic lucent lesion with nonsclerotic rim, centered in metaepiphysis and extending into subarticular bone
- Cortical thinning common; expansion and cortical penetration in 20–50%
- Periosteal reaction unusual
- Can have pseudotrabeculations, which are not true septations
- Soft tissue mass visible in up to 44% (on CT)
- Secondary ABC seen in 14%—if present, tends to appear more aggressive radiographically
- May have pathologic fracture (up to 1/3)
- Occasionally has wide zone of transition
- Campannacci defined three radiographic patterns, but radiographic appearance does not reflect histology or clinical behavior
  - *Type I*—quiescent lesions—well-defined margins, with defined sclerotic rim, rarely cortical involvement
  - *Type II*—active lesions—well-defined, but without sclerotic rim; cortex thinned and expanded; 70–80% of GCTs are Type II
  - *Type III*—aggressive lesions—often with cortical destruction and soft tissue extension
- CT:
  - Shows cortical detail, periosteal new bone, fluid levels, confirms absence of matrix
  - Peripheral sclerosis more commonly seen on CT, in ~20%

- MRI:
  - Best to show extension into joint or surrounding soft tissues
  - Well-defined lesion with thin low signal margins
  - Low to intermediate T1; majority low to intermediate T2 signal (due to hemosiderin or fibrosis), but can be heterogeneous or high T2 signal
  - May have cystic areas and fluid levels (due to ABC) that are high T2 and high or low T1
  - Mild to prominent enhancement of solid components and peripheral rim-enhancement of cystic components
  - Can see high T2 signal and contrast enhancement in marrow surrounding lesion, attributed to inflammatory reaction in lesions with high prostaglandin levels
  - Recurrence—nodular, mass-like marrow replacement (not diffuse)
- Bone scintigraphy:
  - Most show increased blood pool and bone activity
  - "**Donut sign**" in 49%—intense activity around periphery due to reactive new bone or hyperemia
  - Occasionally see activity in an adjacent joint or bone due to hyperemia—should not be mistaken for tumor extension

Malignant potential:

- Majority are benign; 5–10% or less are malignant
- Benign GCTs are locally aggressive and can recur locally
- "**Malignant GCT**" refers to a heterogeneous group of giant-cell containing lesions that are capable of malignant behaviors and of generating pulmonary metastases. These are detailed in the table below; however, the term is most frequently used for de novo malignant transformation of a formerly benign GCT
- Even though histologically benign, 2–3% of benign GCTs are "**benign metastasizing GCTs**" that can have distant metastases to lungs; surgical resection of lung metastases may improve survival. The metastases have no nuclear atypia and may actually be implants
- Clinical behavior cannot be predicted based on clinical, histologic, or radiologic features
- Malignant transformation can occur spontaneously, or after multiple surgical resections for recurrent disease, or after radiation treatment of a benign tumor; may transform to fibrosarcoma, MFH, and osteosarcoma

Treatment:

- GCTs are treated due to subarticular location and risk for pathologic fracture, especially larger lesions
- Curettage and packing (C&P), cryosurgery, or en bloc resection—given subchondral location, the main challenge is to avoid joint replacement
- Recurrence rate with C&P 40–60%, usually seen within 3 years
- Packing of the GCT cavity with methyl methacrylate cement (PMMA) instead of bone graft alone is thought to reduce recurrence, possibly due to cytotoxic effects and/or hyperthermia; radiolucent zone <2 mm about PMMA is normal and does not indicate recurrence
- Recurrence in bone seen as new lytic areas (though early post-op films can show incomplete incorporation or early resorption of graft); recurrence in surrounding soft tissues may appear as calcification of soft tissue mass
- Due to late recurrence/metastases, need long-term surveillance
- Radiation associated with risk of malignant degeneration into sarcoma

Miscellaneous facts:

- Very rarely can be isolated to metaphysis, usually in skeletally immature
- Multifocal tumors very rare (≤1%)—some associated with Paget disease
- Giant cell-rich forms of osteosarcoma, fibrosarcoma, and MFH can occur and should not be confused with malignant GCTs at pathology

Differential diagnosis:

- Primary ABC—can extend into subarticular end of bone after skeletal maturity; usually seen in younger patients; fluid levels are characteristic of ABC, but GCTs can have secondary ABCs; no significant solid component in ABC
- Brown tumors—like GCTs, are also considered "osteoclastomas," look for other lesions and other signs of hyperparathyroidism
- Subchondral cyst or intraosseous ganglion—sclerotic borders; high T2 signal
- Myeloma and metastasis—occur in older patients
- Brodie's abscess—have prominent surrounding sclerosis
- Clear cell chondrosarcoma—are more rounded, have chondroid calcification, and occur in epiphysis (Tables 7.1 and 7.2; Figs. 7.6–7.9)

Table 7.1 Malignant giant cell tumors (5–10% or less of all GCTs)

Entity	Definition	Characteristics
Benign metastasizing GCT	Benign primary GCT, with metastases that are histologically benign (no nuclear atypia)	Pulmonary metastases in up to 2–5% of benign GCTs, 3–4 years after initial diagnosis May be more likely in radiographically aggressive lesions, lesions with soft tissue extension, lesions with ≥1 recurrence, and lesions in distal radius Favorable prognosis, long survival time, resectable, can regress spontaneously, but occasionally cause death
Primary de novo malignant transformation of conventional GCT	Benign primary GCT that undergoes sarcomatous transformation, without ever being treated	Very rare < 1%
Secondary malignant GCT	Sarcoma that develops at site of previously treated benign primary GCT (requires history of prior surgery or radiation)	Occurs with radiation dose >40 Gy in up to 29%, within 5–8 years Worse prognosis than primary malignant GCT
Osteoclastic (giant cell) sarcoma	Sarcoma that contains giant cells	Rare, poor prognosis More common when associated with other processes like severe Paget disease, than de novo

Table 7.2 Lesions that contain secondary giant cell tumors

- ABC
- UBC
- NOF
- CMF
- Brown tumor
- Chondroblastoma
- Fibrous dysplasia and variants
- Osteoblastoma
- Giant cell reparative granuloma

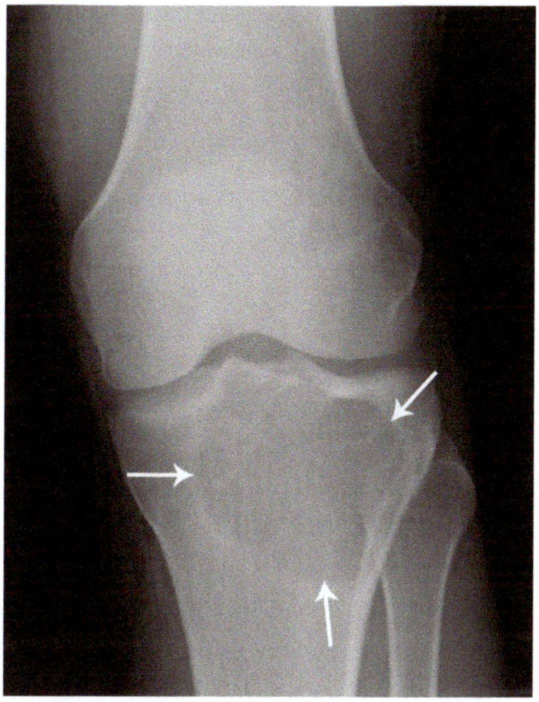

Fig. 7.6 Classic appearance of a giant cell tumor (*arrows*): an eccentric, well-defined geographic lucent lesion, centered in the metaphysis and extending into subarticular bone. The majority of GCTs do not have a sclerotic rim. Note the internal pseudotrabeculations, which are neither true septations nor internal matrix

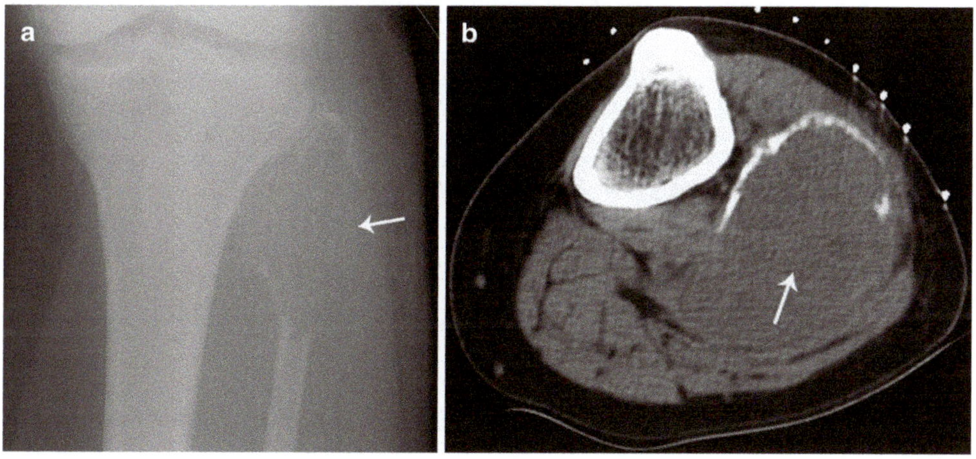

Fig. 7.7 Radiograph (**a**) shows a giant cell tumor in the proximal fibula (*arrow*), with marked bony expansion and cortical destruction. Axial CT image (**b**) better demonstrates the extent of cortical destruction and shows the presence of soft tissue extension (*arrow*). This represents a Campannacci Type III lesion

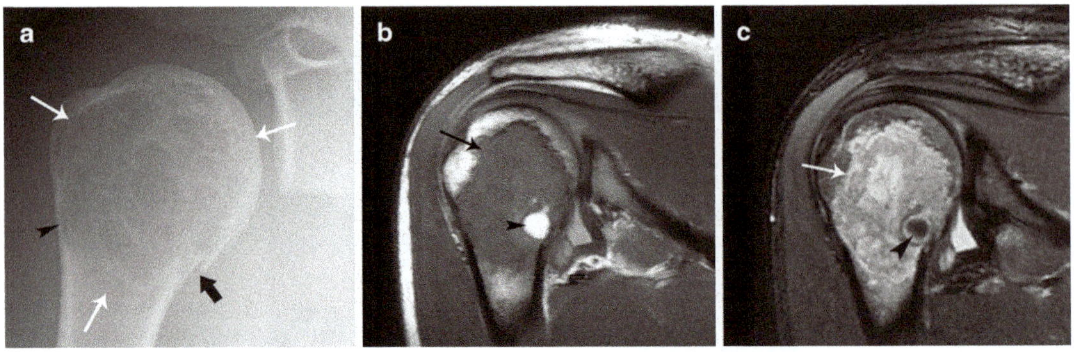

Fig. 7.8 Radiograph (**a**) shows a giant cell tumor (*arrows*)—geographic lucent lesion, centered in the humeral metaphysis and extending into the epiphysis. Although GCT is classically eccentric, large lesions may fill the bone and appear central. Note mild endosteal scalloping (*arrowhead*) and pathologic fracture (*thick arrow*). The GCT (*arrow*) is well-circumscribed and isointense to muscle on the T1-weighted MR image (**b**). A small rounded high T1 focus (*arrowhead*) represents focal fat. On postcontrast fat-saturated T1-weighted MR image (**c**), the GCT demonstrates heterogeneous internal enhancement, with rim enhancement about the small high T1 fatty focus (*arrowhead*)

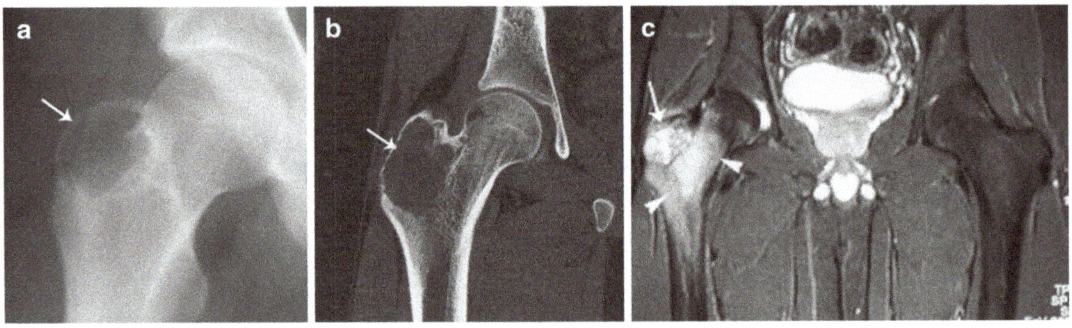

Fig. 7.9 Radiograph (**a**) shows a well-circumscribed lytic lesion centered in the greater trochanter (*arrow*), in a skeletally mature individual. GCTs can occur in apophyses such as the greater trochanter and in other epiphyseal equivalents. The CT (**b**) better delineates the lesion borders and show subtle cortical fenestration (*arrow*). This lesion (*arrow*) is heterogeneously high signal on the fat-saturated T2-weighted MR image (**c**), but GCTs can be lower signal on T2-weighted images due to hemosiderin or fibrosis. Note prominent reactive marrow edema pattern (*arrowheads*), which has been attributed to high prostaglandin levels that occur in some GCTs

Simple Bone Cyst

Synonyms: solitary bone cyst, unicameral bone cyst, juvenile bone cyst, essential bone cyst

Demographics:

- 3% of all biopsied bone neoplasms
- Most <20 years old (85%)
- M:F = 3:1

Origin:

- Single chamber cavity lined by mesothelial cells, filled with serous or serosanguinous fluid
- Pathogenesis uncertain: forms in childhood, possibly due to growth defect at epiphysis or due to obstruction of venous blood flow. Not neoplastic

Location:

- Central metaphysis of long bones; can migrate into diaphysis
- 90% occur in proximal humerus, proximal femur, or proximal tibia
- If over 20 years old—iliac bone, calcaneus, and talus

Clinical symptoms:

- Most are asymptomatic; rarely, pain and swelling
- 50% or more present with pathologic fracture

Imaging characteristics:

- Well-defined, geographic lucent lesion in central metadiaphysis, extending to physeal plate, with little or no bone expansion
- Margins are smooth or slightly lobulated, with thin, if any, sclerotic rim
- No matrix mineralization or extraosseous soft tissue extension
- Unlike ABC, width does not exceed that of neighboring growth plate and there is no periosteal reaction, unless fractured
- "**Fallen fragment**" sign—fracture fragment falls to dependent portion of cyst, indicating fluid-filled lesion; is diagnostic of simple bone cyst
- "**Trap door sign**"—fragment remains attached to periosteum, but folds inward
- Pathologic fracture can lead to growth arrest or femoral head osteonecrosis
- CT:
  - Simple fluid, HU 15–20
  - May have fluid level or fluid-gas level (bubble of gas at the most nondependent margin of a lesion following fracture)
  - CT can help identify fallen fragment
- MRI:
  - Simple fluid signal; may have fluid–fluid level (but usually only one)
  - Low-intermediate T1, homogeneous high T2, with thin low signal rim; thin peripheral rim of gadolinium enhancement
  - If fracture, will look more complex: with hemorrhage and more heterogeneous signal, internal septations, fluid levels, and thicker peripheral enhancement (up to 1 cm)
- Bone scintigraphy:
  - May be normal if no fracture
  - Increased peripheral activity and no activity centrally

Malignant potential: extremely rare

Treatment:

- Can regress, either spontaneously or following fracture
- Curettage and grafting; low recurrence rate (10–20%)
- Intralesional steroids—70–95% effective

Miscellaneous facts:

- Unicameral refers to the fact that the lesion is comprised of a single chamber
- May need multiple radiographic views to accurately identify "fallen fragment" sign, films taken in erect and recumbent position. Flouroscopy or CT are alternative

Differential diagnosis:

- ABC—eccentric, very expansile, typically has solid periosteal reaction, multiple locules and multiple fluid levels
- Enchondroma—lobulated contours, should have chondroid matrix if outside of hands and feet
- Fibrous dysplasia—ground glass density, lacks trabeculation, cannot demonstrate "fallen fragment" sign (caveat: cystic forms of fibrous dysplasia)
- GCT—extends to subchondral bone, physes fused

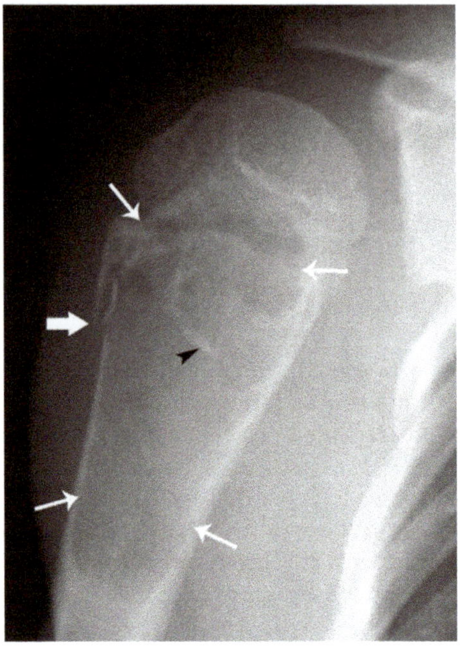

Fig. 7.10 Focal lytic lesion centered in the medullary cavity, with cortical thinning and mild bone expansion (*arrows*). The physis is unfused and there is a pathologic fracture (*thick arrow*). The linear density seen centrally (*arrowhead*) represents a dependent "fallen fragment" in this supine patient

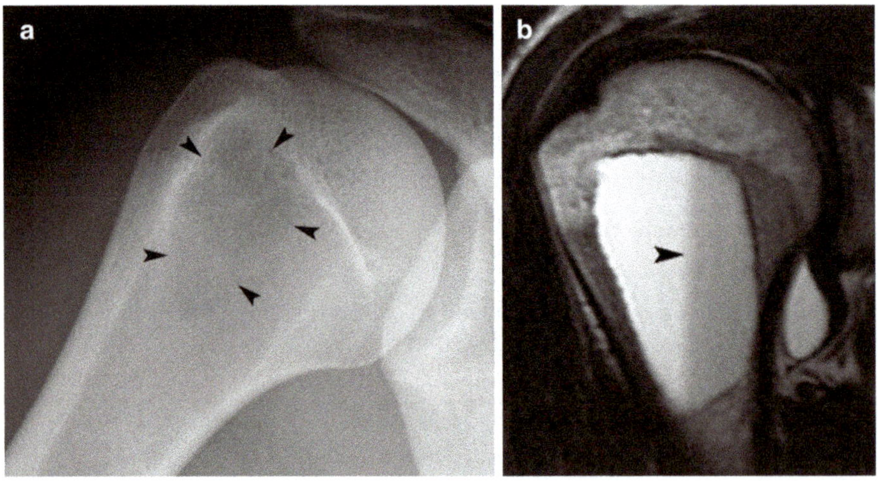

Fig. 7.11 Radiograph (**a**) shows a subtle focal lucency in the proximal humerus with a thin sclerotic rim (*arrowheads*) consistent with a simple bone cyst. On the fat-saturated T2-weighted MR image (**b**), the lesion consists of a single chamber, with a single fluid level (*arrowhead*). The nondependent fluid is simple, with high T2 signal; dependent fluid contains blood or other proteinaceous material and has lower T2 signal. (The patient was lying on his side)

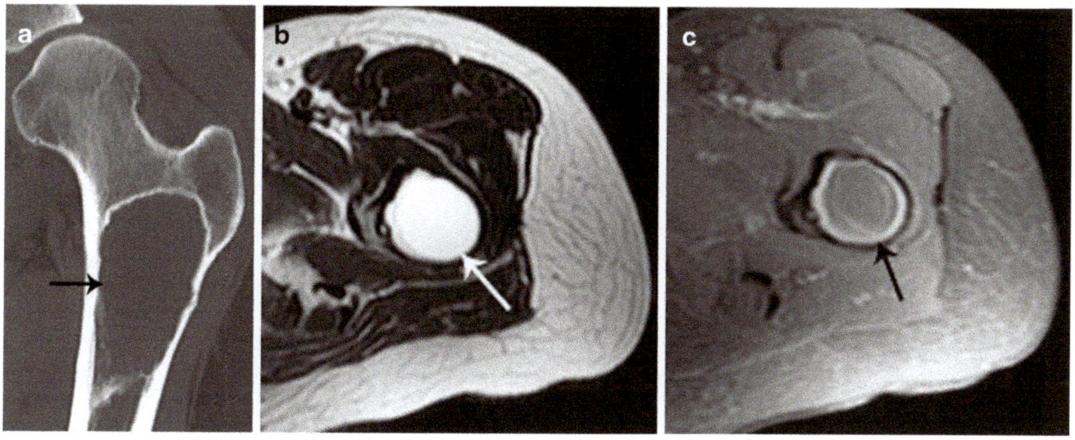

Fig. 7.12 Radiograph (**a**) shows a classic simple bone cyst in the proximal femur (*arrow*), centered in the metadiaphysis of the medullary cavity, with thin sclerotic rim and absence of "matrix" mineralization. The lesion (*arrow*) is uniformly bright on the T2-weighted MR image (**b**). The axial postcontrast fat-saturated T1-weighted image (**c**) demonstrates central nonenhancement and peripheral rim enhancement (*arrow*), consistent with a cyst

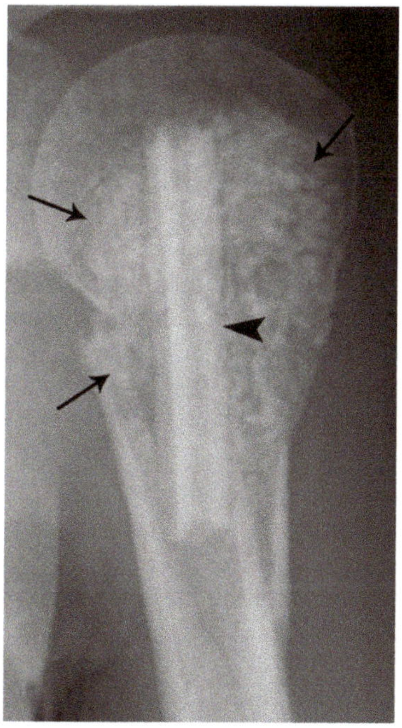

Fig. 7.13 Simple bone cyst treated by curettage and grafting. The cavity is now filled with both morselized bone graft (*arrows*) and a fibular strut graft (*arrowhead*)

Aneurysmal Bone Cyst

Synonyms: multilocular hematic cyst, giant cell reparative granuloma

Demographics:

- 1% of biopsied primary bone neoplasms
- Most 5–20 years old
- M=F

Origin:

- Nonneoplastic, etiology unknown; possibly due to venous obstruction or arteriovenous fistula; may be associated with trauma
- Can be primary (~70% of cases) or can occur as secondary process arising in other benign or malignant bone tumors (Table 7.3)

Location:

- Most are metaphyseal, eccentric
- Majority are in long bones—femur, tibia, and humerus
- Also in spine (usually in posterior elements, T>L>C>S), pelvis, hands

Clinical symptoms:

- Pain and swelling
- Pathologic fracture in 10–20%
- Spinal lesions can lead to cord compression, neurologic symptoms

Imaging characteristics:

- Markedly expansile, multiloculated, geographic lucent lesion with well-defined margins, but little or no sclerotic rim
- Eccentric, but large lesions may appear central
- Cortex markedly thinned; may be intact but not visible on radiograph
- May see (laminated or solid) periosteal new bone in either intact ABC or pathologic fracture
- Rarely, can have extraosseous soft tissue component
- In kids, may extend into/across growth plate, resulting in growth plate closure or angular deformity
- Can cross intervertebral disc to involve more than one vertebra
- If it is a secondary ABC, may show evidence of underlying primary bone lesion
- CT:
  - Can help demonstrate radiographically-occult cortex
  - Internal septations and fluid–fluid levels due to layering blood products
- MRI:
  - Heterogeneous T1 and T2 with multiple fluid–fluid levels—dependent fluid is high T1 due to methemoglobin; gadolinium enhancement of periphery and of internal septations
- Bone scintigaphy:
  - Nonspecific, 64% show peripheral activity, otherwise diffuse, homogeneous activity

Malignant potential:

- Benign lesion with potential for local recurrence
- Rare reports of malignant transformation are controversial
- Can be seen as secondary ABC in malignant sarcomas, especially osteosarcoma. Concern for secondary ABC may prompt biospy

Treatment:

- Rare spontaneous regression
- Curettage or cryosurgery and bone grafting; occasionally marginal or wide excision. Some embolize prior to surgery
- Recurrence after curettage variable (20–70%); recurrence happens in first 2 years
- Rarely, incompletely resectable, aggressive, and/or recurrent ABCs are treated with low-dose radiotherapy, but this risks growth arrest in children

Miscellaneous facts:

- Appearance of "blood-filled sponge" on gross pathology
- Fluid–fluid levels are characteristic of, but not specific for, ABC (Table 7.4)
- Controversial solid variant of ABC is known as giant cell reparative granuloma and tends to occur in short tubular bones of hands and feet

Differential diagnosis:

- GCT—is less expansile, extends to subchondral surface; solid components; rarely sclerotic rim, no periosteal reaction
- SBC—is central rather than eccentric, minimal expansion, single chamber, periosteal new bone only if fractured, fallen fragment and gas bubble signs diagnostic
- NOF—is less expansile, no fluid levels
- Hemophiliac pseudotumor—has other clinical and imaging signs of hemophilia

Table 7.3 Lesions that contain secondary aneurysmal bone cysts

Benign lesions

- Brown tumor
- Chondroblastoma
- Chondromyxoid fibroms
- Langerhans cell histiocytosis
- Fibrous dysplasia
- Giant cell reparative granuloma
- Hemangioma
- GCT
- NOF
- Osteoblastoma
- Simple bone cyst

Malignant lesions

- Angiosarcoma
- Chondrosarcoma
- Fibrosarcoma
- Hemangioendothelioma
- Malignant fibrous histiocytoma
- Telangiectatic osteosarcoma

Table 7.4 Differential diagnosis—lytic lesions with fluid levels

- Simple bone cyst with fracture
- ABC
- GCT—extends to subarticular bone
- Chondroblastoma—centered in epiphysis
- Osteoblastoma—posterior elements of spine
- Telangiectatic osteosarcoma—thick wall, osteoid formation

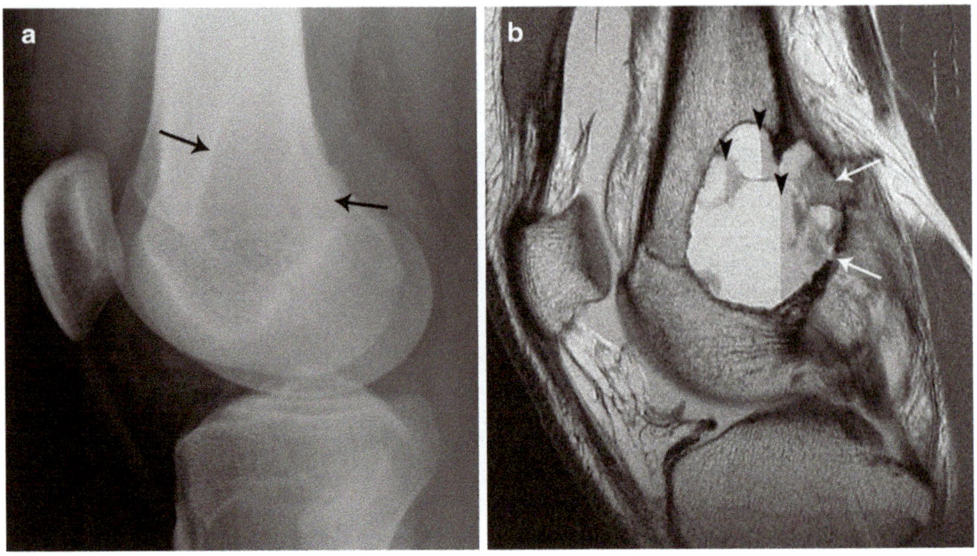

Fig. 7.14 Radiograph (**a**) shows an ABC as a geographic lucent lesion, eccentric in the metaphysis, with a thin sclerotic rim (*arrows*). The PD-weighted MR image (**b**) shows characteristic multiple fluid–fluid levels (*arrowheads*), with aneurysmal bone expansion and thinned posterior cortex (*arrows*)

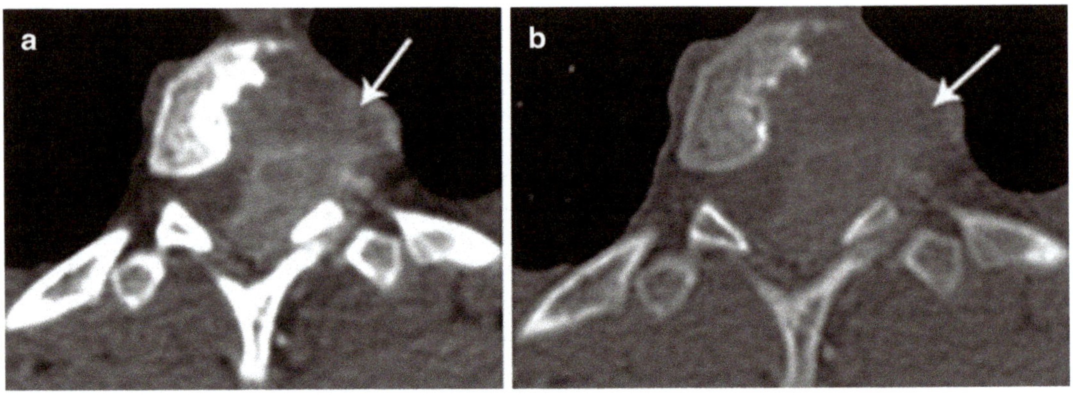

Fig. 7.15 Axial CT, in soft tissue (**a**) and bone (**b**) windows show an ABC in the thoracic spine. The lesion (*arrows*) is a multilocated, geographic, lucent lesion (*arrows*) with some high density due to blood products. ABCs in the spine can cause cord compression and neurologic symptoms. They are more likely to occur in the posterior elements and are most common in the thoracic spine

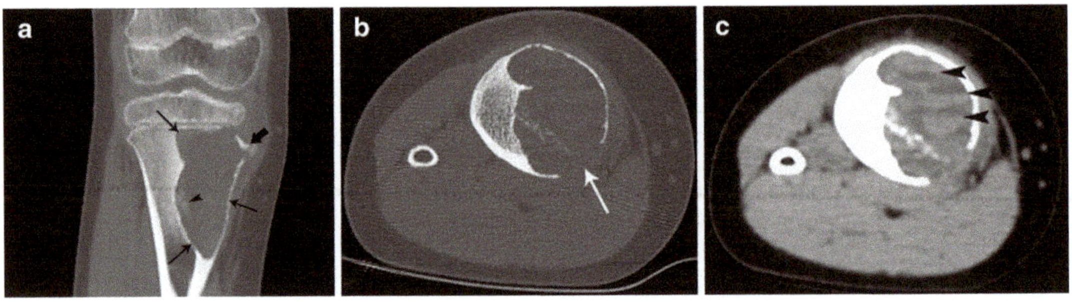

Fig. 7.16 Coronal CT image (**a**) shows an ABC (*arrows*) in a child. There is a thin shell of subperiosteal reactive bone along the inner surface of the rim (*arrowhead*). Note also buckling of metaphyseal cortex consistent with fracture (*thick arrow*). Axial CT image (bone window) (**b**) shows that the cortex is markedly expanded and thinned. In the posteromedial tibia, the cortex is unmineralized (*arrow*), but the periosteum is intact. CT image (soft tissue window) (**c**) show multiple fluid–fluid levels (*arrowheads*), indicating multiple internal loculations

Lipoma of Bone

Synonyms: intraosseous lipoma, ossifying lipoma, parosteal lipoma

Demographics:

- <0.1% of primary bone tumors, but some think much more common
- Second to eighth decades
- M:F 1.6:1
- Parosteal lipoma variant—very rare, 0.3% of all lipomas, most patients are 40–60 years old at time of diagnosis; M:F 9:7

Origin:

- Benign neoplasm of mature adipocytes, may contain fibrous or vascular tissue
- Some argue that many intraosseous lipomas are actually primary bone infarcts or areas of normal dense fat, rather than true neoplasms
- Parosteal (formerly periosteal) lipoma—variant that is identical to soft tissue lipoma, but arises on outer surface of bone, in association with periosteum

Location:

- Medullary cavity; rarely, is intracortical or along bone surface
- Proximal femur, calcaneus, ilium, tibia, fibula are most frequent locations
- Parosteal lipomas usually arise along diaphysis of long bones

Clinical symptoms:

- Usually asymptomatic, incidental finding
- May have achy pain—likely incidental, but may be due to intraosseous pressure and ischemia
- Pathologic fractures rare
- Parosteal lipomas are often asymptomatic, but may present as a mass or cause nerve compression, with secondary muscle atrophy

Imaging characteristics:

- Geographic, lucent lesion with sharply defined borders, narrow zone of transition, surrounded by thin or thick sclerotic rim
- Characteristic central or ring-like calcification or ossification seen in 57%
- Pathognomonic—central or ring-like calcification in body of calcaneus
- Milgram—histopathologic staging with imaging correlates
  - Stage 1—viable fat cells only—radiolucent, well-circumscribed, often with mild focal expansile remodeling, peripheral ridges
  - Stage 2—partial fat necrosis and calcification—central or peripheral calcification or ossification
  - Stage 3—necrotic fat with some calcification, variable cyst formation, fibrous proliferation, reactive woven bone—fibrous proliferation and cystic degeneration surrounded successively by ossific rim, fat, and outermost ossification or fibrous capsule leading to pathognomonic "**bull's eye**" appearance
- CT:
  - Is diagnostic due to fatty attenuation (HU < −60 to −100)
  - May be slightly lower attenuation than normal fatty marrow, due to absence of cellular elements
  - May have central fluid and central or peripheral calcification or ossification

- MRI:
  - Isointense to marrow and subcutaneous fat, with high T1/intermediate T2 signal. No gadolinium enhancement
  - Lipoma sometimes slightly higher T1 signal than marrow fat
  - Need not be pure fat to be diagnostic—presence of high T2 fluid and low signal calcification or ossification is common!
- Bone scintigraphy: absent to moderate activity
- Parosteal lipoma—appearance is diagnostic—a lobulated, exophytic radiolucent fatty mass abutting cortex with variable amounts of cortical thickening or periosteal reaction and bone erosion or bowing. May be visible on radiographs. Unlike osteochondroma, medullary cavity is *not* confluent with the host bone. MRI best for presurgical planning

Treatment:

- No treatment; if symptomatic, then curettage and packing with bone graft
- Parosteal lipoma—complete surgical resection; if nerve entrapment, avoid delay due to potential irreversible damage; recurrence unusual

Malignant potential:

- Negligible; sarcomatous transformation is extremely rare (case reports)
- Parosteal lipoma—no reports of malignant transformation

Miscellaneous facts: case reports of multiple intraosseous lipomas, sometimes in association with hyperlipoproteinemia

Differential diagnosis:

- Bone infarct—no bone expansion; serpentine (as opposed to rounded)
- SBC (calcaneus)—no central calcification; fluid content, not fat
- ABC (calcaneus)—more expansile, more posterior and plantar
- Chondroblastoma (calcaneus)—usually abuts subtalar joint
- Pseudotumor (calcaneus)—no cystic component or central calcification

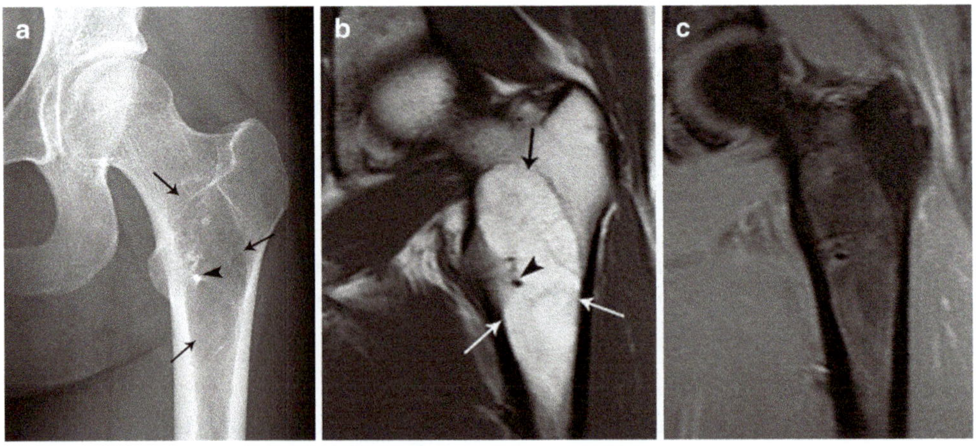

Fig. 7.17 Radiograph (**a**) shows an intraosseous lipoma in the proximal femur (*arrows*) as a well-circumscribed, geographic lucent lesion, with a thin sclerotic rim. Note the characteristic central calcification (*arrowhead*). The lesion (*arrows*) has high signal on the T1-weighted MR image (**b**) and a central low signal calcification (*arrowhead*) from fat necrosis. Signal from intralesional fat is selectively suppressed on the frequency-selective fat-saturated T1-weighted image (**c**), confirming that the high T1 signal is due to fat, rather than hemorrhage or proteinaceous fluid

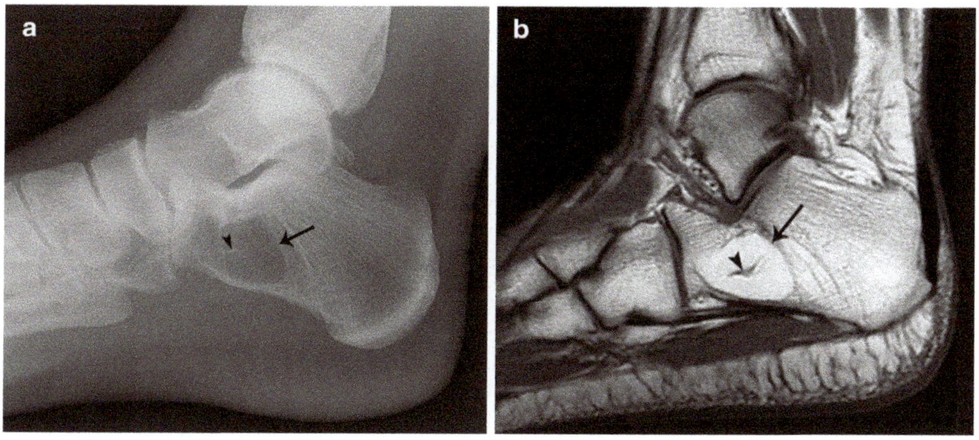

Fig. 7.18 Radiograph (**a**) shows an intraosseous lipoma in the body of the calcaneus (*arrow*), a common location. Central density (*arrowhead*) is consistent with the central calcification or ossification from fat necrosis. Differential diagnosis includes simple bone cyst and ABC. The lipoma (*arrow*) is high signal on the T1-weighted MR image (**b**). A frequency-selective fat-saturated T1-weighted image could confirm that this lesion contains fat and not hemorrhage or proteinaceous fluid

Ewing Sarcoma

Synonyms: Ewing tumor, peripheral neuroepithelioma, peripheral neuroblastoma, Askin tumor

Demographics:

- Second most common sarcoma of bone and soft tissue in children, after osteosarcoma
- Almost 80% of pts are <20 years old; peak 10–15 years
- M = F
- Most are caucasian, extremely rare in black or asian children

Origin:

- Round cell sarcoma with varying degrees of neuroectodermal differentiation (none in Ewing sarcoma, present in Primitive Neuroectodermal Tumor or PNET)
- Ewing sarcoma family of tumors (Ewing sarcoma, atypical ES, PNET, Askin tumor or malignant small cell tumor of the thoracopulmonary region) all share the same chromosomal translocation

Location:

- Metadiaphysis > diaphysis
- Any bone with red marrow: femur, ilium, humerus, and tibia; fibula; ribs and axial skeleton
- Usually solitary at presentation (90%)

Clinical symptoms:

- Pain, swelling, and sometimes local warmth
- May have constitutional symptoms, particularly if metastatic: fever, increased ESR, weight loss, anemia, and leukocytosis
- Can be mistaken for osteomyelitis

Imaging characteristics:

- Radiographs often underestimate extent
- Permeative or moth-eaten lytic lesion in diaphysis or metadiaphysis of long bone or in flat bone, with aggressive periosteal reaction and large soft tissue mass
- Can see reactive bone, leading to mixed lytic-and-sclerotic or, occasionally, a markedly sclerotic appearance
- Irregular cortical thinning and destruction common
- Periosteal reaction in 85%, classically laminated or onion-skin, also hair-on-end/sunburst, Codman's triangle
- Pathologic fracture in 10–15%
- "**Saucerization of cortex**" secondary to extrinsic pressure by soft tissue mass and destruction of periosteal surface of bone; together with permeative lesion and mass, saucerization is highly suggestive of Ewing
- PNET—epiphyseal involvement, pathologic fractures, and metastases more common than in Ewing
- CT:
  - Depicts bone destruction, changes in marrow density, periosteal new bone formation, and soft tissue mass
- MRI:
  - Best modality for showing intramedullary extent, soft tissue mass, predicting respectability, skip metastases in same or adjacent bone (less common than osteosarcoma), and for assessing response to therapy
  - Lesions are low-intermediate on T1/heterogeneously intermediate to high on T2
  - Margins are ill-defined. Prominent reactive edema can lead to overestimation of medullary involvement
  - Hair-on-end periosteal new bone appears as low T2 striations
  - Dynamic contrast enhancement can help distinguish rapidly enhancing tumor (high mean initial slope) from reactive intramedullary and nonneoplastic soft tissue edema
  - After treatment, dynamic contrast can help to distinguish remaining viable tumor (early rapid enhancement) from necrosis
- Bone scintigraphy:
  - Nonspecific increased activity (even when radiographic sclerosis is not impressive); can help detect metastases; soft tissue component visible on blood pool
  - Increased activity on gallium-67-citrate, which may demonstrate soft tissue component; can be used to monitor response
  - FDG PET has high sensitivity for detecting metastases and can demonstrate response
- Staging workup: radiographs and MRI of primary site; chest radiographs and chest CT; bone scan; bone marrow biopsy; as well as CBC, ESR, and chemistry

Malignant potential:

- Highly malignant, but survival and limb-sparing surgery rates have improved
- At presentation, approximately 25% have macroscopic metastases (lung>bone, marrow) and nearly all have micrometastases
- 5-year survival—55–70% for localized disease at diagnosis, ~25% for metastases at diagnosis
- Increased risk for secondary bone sarcomas developing in radiation field, at 20 years post-therapy (10–30%)

Treatment:

- Neoadjuvant chemotherapy, resection of primary tumor (limb-sparing, when possible), post surgical chemotherapy; radiation pre- or post-op if concerned about margins
- 30–40% of patients who present with local Ewing sarcoma develop recurrent disease

Miscellaneous facts:

- Ewing sarcoma can cross sacroiliac joint
- Rarely, a soft tissue variant of Ewing sarcoma can arise outside the bone

Differential diagnosis:

- PNET—epiphyseal involvement, pathologic fractures, and metastases more common than in Ewing, otherwise, indistinguishable at imaging
- Osteomyelitis, Langerhans cell histiocytosis—essentially indistinguishable at imaging and can be similar clinical presentations; less likely than Ewing to have large soft tissue mass
- Osteosarcoma—usually metaphyseal, not diaphyseal; Codman's triangle and sunburst periosteal reaction are more common; demonstrates osteoid matrix (except telangiectatic OS); less likely to occur in flat bone or rib or to have large soft tissue mass
- Lymphoma—hard to distinguish, can occur at same age, and often has soft tissue mass
- Metastatic neuroblastoma—occurs in younger patients, <5 years old

Table 7.5 Small round cell tumors

• Dedifferentiated synovial sarcoma
• Desmoplastic small round cell tumors
• Ewing/PNET
• Medulloblastoma
• Mesenchymal chondrosarcoma
• Neuroblastoma
• Non-Hodgkin lymphoma
• Rhabdomyosarcoma
• Small cell osteosarcoma

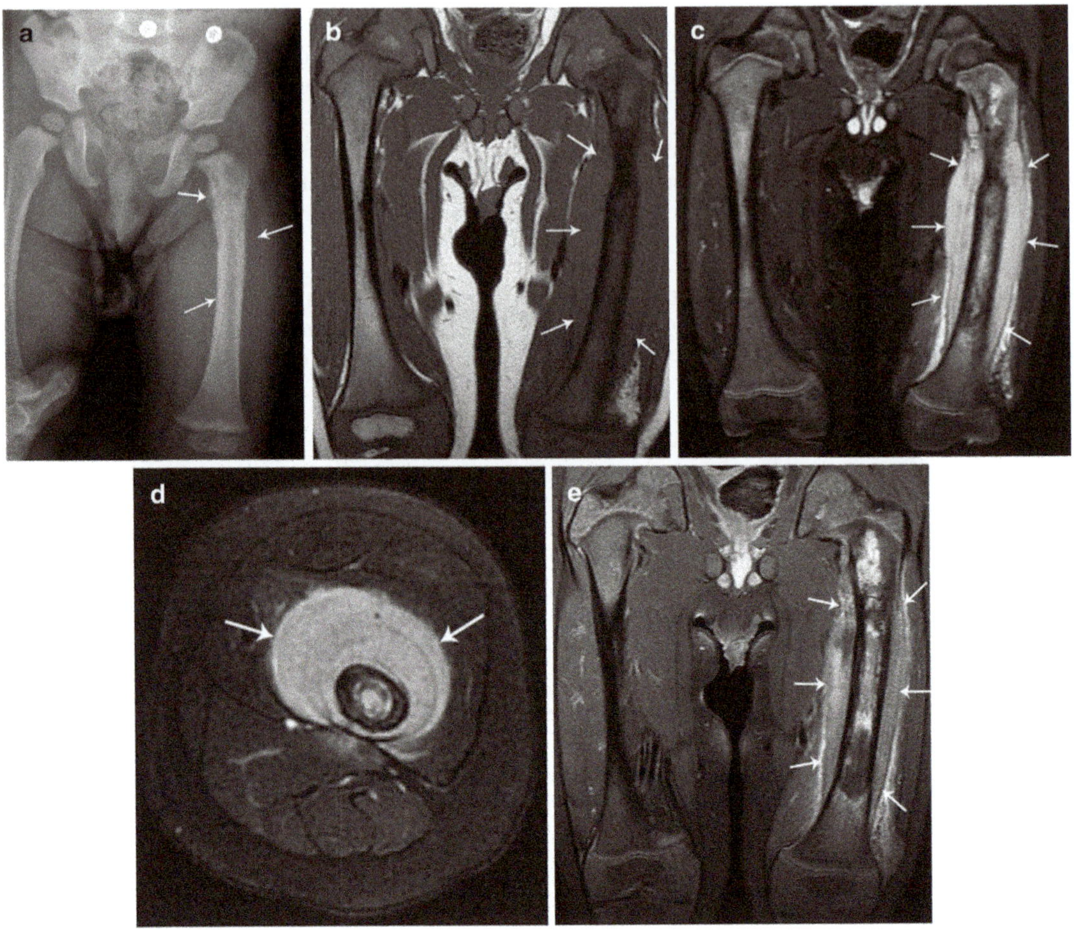

Fig. 7.19 Ewing sarcoma, Radiograph (**a**) shows a permeative mixed lucent and sclerotic lesion (*arrows*) in the femoral diaphsysis of this skeletally immature patient. Coronal T1-weighted (**b**) and fat-saturated T2-weighted (**c**) MR images show extensive replacement of the normal marrow signal and a large soft tissue mass emanating from the bone (*arrows*). As with other round cell lesions (lymphoma, osteosarcoma), a large soft tissue mass can develop (*arrows*), even without much cortical destruction, as seen on the axial fat-saturated T2-weighted MRI (**d**). Coronal postcontrast MR image (**e**) shows heterogeneous enhancement of the bone and soft tissue components (*arrows*). (Images courtesy of Dr. Daniel Siegal, Detroit, Michigan)

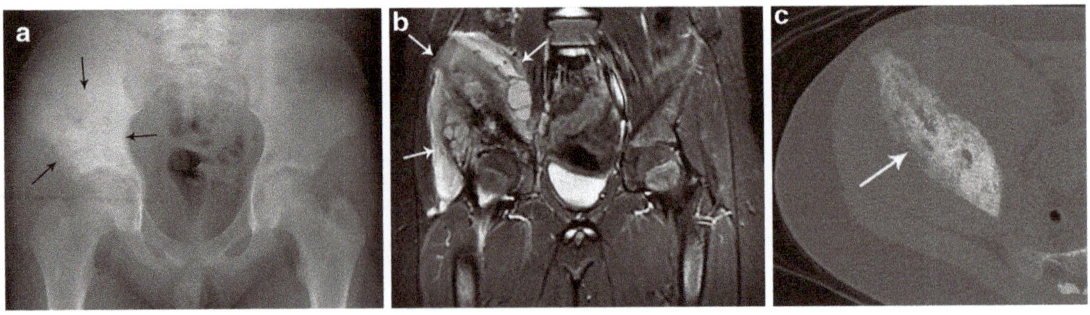

Fig. 7.20 Radiograph (**a**) shows an Ewing sarcoma presenting as a large mixed lytic and sclerotic lesion in the right iliac bone (*arrows*), with aggressive periosteal new bone formation. The extent of the soft tissue mass (*arrows*) is best demonstrated on the fat-saturated T2-weighted MR image (**b**). The axial CT image (**c**) better demonstrates the extent of bone permeation and destruction. (Images courtesy of Dr. Daniel Siegal, Detroit, Michigan)

Adamantinoma

Synonyms: extragnathic adamantinoma, adamantinoma of long bones, juvenile intracortical adamantinoma, and angioblastoma

Demographics:
- Rare, 0.1–0.5% of all primary bone tumors
- Median age 25–35 years old
- M>F (slight)

Origin:
- Low grade malignant neoplasm consisting of epithelial cells in fibrous and fibroosseous stroma
- Two forms: (1) classic and (2) osteofibrous-dysplasia-like
- Pathogenesis: epithelium trapped in bone or periosteum during fetal development

Location:
- 90% occur in tibia, almost always in anterior cortex
- Up to 10% present with ipsilateral fibular lesions
- Diaphyseal to metadiaphyseal

Clinical symptoms:
- Swelling, with or without pain, for months to years
- Tender, firm, and fixed mass

Imaging characteristics:
- Radiographs
  - Elongated, well-circumscribed, mixed lytic-and-sclerotic lesion, centered in anterior tibial cortex, along diaphysis or metadiaphysis with lobulated borders
  - Lesions are large. 80% are >5 cm long
  - Most extend into medullary bone; can have soft tissue extension (seen in 9%)
  - May have internal septation, peripheral sclerosis, cortical thickening, expansile remodeling, and lamellated or solid periosteal reaction
  - Rounded "lucent" foci may have ground glass opacity
  - "**Sawtooth**" cortical destruction is characteristic
  - Multifocal satellite lesions may occur within same bone (appear separated by intervening cortex, but histologically continuous)
  - Rate of growth can be slow
- CT: better delineates lucent and sclerotic areas and cortical abnormalities
- MRI:
  - Demonstrates intramedullary and soft tissue extension for surgical planning
  - Low-intermediate T1, homogeneous or heterogeneous high T2, can have focally intense gadolinium enhancement
  - When multinodular, tumor foci are separated by low signal cortical bone
- Bone scintigraphy: increased activity

Malignant potential:
- Low-grade malignancy, locally aggressive
- Classic form—12–29% have metastases to regional lymph nodes and lungs
- OFD-like adamantinomas do not metastasize, but can convert to classic form when they recur and may then metastasize
- 10-year survival rates 10–65%

Treatment:

- Wide en bloc excision and bone grafting
- Local recurrence and lung metastasis may develop years after surgery, so that long-term clinical and imaging follow-up is required

Miscellaneous facts:

- Adamantinoma and mandibular ameloblastoma are now felt to be separate entities
- Consider adamantinoma in differential for any pretibial cortical lesion, even if small, nonaggressive appearance, mild symptoms, or indolent growth
- At biopsy, important to sample central tumor, in order to distinguish classic and OFD forms, due to zonal histology of classic adamantinoma (abundant epithelium at center and sparser epithelium at periphery)

Differential diagnosis:

- Osteofibrous dysplasia—is seen in younger patients (adamantinoma rarely occurs before physes fuse); is usually well-defined and less destructive, unless large
- Fibrous dysplasia—is more central within medullary cavity
- Non-ossifying fibroma—is seen in younger patients, bulk of the lesion appears to lie in medullary cavity
- Osteomyelitis—can have similar appearance, but look for sequestrum and periosteal new bone formation

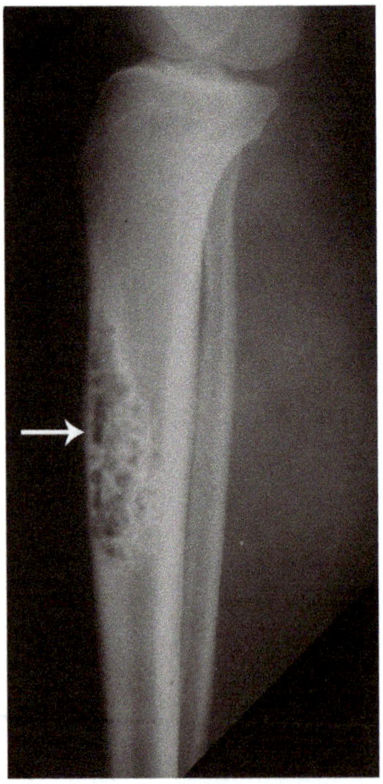

Fig. 7.21 Typical adamantinoma (*arrow*) appearing as elongated, well-circumscribed, mixed lytic-and-sclerotic lesion, centered in anterior tibial cortex. The lesion consists of multiple rounded "lucent" foci, with ground glass opacity and "sawtooth" cortical destruction

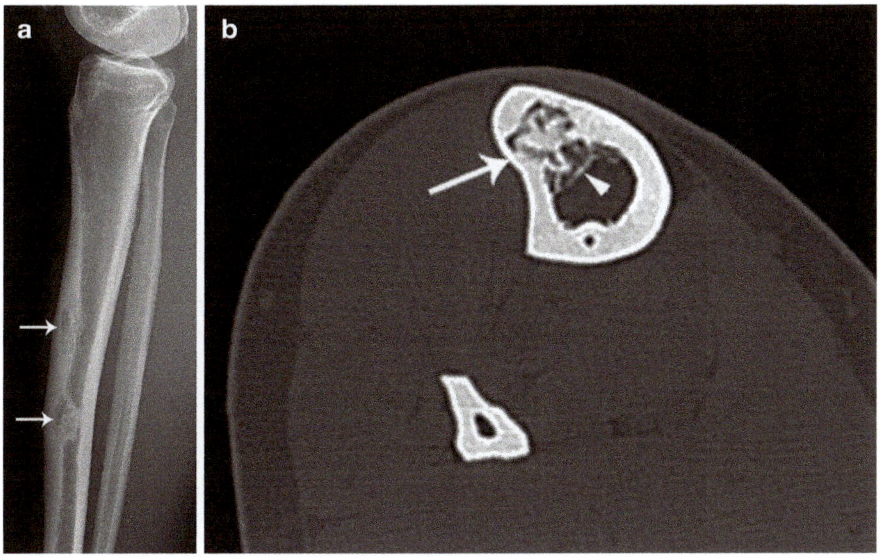

Fig. 7.22 Adamantinoma. Radiograph (**a**) show two mixed lytic and sclerotic lesions in the anterior tibial cortex. Multifocal lesions within same bone (*arrows*) appear separate, but are histologically continuous. The axial CT image shows that the lesion (*arrow*) is centered in the anterior cortex and extends into the medullary bone (*arrowhead*)

Chordoma

Demographics:

- 1–4% of all primary malignant bone tumors
- Most often diagnosed in fifth to seventh decades
- M:F = 2:1

Origin:

- Low to intermediate grade malignant tumor that arises from remnants of embryonic notochord, consists of vacuolated "physaliphorous" cells and intracellular mucoid material
- Three forms—conventional, chondroid, and dedifferentiated

Location:

- Favors axial spine, at any point along the notochordal track
- Sacrococcygeal 60%; spheno-occipital-nasal (mainly clivus) 25%
- Centered in vertebral body; tends to spare posterior elements and disc, usually extradural

Clinical symptoms:

- Symptoms relate to site and spread
- Slow growing, often nonspecific symptoms for months to years
- Spheno-occipital—headache, ocular and cranial nerve palsies, endocrine dysfunction secondary to pituitary gland compression; can mimic cerebellopontine angle tumor or cause nasal obstruction and bleeding
- Spine—nerve or cord compression
- Sacrococcygeal—lower back pain and paresthesias, anorectal or bladder dysfunction, may be palpable on rectal exam

Imaging characteristics:

- Solitary, expansile, highly destructive lytic lesion of axial skeleton, in midline, with soft tissue mass and often with bony debris
- Borders irregular, scalloped
- May see sclerotic rim, matrix calcification, pathologic fracture
- Often with large, lobulated soft tissue mass and local soft tissue infiltration; mass can span several vertebral segments and spares intervertebral discs
- Can be paramedian; can be osteosclerotic
- CT: best for demonstrating bony margins and osseous fragmentation
- MRI:
  - Large destructive lesion with soft tissue mass, lobulated borders, displacing (rather than invading) bowel and or bladder
  - Nonspecific low-intermediate T1, heterogeneously high T2; may have high T1 foci and low T2 septae; heterogeneous gadolinium enhancement
  - If myxoid, very high T2 signal
- Bone scintigraphy: Photopenic centrally, increased activity at periphery

Malignant potential:

- Slow growing, locally aggressive, with frequent local recurrence
- Long-term prognosis is poor

Treatment:

- Aggressive surgical resection and radiation; chemotherapy for metastases
- Complete excision is difficult, due to location and infiltrative borders
- Distant metastases occur late—lung, bone, lymph nodes, liver, and skin

Miscellaneous facts:

- Rarely, chordoma presents as soft tissue mass, without bone involvement

Differential diagnosis:

- Chondrosarcoma—may demonstrate "arcs and rings" of chondroid calcification (but chordoma also has rare chondroid form)
- Metastases—soft tissue mass is less common in metastases
- Plasmacytoma—is less likely to be positive on bone scan
- Osteomyelitis, lymphoma—have similar imaging, clinical information may be helpful

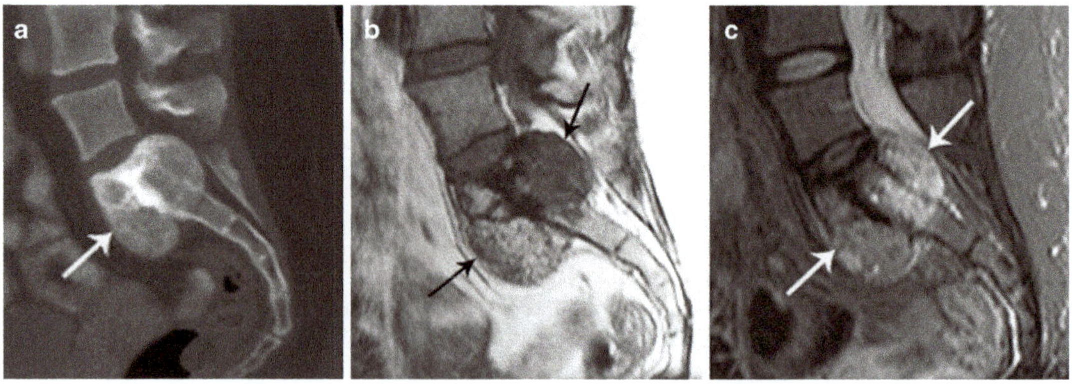

Fig. 7.23 Chordoma, there is a chordoma centered in the sacrum at S1 and expanding out anteriorly and posteriorly on the sagittal CT image (**a**). The lesion is typically lytic, with bone destruction, but can be sclerotic, as seen here. The lesion location, expansion, and signal heterogeneity on T1-weighted (**b**) and fat-saturated T2-weighted (**c**) MR images are in keeping with the diagnosis. In general, enhancement can vary from mild to avid

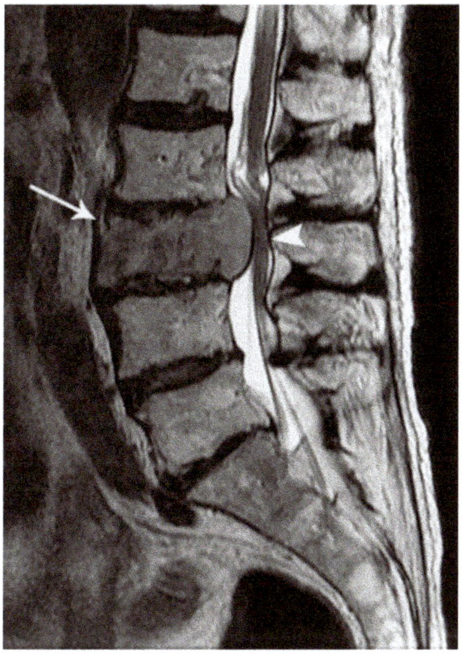

Fig. 7.24 Although most common in the clivus and sacrum, chordomas can occur anywhere along the course of the notochordal remnants, here, in the L3 vertebral body (*arrow*). Note the bone expansion and compression of the lumbosacral nerve roots (*arrowhead*)

Lymphoma

Synonyms: reticulum cell sarcoma, lymphosarcoma, primary non-Hodgkin lymphoma, Hodgkin lymphoma, malignant lymphoma of bone, osteolymphoma

Demographics:

- Primary non-Hodgkin lymphoma of bone is rare, less than 5% of all primary malignant bone tumors
  - Most are diffuse large cell B cell lymphomas; older patients, M>F
  - Diagnosis requires evidence of no distant soft tissue or lymph node involvement and, according to some, no extra-osseous or nodal involvement for 6 months after diagnosis
- Secondary involvement (metastases) of skeletal system in NHL occurs in 10–20% of adults and 20–30% of children, usually after initial presentation
- Primary Hodgkin lymphoma of bone is extremely rare, but secondary involvement can occur in widespread disease
- Primary NHL of bone ≫ primary Hodgkin lymphoma of bone

Origin:

- NHLs are a heterogeneous spectrum of neoplasms, most are large cell
- Hodgkin lymphoma usually arises within lymph node tissue, with late hematogenous dissemination; characterized by Reed–Sternberg cells

Location:

- Primary NHL-long bone (femur, tibia), pelvis, ribs, and vertebrae
- Usually diaphyseal, near metaphysis
- Secondary NHL—axial skeleton

Clinical symptoms:

- Asymptomatic
- Pain and swelling
- Systemic symptoms (fever, weight loss)—rare with primary NHL
- Pathologic fractures in 25%

Imaging characteristics:

- Primary NHL
  - Can be radiographically near-normal if no cortical destruction
  - Lytic lesion near end of long bone most common, often large and poorly defined; can also be mixed lytic–blastic
  - Pathologic fracture and soft tissue extension are common
  - Periosteal reaction common, both aggressive and nonaggressive
  - Bony sequestra seen in 16% of primary lymphomas of bone
  - Can spread across joints—one of few neoplasms that do
- Secondary NHL
  - Single or, more commonly, multiple lytic lesions with poorly defined margins and moth-eaten or permeative bone destruction
  - May have adjacent soft tissue extension
  - Sclerosis rare (more common in Hodgkin lymphoma)
- Hodgkin lymphoma
  - Radiographic findings present in 10–25% of cases
  - Spine, pelvis, ribs, femora, sternum; multifocal or solitary
  - Sclerotic, lytic, or mixed
  - **"Ivory vertebra"**—diffuse sclerosis
- Burkitt lymphoma: Characteristically involves facial bones
- Musculoskeletal complications of therapy:
  - Osteonecrosis due to chemotherapy (which can include steroids), 1–3 years after therapy initiated
  - Methotrexate osteoarthropathy—pain, osteopenia, growth recovery lines, dense metaphyseal bands and fractures; cause unknown
- CT: Shows bone destruction, early cortical erosion, sequestra, soft tissue mass
- MRI
  - Most accurate for determining extent of marrow and soft tissue disease
  - Focal or diffuse marrow involvement (can be extensive even with normal radiographs), with or without soft tissue extension
  - Isointense or slightly hyperintense to muscle on T1; often hyperintense to muscle and isointense to fat on T2, but can see lower and heterogeneous T2 signal; peritumoral and reactive marrow edema; variable enhancement
  - Tumor permeating or "oozing" through cortex into soft tissues, with only limited cortical disruption, is highly suggestive of lymphoma or other round cell tumors (possibly due to spread along transcortical vessels or due to osteoclastic cytokines)
- Bone scintigraphy: usually positive, even when radiographs are negative

Malignant potential:

- Malignant; cortical breakthrough, pathologic fractures, and soft tissue masses suggest poorer prognosis

Treatment:

- Primary lymphoma of bone usually responds well to combined radiation and chemotherapy (overall response rate 94%), with 61% 5-year survival

Miscellaneous facts:

- A truly primary bone lesion is considered stage I non-Hodgkin lymphoma, whereas a bone lesion associated with disease at other sites is considered stage IV
- Primary multifocal osseous lymphoma—controversial entity with predilection for bones about the knee; consider this diagnosis if lesions in distal femur, proximal tibia, and skull (unusual pattern for metastases)

Differential diagnosis:

- Ewing sarcoma, osteomyelitis, Langerhans cell histiocytosis—round cell lesions that may be hard to differentiate
- Metastases, plasmacytoma—permeative or moth-eaten pattern and periosteal reaction less common in these
- Paget disease ("ivory vertebra")—vertebral enlargement, thickened cortex and trabeculae

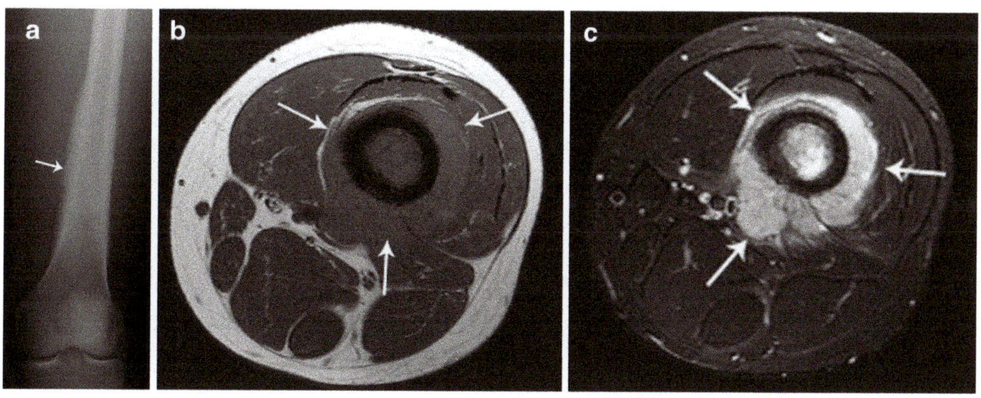

Fig. 7.25 AP radiograph of the distal femur (**a**) shows increased density in the distal diaphysis and aggressive periosteal new bone formation (*arrow*). The majority of lymphomas are lytic, though a small percentage can appear sclerotic. Here, density may also be due to superimposed periosteal new bone formation along the anterior and posterior surfaces of the bone. Axial T1-weighted (**b**) and fat-saturated T2-weighted (**c**) MR images show replacement of normal medullary fat by the tumor (*arrows*). The tumor "oozes" concentrically out of the bone, into the surrounding soft tissues. Soft tissue extension with minimal cortical disruption is a feature of lymphoma and can also be seen in other round cell processes

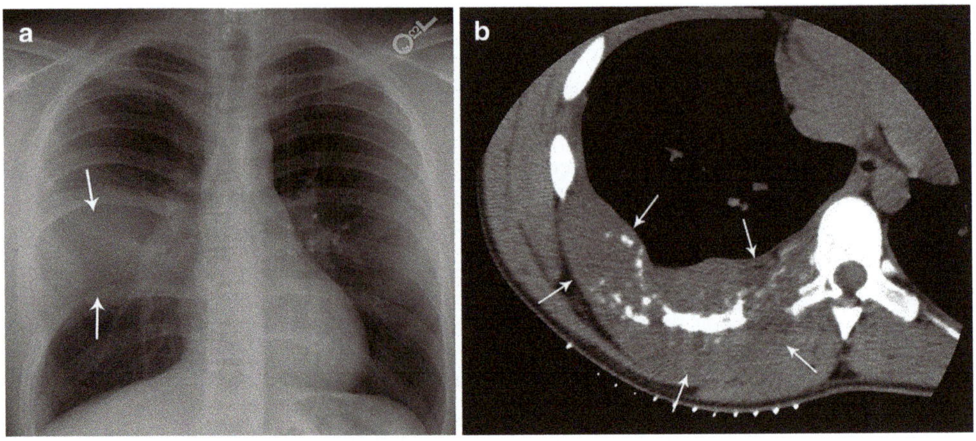

Fig. 7.26 On the radiograph (**a**) the right eighth rib has been destroyed (*arrows*) and there is increased soft tissue density overlying the right mid-lung due to the associated soft tissue mass. Axial CT (**b**) through the eighth rib shows extensive bone destruction, with surrounding soft tissue mass (*arrows*)

Leukemia

Demographics:

- ALL (acute lymphoblastic)—children and adolescents
- AML (acute myelogeneous)—adolescents and young adults
- CLL (chronic lymphocytic)—adults
- CML (chronic myelogenous)—adults >25 years
- Hairy cell leukemia—rare B cell neoplasm that accounts for 2% of all leukemias; typically affects middle-aged men
- All types slightly more common in men

Origin:

- Diverse group of lymphoid neoplasms with involvement of marrow and peripheral blood

Location:

- Variable; in myelogeneous leukemia, chloromas can cause lytic lesions in skull>spine>ribs>sternum

Clinical symptoms:

- Fever, bleeding, fatigue, lymphadenopathy, hepatosplenomegaly, alterations of cell population in marrow and CBC, susceptible to infection

Imaging characteristics:

- ALL
  - Diffuse osteopenia
  - Focal moth-eaten or permeative lytic lesions with periosteal new bone due to subperiosteal leukemic cells
  - In children—thin radiolucent metaphyseal bands due to either osteoporosis (narrow, sharply defined) or leukemic infiltration (broad, irregular, and poorly demarcated) and growth arrest
  - Pathologic fractures and bone infarcts

- AML, CLL, and CML
  - Diffuse osteopenia and focal lytic lesions
  - Chloroma (granulocytic sarcoma)—mass of myelogeneous cells that can cause lytic lesions or soft tissue masses (AML>CML)
  - Myelofibrosis causing myelosclerosis—typically seen as precursor to leukemia in myelogeneous and megakaryocytic lines, rare in childhood
- MRI:
  - Marrow replacement with diffuse or focal ill-defined low-intermediate T1 and intermediate to high fat-saturated T2 signal, usually with some contrast enhancement
  - Assessment can be difficult when there is baseline erythropoietic marrow (children) and normal marrow enhancement (vertebrae in children less than 7 years old)
  - Response to chemotherapy has been monitored using T1, STIR, and contrast enhancement pattern
  - Chloromas: variable appearance, well or poorly circumscribed, low-intermediate T1, intermediate to high T2, prominent contrast enhancement

Treatment:
- All forms are treated with chemotherapy; AML and CML with marrow transplant
- ALL—5-year survival >70%; AML—can achieve good remission, but only a minority still disease free after 5 years; CLL—chemotherapy, variable results, can progress to blast crisis

Differential diagnosis: hard to differentiate from other round cell lesions on imaging

Table 7.6 Differential diagnosis—radiolucent metaphyseal bands

- Normal variant
- Leukemia
- Metastatic neuroblastoma
- Metabolic disease—rickets and scurvy
- Transplacental infection (syphilis)

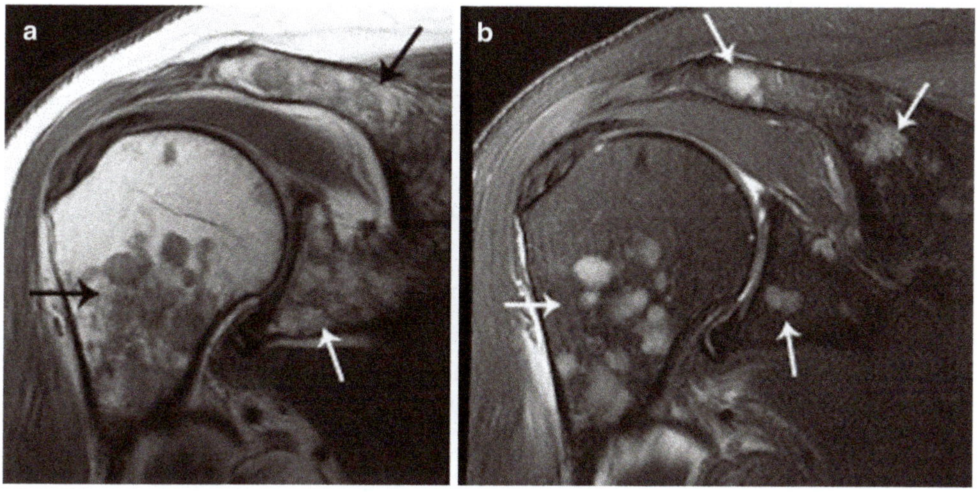

Fig. 7.27 Leukemic deposits are seen as multiple focal lesions in the marrow (*arrows*) that are isointense to muscle on T1-weighted (**a**) and hyperintense on fat-saturated T2-weighted (**b**) MR images. Leukemia can also cause more diffuse infiltration. Assessment can be difficult when there is baseline erythropoietic marrow

Angiosarcoma

Synonyms: hemangioendothelioma, malignant hemangioendothelioma, high-grade hemangioendothelioma, hemangiosarcoma, hemangioendothelial sarcoma, angioendothelioma, angiofibrosarcoma, hemangioendotheliosarcoma, epithelioid angiosarcoma, vascular sarcoma

Demographics:
- Very rare in bone (much less common than in soft tissue)
- Nearly equal distribution second to eighth decade; M:F=1:1

Origin:
- Neoplastic blood vessels with malignant endothelial lining cells

Location:
- Most common in long bones (60%) and axial skeleton (mainly spine)
- Approximately 1/3 are multifocal

Clinical symptoms:
- Local pain and swelling; occasionally pathologic fracture

Imaging characteristics:
- Nonspecific; cannot distinguish benign from malignant
- One or more lytic lesions of varying sizes at or near ends of bone, often aggressive, with soft tissue mass
- Clustered multicentric lesion with "**honeycomb**" or "**hole-in-hole**" appearance suggests vascular neoplasm
- Smaller, lower grade lesions tend to be better defined, have sclerotic rim
- AS can be associated with bone infarct, site of prior radiation
- Skeletal survey is recommended, given high incidence of multifocal lesions and risk of pathologic fracture
- Angiograms: dense well-circumscribed areas of staining with early draining veins and shunting
- CT: nonspecific
- MRI:
  - Nonspecific infiltrative lesion; unlike hemangioma, no fatty component
  - May see prominent serpentine high flow (low signal on all sequences) or low flow (high T2) vessels, more often in periphery, which is highly suggestive of vascular lesion
- Bone scintigraphy: increased activity

Malignant potential:
- AS is aggressive malignancy, with frequent local recurrence and distant metastases (lung, bones, and nodes); ~20% overall survival when high-grade

Treatment:
- Treated with surgical resection, radiation, and adjuvant chemotherapy

Miscellaneous facts:
- Kasabach–Merritt syndrome—association of hemangioma, hemangioendothelioma, or angiosarcoma with thrombocytopenia and purpura, with intravascular coagulation, bleeding diathesis, and arthropathy secondary to repetitive hemarthrosis
- Needle aspiration or biopsy of vascular lesions is often nondiagnostic and risks bleeding

Differential diagnosis:

- Hemangioma—has less infiltrative borders, and demonstrates fat overgrowth
- Kaposi sarcoma, metastases, myeloma—lack prominent vessels on MRI
- Bacillary angiomatosis—seen in AIDs, commonly has associated cutaneous lesions, systemic symptoms, periosteal reaction
- Cystic angiomatosis—has similar findings, but visceral involvement is common; favors spine

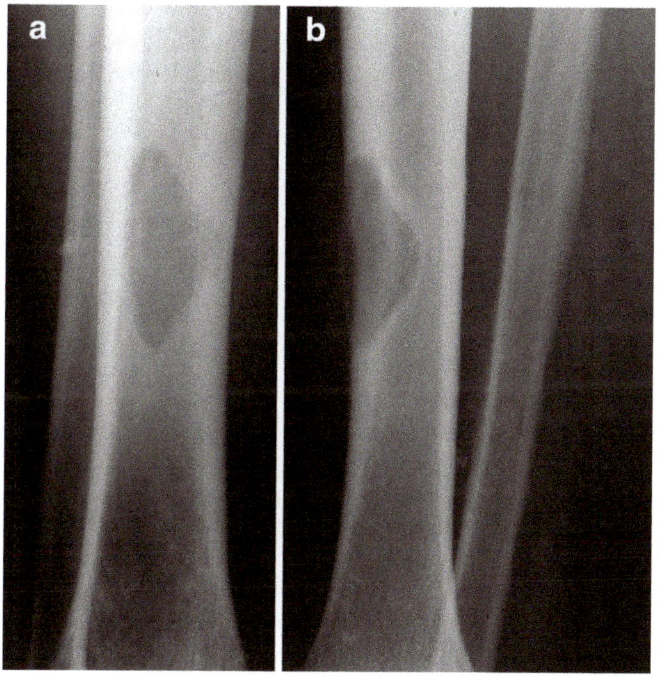

Fig. 7.28 AP (**a**) and lateral (**b**) radiographs show an angiosarcoma in the distal tibia. Smaller lesions tend to better defined and, when low grade, can have peripheral sclerosis, but larger lesions can appear very aggressive. Angiosarcomas can also occur as clustered multicentric lesions with a "honeycomb" or "hole-in-hole" appearance similar to intraosseous hemangioma

Multiple Myeloma

Symptoms: Plasma cell myeloma, solitary plasmacytoma of bone, sclerotic myeloma, POEMS

Demographics:

- Most common primary malignant tumor of bone
- Most patients are in the sixth and seventh decades
- Rare (<10%) in individuals <40 years old
- M=F

Origin:

- Neoplastic monoclonal proliferation of plasma cells, that originates in bone marrow, but can infiltrate other tissues; myeloma cells produce osteoclast stimulating factor causing bone resorption

Location:

- Can involve any bone, but axial skeletal most common
- Predominantly in bones with adulthood hematopoietic marrow—vertebrae, ribs, skull, pelvis, femur, clavicle, and scapula
- Rare distal to elbow and knee (only 10%)

Clinical symptoms:

- Bone pain, most often lumbar and thoracic
- Often present with pathologic fracture
- Weakness, fatigue, fever, weight loss, bleeding, bacterial infection, neurologic symptoms due to compression fracture or soft tissue extension of plasma cells
- Renal insufficiency, hyperviscosity, and symptoms from amyloidosis
- Anemia, hypercalcemia, elevated alkaline phosphatase, monoclonal M component spike in serum or urine in 99% of patients, monoclonal light chain (Bence Jones protein) in serum in 75%
- *Solitary plasmacytoma of bone (SBP)*—solitary myeloma lesion; mean patient age is 10–15 years younger than for multiple myeloma; twice as common in men; 50–60% of patients with SPB develop multiple myeloma after initial radiation therapy, most within 4 years; serologic tests may be negative at presentation; initial workup should include MRI of the spine or whole body PET/CT to assess for multiple lesions
- *POEMS syndrome* (**p**olyneuropathy, **o**rganomegaly, **e**ndocrinopathy, **m**onoclonal gammopathy and **s**kin changes)—M>F; younger onset than MM; also known as osteosclerotic myeloma: bone lesion may be single or multiple; 97% show some osteosclerotic component on radiographs, though lesions may be mixed-lytic sclerotic, very small sclerotic, or have as little sclerotic component as a thin sclerotic rim; longer survival than myeloma; treated with radiation or chemotherapy, depending on extent
- *MGUS* (**m**onoclonal **g**ammopathy of **u**ndetermined **s**ignificance)—patients with elevated monoclonal protein in blood, but no other findings or symptoms; 19% progress to an aggressive form, within 10 years

Imaging characteristics:

- Four radiologic presentations: diffuse osteopenia, diffuse myelomatosis (multiple lytic lesions), sclerosing myeloma, and plasmacytoma
- At presentation, 12–25% have generalized osteopenia, but no detectable focal lytic bone lesion
- Classic-multiple small, uniform, sharply demarcated "**punched out**" lytic lesions, up to 5 cm diameter; may cause endosteal scalloping (rat bites) or expansion of small diameter bones; no sclerotic rim or periosteal new bone formation
- 80% have abnormal skeletal survey
- Vertebral body compression fractures; if severe, "**vertebra plana**"

- <3% of the lesions are pure sclerotic, typically, but not always, associated with POEMS syndrome
- <3% have diffuse sclerosis, which can mimic osteoblastic metastases, lymphoma, mastocytosis, renal osteodystrophy, and myelofibrosis
- Solitary plasmacytoma—single large expansile bubbly lytic lesion, any margin, sometimes with thickened trabeculae, sclerosis, calcification, or ossification and associated soft tissue mass; in spine, can collapse, extend into spine, or cross into adjoining vertebral body
- Workup—radiographic skeletal survey including humeri and femurs, bone marrow aspirate/bx, and, in patients with bone pain, but negative radiographs, CT, MRI, or PET/CT
- CT: can show some radiographically occult lesions
- MRI:
  - Overall more sensitive than radiographs, bone scan, or CT (but less sensitive than radiographs in ribs)
  - Four patterns (may coexist):
    - Normal
    - Focal lesions—T1 signal usually is equal to or lower than muscle, unless higher due to hemorrhage; individual lesions can be either low or high T2 signal; lesions show diffuse enhancement; identical to metastases
    - Variegated—heterogeneous due to innumberable low T1 foci
    - Diffuse replacement—homogeneous abnormal narrow signal
  - Response to treatment: (1) nonenhancement, with or without lesion resolution; (2) conversion of lesion from high T2 to low T2
- Bone scintigraphy: Usually normal, only small percentage of lesions detected
- FDG PET/CT Scan:
  - Lytic lesions with increased activity
  - Highly sensitive; activity decreases in response to therapy

Malignant potential:

- Malignant, incurable
- Some patients progress rapidly despite treatment, others do not
- Median survival 3 years; 10-year survival is 10%
- Better prognosis for solitary lesions

Treatment:

- Autologous hematopoietic cell transplantation
- Chemotherapy, often including steroids
- Bisphosphonate used to treat clastic resorption

Miscellaneous facts:

- Durie–Salmon staging system includes skeletal survey results as a measure of tumor cell mass, together with other criteria: Stage I—no generalized bone lesions; Stage II—either I or III, Stage III—advanced lytic bone lesions. The newer International Staging System is now used for patients with overt, symptomatic myeloma
- Involvement of distal clavicle, acromion, glenoid, and olecranon and multiple discrete lesions in skull more common in myeloma than metastasis

Differential diagnosis:

- Lytic metastases—are less likely to be discrete and uniform in size and do not create same kind of discrete endosteal scalloping as multiple myeloma, favor pedicle as opposed to vertebral body in spine, more likely positive on bone scan
- Brown tumors—are accompanied by other findings of hyperparathyroidism
- Giant cell tumor, ABC, osteoblastoma—are seen at younger age; osteoblastoma may have matrix mineralization

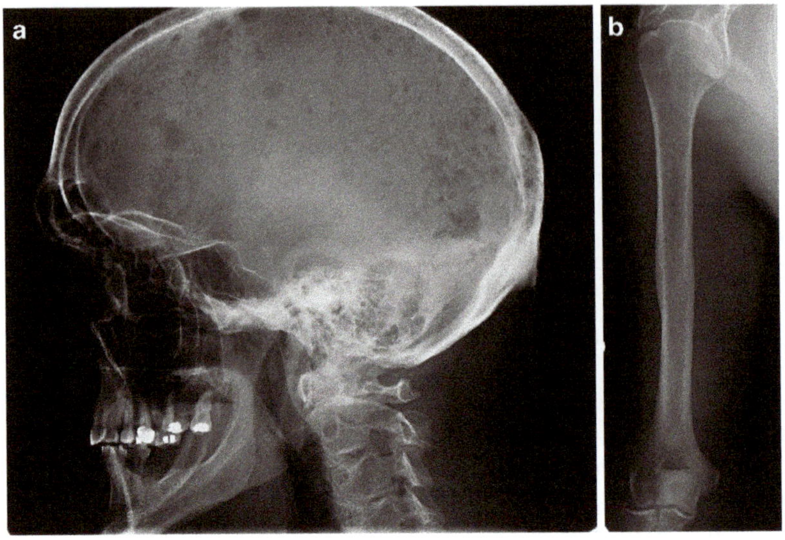

Fig. 7.29 Skull radiograph (**a**) demonstrates multiple small, sharply demarcated "punched out" lytic lesions, without sclerotic rim, a classic appearance for multiple myeloma. The AP humerus radiograph (**b**) shows innumerable small, "punched out" lytic lesions due to myeloma. The appearance here might be hard to distinguish from severe osteoporosis, with intracortical tunneling, but should prompt consideration of laboratory analysis for myeloma

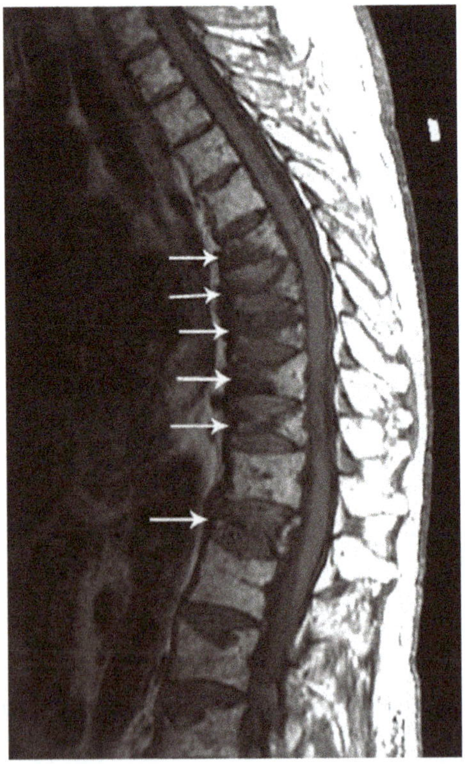

Fig. 7.30 Sagittal T1-weighted MR image shows extensive marrow infiltration and multiple compression fractures (*arrows*), including some completely flattened vertebrae plana. Normal marrow should be high signal on T1-weighted in someone of this age. Subtle low signal stippling seen in all the imaged vertebral bodies is related to multiple myeloma

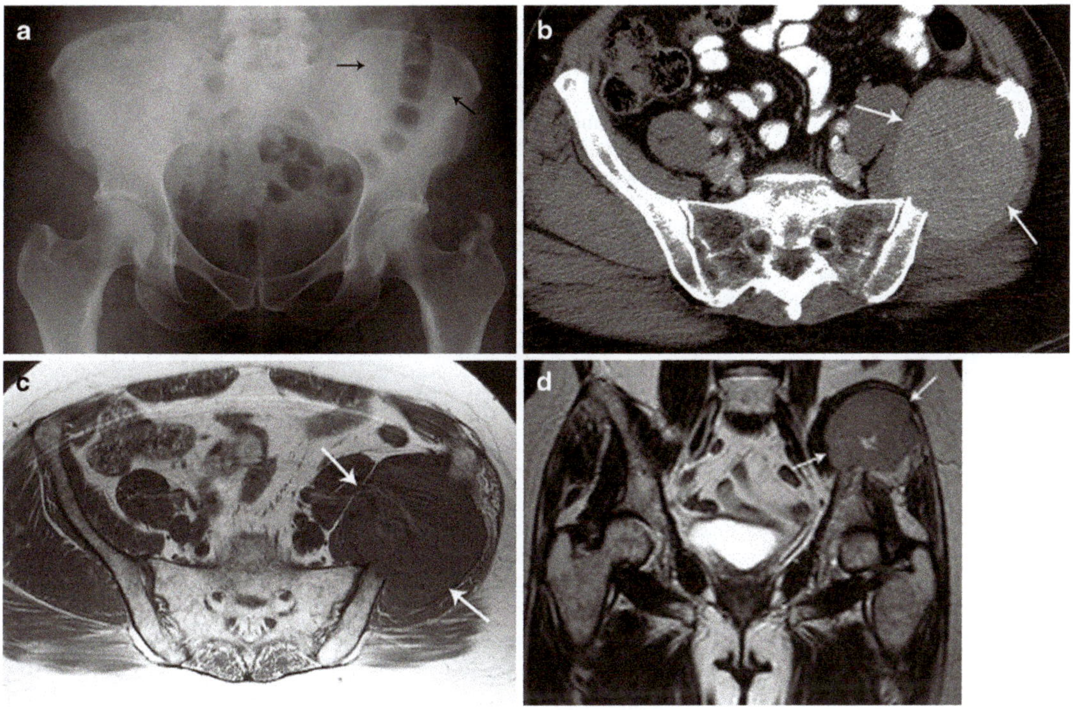

Fig. 7.31 On the radiograph (**a**) the plasmacytoma (*arrows*) in the left iliac bone is large, but difficult to detect. The axial skeleton is a common site for plasmacytoma, due to persistent red marrow. The axial CT image (**b**) shows the full extent of the plasmacytoma, a well-demarcated mass, hyperintense to muscle (*arrows*). Note well-defined "punched out" borders in the bone, without a sclerotic rim. The plasmacytoma (*arrows*) is isointense to muscle on T1-weighted (**c**) and relatively hypointense on the T2-weighted (**d**) MR images, with minimal heterogeneity

Suggested Reading

1. Antonescu CR, Erlandson RS, Huvos A. Primary leiomyosarcoma of bone: a clinicopathologic, immunohistochemical, and ultrastructural study of 33 patients. Am J Pathol. 1997;21(11):1281–94.
2. Delorme S, Baur-Melnyk A. Imaging in multiple myeloma. Eur J Radiol. 2009;70(3):401–8.
3. Grier HE. The Ewing family of tumors. Pediatr Clin North Am. 1997;44:4.
4. Guermazi A, Feger C, Pusselot P, et al. Granulocytic sarcoma (chloroma): imaging findings in adult leukemia. AJR Am J Roentgenol. 2002;178:319–25.
5. Hecht AC, Gebhardt MC. Diagnosis and treatment of unicameral and aneurysmal bone cyst in children. Curr Opin Pediatr. 1998;10:87–94.
6. Ishida T, Iijima T, Kikuchi F, et al. A clinicaopathological and immunohistochemical study of osteofibrous dysplasia, differentiated adamantinoma, and adamantinoma of long bones. Skelet Radiol. 1992;21:493–502.
7. Kleer CG, Unni KK, McLeod RA. Epithelioid hemangioma of bone. Am J Surg Pathol. 1996;20(11):1301–11.
8. Mankin HJ, Hornicek FJ, Ortiz-Cruz E. Aneurysmal bone cyst: a review of 150 patients. J Clin Oncol. 2005;23:6756–62.
9. McClain KL. Langerhans cell histiocytosis, Juvenile xanthogranuloma and Erdheim-Chester disease. Basow DS, editor. UpToDate. Waltham, MA: UpToDate; 2011.
10. Meyers SP, Hirsch Jr WL, Curtin HD, et al. Chordomas of the skull base: MR features. AJNR Am J Neuroradiol. 1992;13:1627–36.

11. Mulligan ME, McCrae GA, Murphey MD. Imaging features of primary lymphoma of bone. AJR Am J Roentgenol. 1999;173:1691–7.
12. Murphey MF, Faribarn KJ, Parman LM, et al. Musculoskeletal angiomatous lesions: radiologic–pathologic correlation. Radiographics. 1995;15:893–917.
13. Murphey MD, Nomikos GC, Fleming D, et al. Imaging of giant cell tumor and giant cell reparative granuloma of bone: radiologic pathologic correlation. Radiographics. 2001;21:1283–309.
14. Propeck T, Bullard MA, Lin J. Radiologic-pathologic correlation of intra-osseous lipomas. AJR Am J Roentgenol. 2000;175:673–8.
15. Stull MA, Kransdorf MJ, Devaney KO. Langerhans cell histiocytosis of bone. Radiographics. 1992;12(4):801–23.

8 Bone Metastases

Metastases represent the most common bone tumor and outnumber primary bone tumors 20-to-1. Moreover, bone metastases have an extremely varied imaging appearance and are difficult to exclude from many differentials. This is especially true in patients over 40 years of age and in those with a known primary malignancy. Metastatic lesions develop when cells from the primary tumor separate and travel to distant sites, where they adhere and grow. Most often, malignant cells spread hematogenously, but they can also spread via the lymphatic system or by direct extension. The tumor cells must be able to (1) survive the transit from the primary site and (2) once at the secondary site, develop their own blood supply, in order to grow. Thus, the vast majority of bone metastases occur in the spine and pelvis, where there is richly vascularized red marrow. Conversely, metastases are rarely found in the bones of the hands and feet, as these areas are filled with fatty marrow. Besides a rich blood supply, several growth factors are produced or stimulated by the tumor in order to optimize its establishment, survival, and growth at the secondary site.

Bone metastases can be categorized as lytic, sclerotic, or mixed, based on the relative amounts of bone resorption and bone formation they generate. When resorption predominates, a lytic lesion is produced and this is seen in 75% of metastases. Conversely, when bone formation predominates, a sclerotic lesion is produced. Both bone resorption and formation occur simultaneously within most lesions; however, one process is typically dominant. For sclerotic lesions, the visualized density can be a combination of stromal bone formation by the underlying tumor and reactive bone formation resulting from the repair mechanisms of the host bone. Reactive bone formation occurs to some extent in all bone metastases, including lytic metastases; however, in highly destructive and rapidly growing tumors, there is not enough time to form sufficient reactive sclerosis to be visible on radiographs.

The text below describes the most common appearances and features of bone metastases due to various malignancies; however, as with many things in medicine, exceptions exist. For instance, although prostate carcinoma typically produces sclerotic (osteoblastic) metastases and renal cell carcinoma typically produces lytic (osteolytic) lesions, on rare occasions, the converse can occur in both. Also, at times, lytic lesions can become sclerotic following treatment.

J.S. Wu and M.G. Hochman, *Bone Tumors: A Practical Guide to Imaging*,
DOI 10.1007/978-1-4419-0808-7_8, © Springer Science+Business Media, LLC 2012

Lytic metastases (75%)
Kidney
Lung
Breast
Thyroid
GI tract

Sclerotic metastases (15%)
Prostate
Seminoma
Breast
Cervix
Ovarian
Carcinoid
Bladder
Osteosarcoma

Mixed lytic and sclerotic metastases (10%)
Breast
Lung

General Features/Considerations

Demographics:

- Typically >40 years of age
- 1.5 million new cancer cases annually in the USA
- 600,000 cancer deaths annually, 2/3 have osseous metastases
- 30% of patients with malignancy will develop bone metastases
- Breast, prostate, lung, renal, and thyroid metastases account for 80% of all metastatic bone lesions
- Prostate carcinoma accounts for 60% of osseous metastases in men
- Breast carcinoma accounts for 70% of osseous metastases in women
- Most metastases develop within 2 years of primary malignancy diagnosis

Origin:

- "**Seed-and-soil**" hypothesis: certain cancer cells (seed) will grow in favorable organ environments (soil)
  - "*Good seeds*"—malignancies that commonly go to bone: breast, prostate, lung, renal, thyroid, and colon
  - "*Bad seeds*"—malignancies that rarely go to bone: head and neck tumors, pancreas, liver, esophagus, stomach, uterus, and ovary
  - "*Good soil*"—favorable sites for metastases: red marrow (ribs, spine, pelvis, and proximal long bones), lung, and liver
  - "*Bad soil*"—unfavorable sites for metastases: fatty marrow (distal bones), irradiated bone, muscle, heart, GI viscera, and uterus

- Growth factors and rich blood supply needed
  - Angiogenesis needed for metastases >2 mm
  - VEGF, TGFβ, and parathyroid hormone related protein can stimulate osteoclasts

Location:

- Metastases prefer areas of rich hematopoietic marrow. They rarely develop in fatty marrow or irradiated bone due to poor blood supply in those locations
- In prostate cancer, metastases spread via valveless Batson's plexus to pelvic bones and spine
- The spine, ribs, skull, and pelvic bones are the most common sites for metastatic spread. Femur and humerus are next most common
- Metastasis in the spine: lumbar>thoracic>cervical
- Vertebral pedicle involvement is highly suspicious for metastasis, but this is usually due to extension of the metastasis from the vertebral body
- Solitary metastases distal to the knee or elbow joint are rare
- 50% of metastases in the hands or feet are due to lung, renal, or breast carcinoma
- Gynecologic malignancy can spread into bone via direct invasion
- Lesions occurring in the lesser trochanter and sternum are highly suspicious for metastatic disease

Clinical symptoms:

- Pain, described as dull and aching
- Weight loss
- Can be asymptomatic, discovered incidentally, or at follow-up imaging for known malignancy
- In a person with known malignancy, any fracture that develops following minor trauma should raise the suspicion for an underlying metastasis
- Pathologic fracture risk should be assessed and reported in order to assess the need for prophylactic fixation
- Assessing the risk for pathologic fracture is not straightforward, although several criteria for long bones exist:
  - Fidler (1981): fracture risk increases with greater circumferential cortical involvement: If cortical involvement is <50% then fracture risk = 2.3%, 50–70% = 60% fracture risk, >75% = 80% fracture risk
  - Harrington (1986): recommends fixation for lytic lesions, with >50% of the diameter of the bone involved by tumor, >2.5 cm in diameter, or associated with persistent pain or growth after irradiation
  - Mirels rating system for impending pathologic fractures (1989): based on four radiographic and clinical factors (site, pain, lesion, and size) where each is scored on a scale of 1–3 (score range 4–12). Lesions with a score of ≤7 do not need prophylactic fixation, whereas lesions with a score ≥8 should be stabilized with hardware to prevent fracture
  - Lesions in the femoral neck, peritrochanteric region, and humeral neck are at especially high risk for fracture
  - Newer methods for fracture risk involve biomechanical analysis with CT
- Neurologic symptoms can occur if tumor compresses spinal cord or nerve roots
- Lesions close to joints can mimic osteoarthritis, potentially delaying diagnosis
- Hypercalcemia can occur with osteolytic lesions due to increased bone resorption
- Hypocalcemia can occur due to excessive uptake of calcium from osteoblastic metastases (prostate)

Imaging characteristics:

- Metastases have a varied appearance depending on the amount of bone resorption (lytic) versus bone formation (sclerotic). Seventy-five percent of metastases are lytic
- In general, osseous metastases have limited periosteal reaction and lack the sclerotic margin that is more commonly seen in benign primary bone neoplasms
- Most metastases are intramedullary
- Some metastatic lesions have a characteristic appearance
  - Bubbly, expansile, lytic lesions are characteristic of renal cell or thyroid carcinoma
  - Multifocal, nonexpansile, dense sclerotic lesions are typical of prostate carcinoma metastases
  - Aggressive periosteal reaction (sunburst pattern) is rare, but most commonly seen with prostate carcinoma, carcinoid, or neuroblastoma metastases
  - Metastases with internal calcifications include colon and thyroid
  - Cortically based lesions suggest breast or lung cancer metastases
- Radiographs
  - Not the most sensitive modality for detection of metastases, but easy to obtain
  - >30–50% of the cortical thickness must be lost before changes are evident on conventional radiography
  - Metastases in the pelvis, even large ones, can be difficult to visualize and assess due to overlying bowel gas. CT or MRI should be considered
  - Skeletal survey useful for multiple myeloma and renal cell, as lesions may not show activity on bone scintigraphy, due to limited reactive bone formation
- Bone scintigraphy
  - Provides whole body imaging; helps to assess overall tumor burden
  - Good sensitivity, >90% of metastases have uptake
  - Poor specificity, as many nonneoplastic processes can also have uptake
  - False negatives can occur (1) when there is decreased blood flow, (2) in mostly osteoclastic (lytic) lesions, or (3) in lesions with low level of osteoblastic activity
  - False positives can occur due to degenerative changes, fractures, infection, and benign or primary malignant bone lesions
  - Radiotracer uptake in contiguous ribs suggest fractures instead of metastases
  - If the sentinel lesion is in a difficult location for biopsy (e.g., cervical spine, rib, and sternum), bone scintigraphy can help identify other lesions in locations more amenable to biopsy
  - May not detect certain osteolytic metastases (multiple myeloma, renal, lymphoma, and thyroid) due to the lack of significant bone turnover
  - Metastases can present as cold lesions (absence of radionuclide activity), so do not limit search to areas of tracer uptake only
  - Sensitivity increases when combined with single photon emission computed tomography (SPECT)
  - If the metastatic disease burden is extensive, a "**superscan**" appearance can occur. In a superscan, there is absence of activity in the kidneys and soft tissues, because the majority of radiotracer is taken up by the bones
    - Most commonly seen in prostate and breast carcinoma
    - Gives false impression of normal scan
  - "**Flare phenomenom**" may occur when there is paradoxical increased tracer uptake following treatment
    - Represents good response due to healing and sclerosis of the osseous lesions
    - Occurs within 3 months of treatment and should resolve in 3–6 months
    - Higher association with chemotherapy or hormonal therapy versus radiation

- CT
  - Helps identify amount of cortical destruction, especially if high risk for pathologic fracture
  - Helpful in assessing areas difficult to evaluate on radiographs: skull, sternum, ribs, pelvis
  - Attenuation difference of >20 Hounsfield units in the marrow between right and left sides should be considered abnormal
  - Helpful in demonstrating degree of sclerosis in treated metastases, thus indicating good response to treatment
- MRI
  - Likely most sensitive modality for demonstrating metastatic disease
  - Excellent for showing changes in fatty marrow, degree of soft tissue component, and relationship to adjacent structures
  - Useful for lesions that are occult on radiographs and CT
  - Lytic metastases are usually low signal on T1-weighted and high on T2-weighted MR images, whereas sclerotic metastases are usually low on both T1 and T2 weighted images
  - "**Target (halo) sign**"—many metastases have a rim of bright T2 signal surrounding the lesion
  - In- and out-of-phase T1-weighted images can help distinguish between benign versus malignant lesions. Metastases should not contain microscopic fat, so will not lose signal on out-of-phase images (unlike normal red marrow, which is admixed with small amounts of fat)
  - Diffusion imaging can be helpful in distinguishing benign osteoporotic vertebral body compression fractures from those due to metastases
    - Metastases are hyperintense to normal marrow due to restricted diffusion
    - Apparent diffusion coefficient (ADC) values are lower in metastatic than benign vertebral body fractures
  - Intravenous contrast can help assess degree of tumor necrosis and help identify areas of enhancing tumor as targets for percutaneous biopsy
- ^{18}FDG-PET/CT
  - Good for detection of skeletal metastases arising from most solid tumors, especially cancers with high metabolic activity (breast, lung, colon, and lymphoma)
  - Not so good for cancers with decreased metabolic activity (prostate, carcinoid, and bronchoalveolar)
  - Complementary role with bone scintigraphy
  - May be as good or better than bone scintigraphy for early, small lesions that are yet to create an osteoblastic response
  - Sclerotic metastases (often prostate) may have increased activity on bone scintigraphy, but lack activity on ^{18}FDG-PET/CT. These lesions have prominent osteoblastic activity, but a relative lack of tumor cellularity and therefore, a relative lack of ^{18}FDG activity
  - In general, higher standardized uptake value (SUV) is more suspicious for metastases
  - Comparing intensity of uptake in the lesion with uptake in the liver or mediastinal blood pool can help control for issues with SUV calibration
  - False positives for metastases can occur when nonneoplastic processes in bone demonstrate increased uptake on ^{18}FDG-PET/CT: fractures, degenerative changes, infection, Paget disease, chemotherapy or G-CSF use

Treatment:

- Surgical stabilization with hardware, if bone is at risk for pathologic fracture
- Bisphosphonates can diminish pain and possibly reduce tumor burden by inhibiting osteoclasts
- NSAIDS and/or opiates for pain management
- Radiotherapy (XRT or radionuclide therapy) and/or chemotherapy
- Hormonal therapy for some breast and prostate cancer patients

- Adult patients presenting with osseous lesions without a known primary malignancy should have a metastatic workup (mammography, chest CT, abdominal/pelvic CT, consider bone scintigraphy, and PET/CT)
- Prognosis is very poor with multiple metastases, about 5-month mean survival from time of diagnosis for most primary cancers

Differential diagnosis: Bone metastases have a variable appearance and can mimic many disease processes

- Primary benign neoplasm
  - Usually have a well-defined sclerotic border
  - No perilesional edema on MRI
- Primary malignant neoplasm
  - Are often >10 cm, whereas most metastases are less than 4 cm
  - Have a larger soft tissue component than most metastases
  - Multiple myeloma is typically cold on bone scintigraphy
  - Have more periosteal reaction than most osseous metastases (exceptions are prostate, carcinoid, retinoblastoma, and neuroblastoma)
- Osteomyelitis
- Stress fracture
- Brown tumors of hyperparathyroidism

Features That Support a Diagnosis of Bone Metastasis

- Patient has a primary malignancy
- Multiple lesions
- Older patient; risk increases with increasing age over 40
- Located in the axial skeleton, especially spine and pelvis
- Metastatic lesions more likely to be variable in size than myeloma
- Less periosteal reaction and soft tissue component than primary bone malignancies

Carcinoma of Unknown Primary

- Accounts for 2–6% of all malignancies
- Poor prognosis, 11-month mean survival
- Primary site not found in about 25% of patients with osseous metastasis, even at autopsy
- Lesions that are not clearly benign should undergo a metastatic workup for a primary source, taking into account the most common primary malignancy to spread to bone
- Laboratory data: CBC, urinalysis, LFTs, renal function tests, stool for occult blood, and PSA
- Imaging workup:
  - Chest/abdominal/pelvic CT
  - Mammography in women
  - Consider PET/CT
  - Consider bone scintigraphy to assess for multifocal disease

Common Bone Metastases

Breast

- Leading cause of bone metastases overall
- Most patients dying from breast cancer have osseous metastases
- Most are lytic, but can be sclerotic or mixed
- Axial skeleton and ribs are the most common sites
- Small subset of patients can have metastases in the bone for long periods without spread to other organs
- Hypercalcemia caused by the lytic lesions occurs in 30% of breast cancer patients

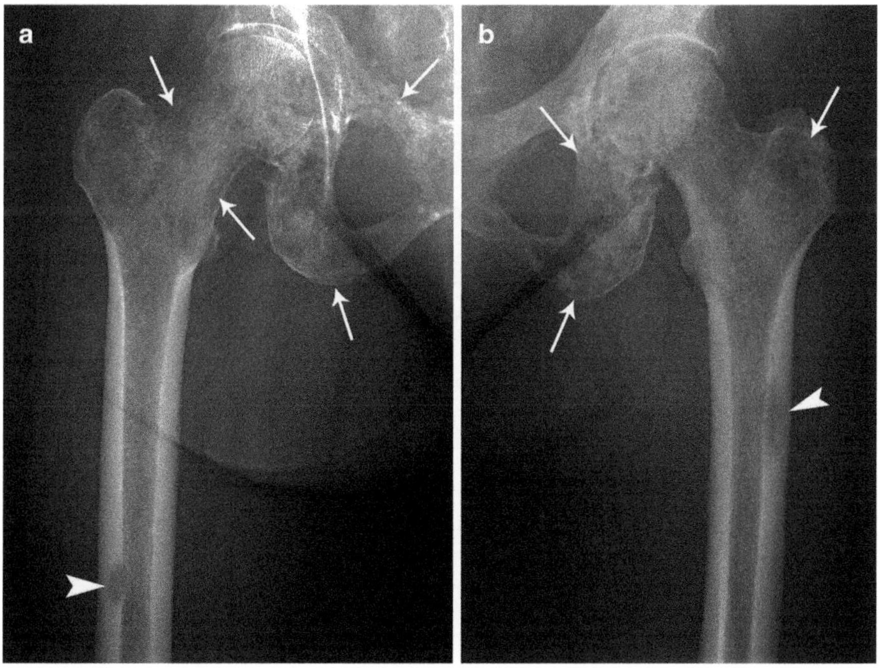

Fig. 8.1 Bilateral femur radiographs (**a**, **b**) show multiple lytic lesions (*arrows*) in the femurs and ischial tuberosities from breast cancer metastases. Cortically based metastases (*arrowheads*) can be seen in breast and lung cancer

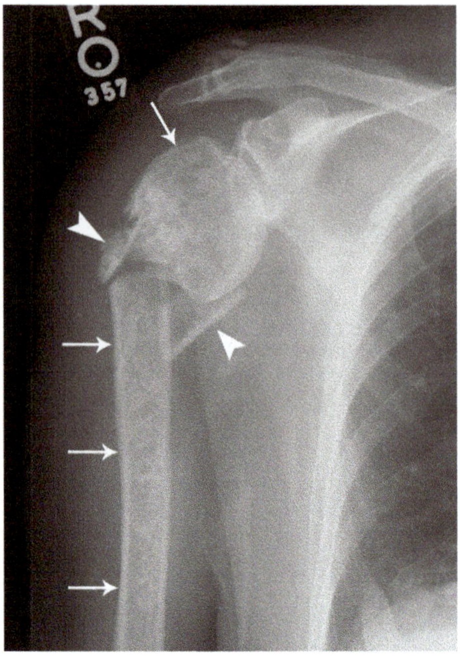

Fig. 8.2 Sclerotic breast metastases (*arrows*) with pathologic fracture (*arrowheads*) in the proximal humerus

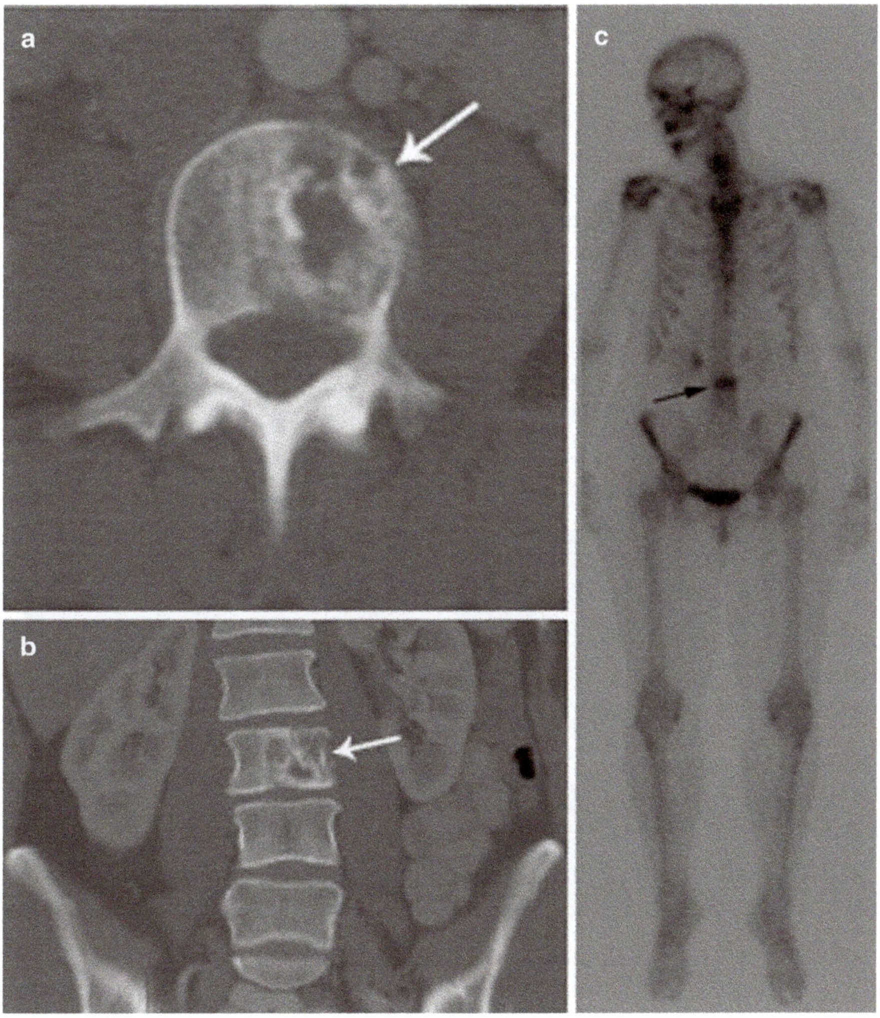

Fig. 8.3 Mixed lytic and sclerotic breast metastases (*arrows*) in the L3 vertebral body on axial (**a**) and coronal (**b**) CT images. There is avid tracer uptake in L3 (*arrow*) on the bone scintigraphy exam (**c**)

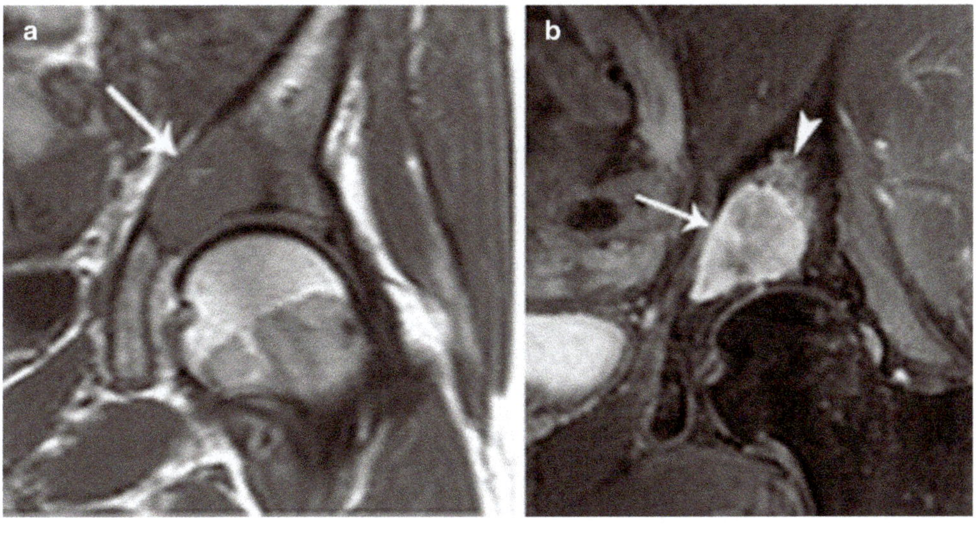

Fig. 8.4 Breast cancer metastasis in the left acetabulum. The lesion (*arrow*) is isointense to skeletal muscle on the T1-weighted MR image (**a**). On the fat-saturated T2-weighted MR image (**b**) the lesion (*arrow*) is bright and has perilesional edema (*arrowhead*)

Prostate

- Leading cause of osseous metastases in men
- Bone metastases are present in 25–35% of patients with prostate cancer
- Most metastases are sclerotic (75%)
- Prostate metastases can have aggressive sunburst periosteal reaction
- Spread into pelvis and lumbar spine from valveless Batson's venous plexus
- Can cause an "**ivory vertebral body**" appearance
- Extensive metastatic disease can mimic Paget disease
- In patients with osseous metastases, PSA >10 ng/mL and often >20 ng/mL
- Can lead to a "**superscan**" appearance on bone scintigraphy

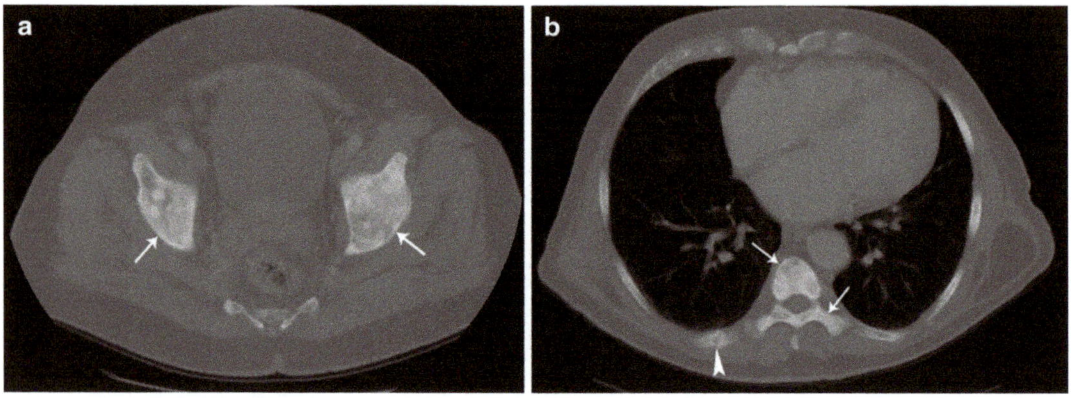

Fig. 8.5 There are diffuse sclerotic metastases (*arrows*) from prostate cancer on the axial CT images of the pelvis (**a**) and chest (**b**). Note the pathologic fracture (*arrowhead*) of a right posterior rib

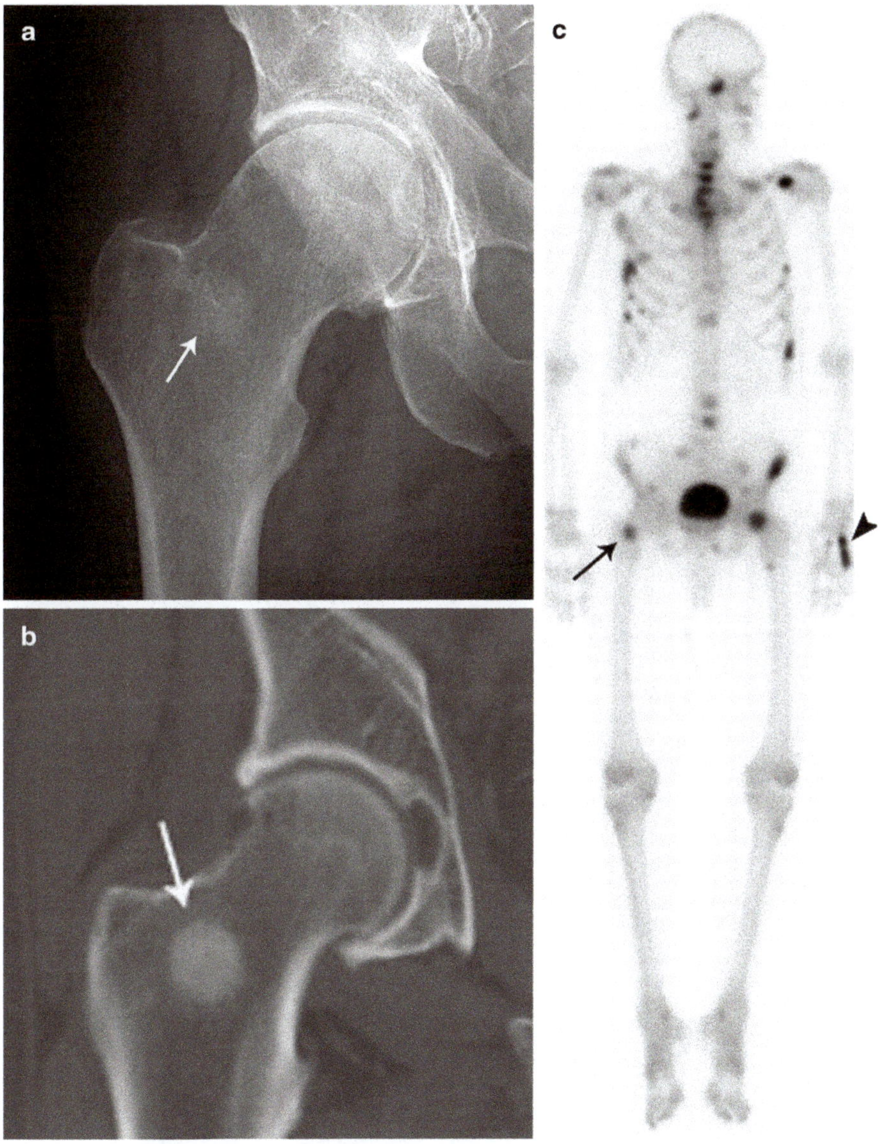

Fig. 8.6 There is a sclerotic prostate metastasis (*arrows*) in the proximal right femur which is better seen on the coronal CT image (**b**) versus the radiograph (**a**). The bone scintigraphy exam (**c**) shows corresponding uptake in the right proximal femur lesion (*arrow*) as well as other lesions in the pelvis, spine, and ribs. Note the lack of lesions distal to the knee or elbows. Activity in the left hand is from the IV catheter (*arrowhead*)

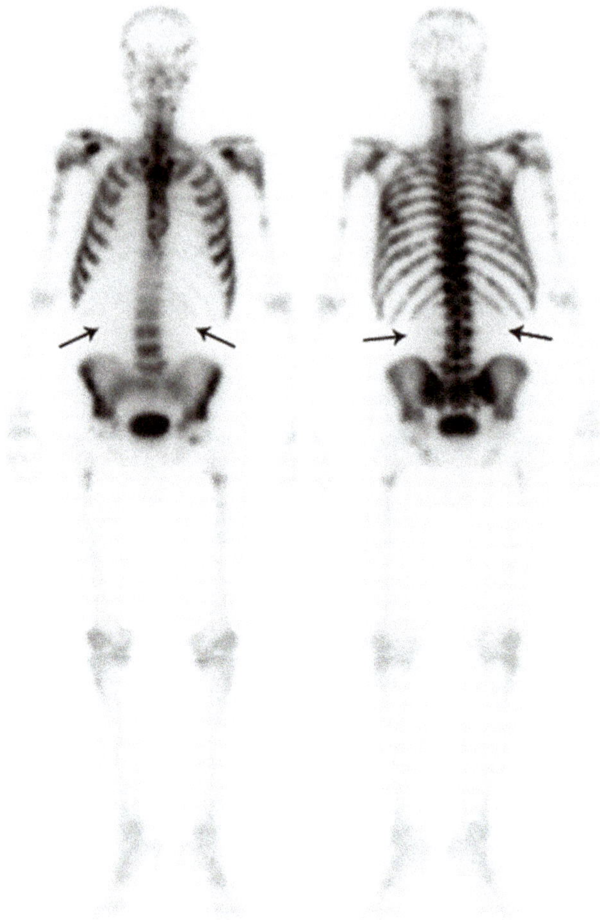

Fig. 8.7 Prostate cancer metastases. "Superscan" appearance on bone scintigraphy can be mistaken for a normal study. There is a lack of radiotracer in the kidneys (*arrows*) and soft tissues, as most of the radiotracer has been taken up by the diffuse osseous metastatic disease. (Images courtesy of Dr. J. Anthony Parker, Boston, MA)

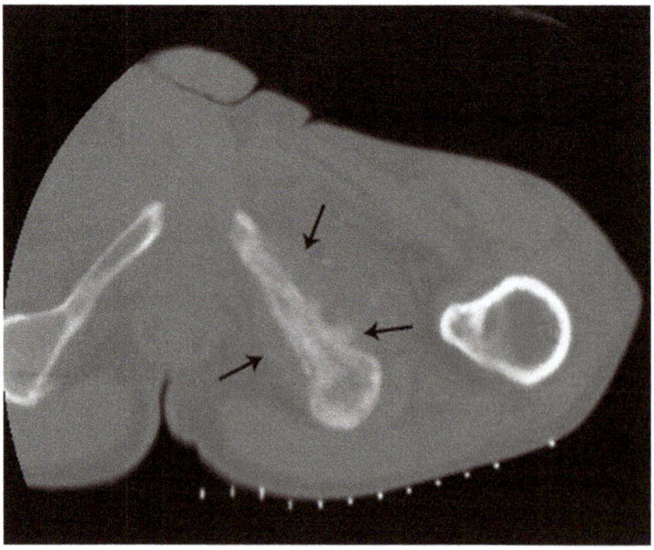

Fig. 8.8 Axial CT of the pelvis shows aggressive sunburst periosteal reaction (*arrows*) in the left inferior pubic ramus from a prostate carcinoma metastasis

Lung

- Most metastases are lytic (80%)
- Four major subtypes: squamous cell, small cell, large cell, adenocarcinoma
- Small cell has a higher percentage of osteoblastic metastases
- Squamous cell can metastasize to the hands and feet
- Ribs and chest wall may be involved by direct extension from the primary lung cancer
- Can have an eccentric "**cookie-bite**" appearance in the bone cortex, with soft tissue component

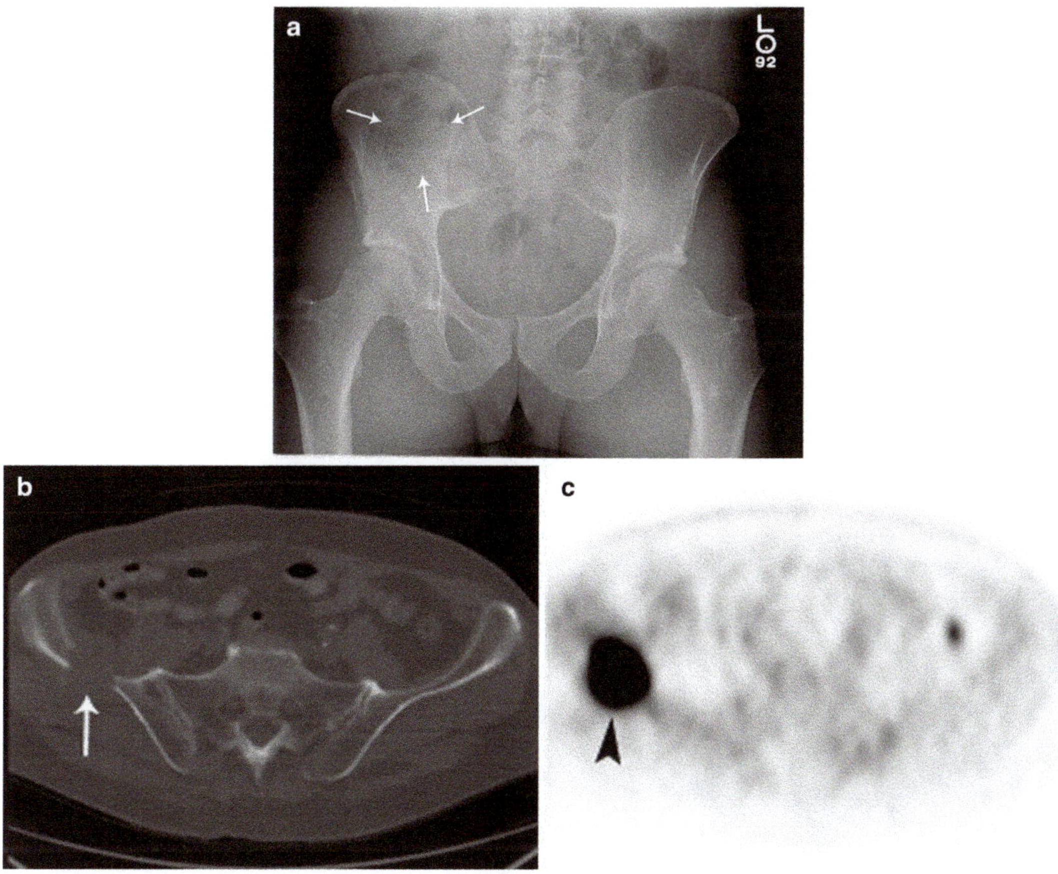

Fig. 8.9 The lung cancer metastasis in the right iliac bone is obscured by the overlying bowel pattern (*arrows*) on the pelvis radiograph (**a**). There is cortical destruction (*arrow*) and avid uptake (*arrowhead*) in the right iliac bone on the ^{18}FDG-PET/CT images (**b**, **c**)

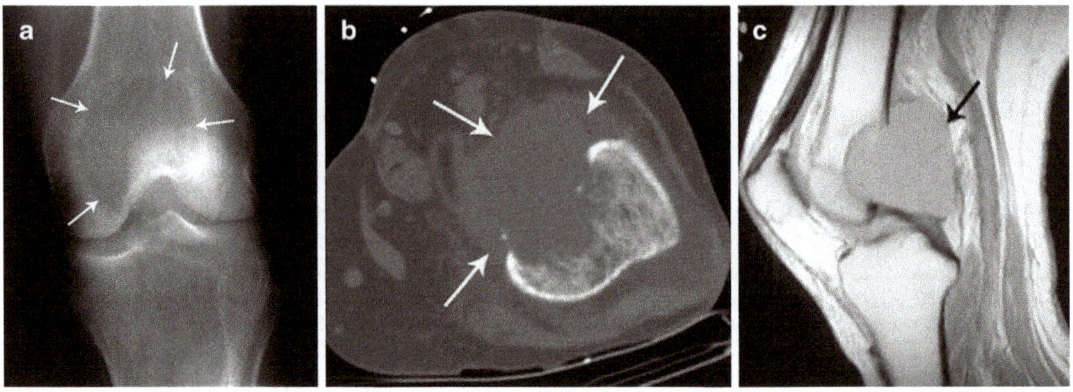

Fig. 8.10 “Cookie-bite” appearance of bronchogenic carcinoma metastasis. There is a large lytic area (*arrows*) in the distal femur with nonsclerotic margin on the knee radiograph (**a**). The large soft tissue component (*arrows*) and cortical destruction is well seen on the axial CT image (**b**) and T1-weighted MR image (**c**). This lesion is at high risk for pathologic fracture with a Mirels score of 10 (site—2, pain—3, lesion—3, and size—2)

Table 8.1 Mirels scoring system for diagnosing impending pathologic fractures in long bones

	Score		
Variable	1	2	3
Site	Upper limb	Lower limb	Peritrochanter
Pain	Mild	Moderate	Functional[a]
Lesion	Blastic	Mixed	Lytic
Size (lesion/diameter of bone)	≤1/3	1/3–2/3	≥2/3

Each of the four variables is scored 1–3. The summed total range: 4–12
Lesions with combined score of 8–12 require prophylactic hardware fixation
[a]Severe pain with decrease in mechanical strength

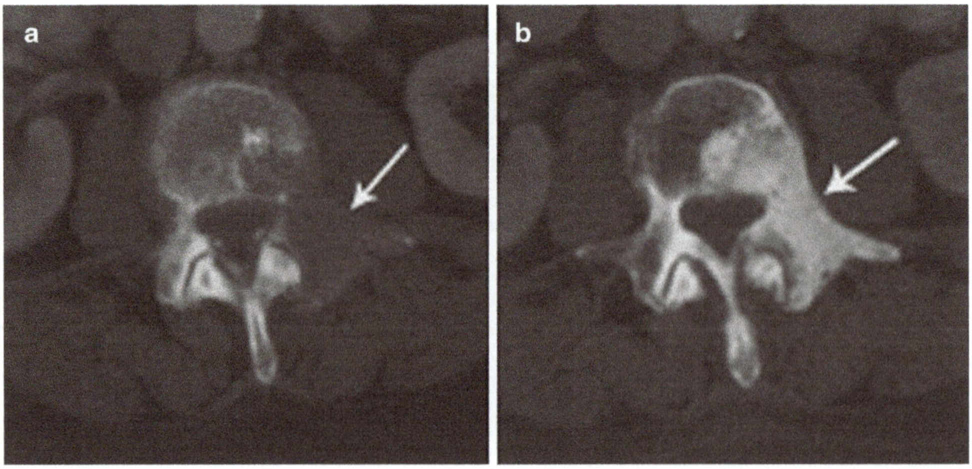

Fig. 8.11 Treated lung cancer metastasis. Axial lumbar spine CT images before (**a**) and after (**b**) radiation treatment demonstrate how the metastasis (*arrows*) changes from a lytic to a sclerotic appearance due to bone healing

Renal

- Most metastases are lytic (90%)
- Osseous metastases are very common and often hypervascular
- Solitary lesions are not infrequent
- Lesion can be expansile, septated, and associated with a soft tissue mass
- Higher risk of pathologic fracture than other primary malignancies due to destructive and expansile nature
- Preoperative embolization can significantly reduce blood loss and the need for RBC transfusions during surgery

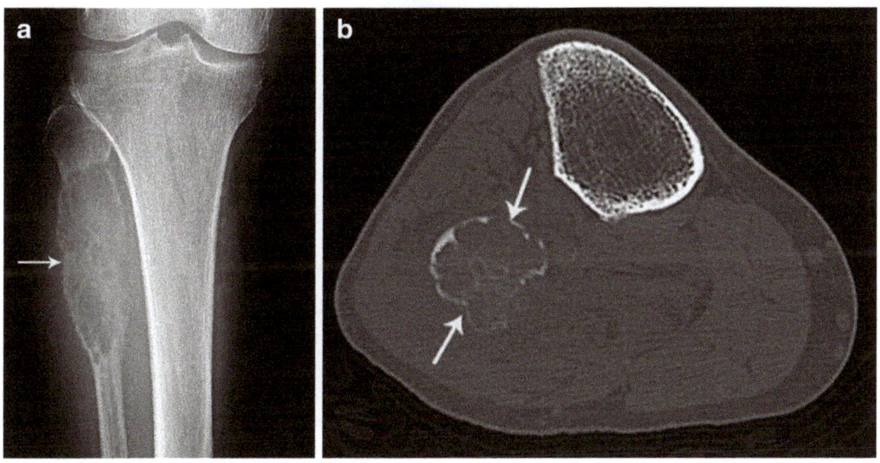

Fig. 8.12 AP radiograph (**a**) and axial CT image (**b**) shows an aggressive, expansile, lytic lesion (*arrows*) in the proximal fibular shaft from a renal cell metastasis

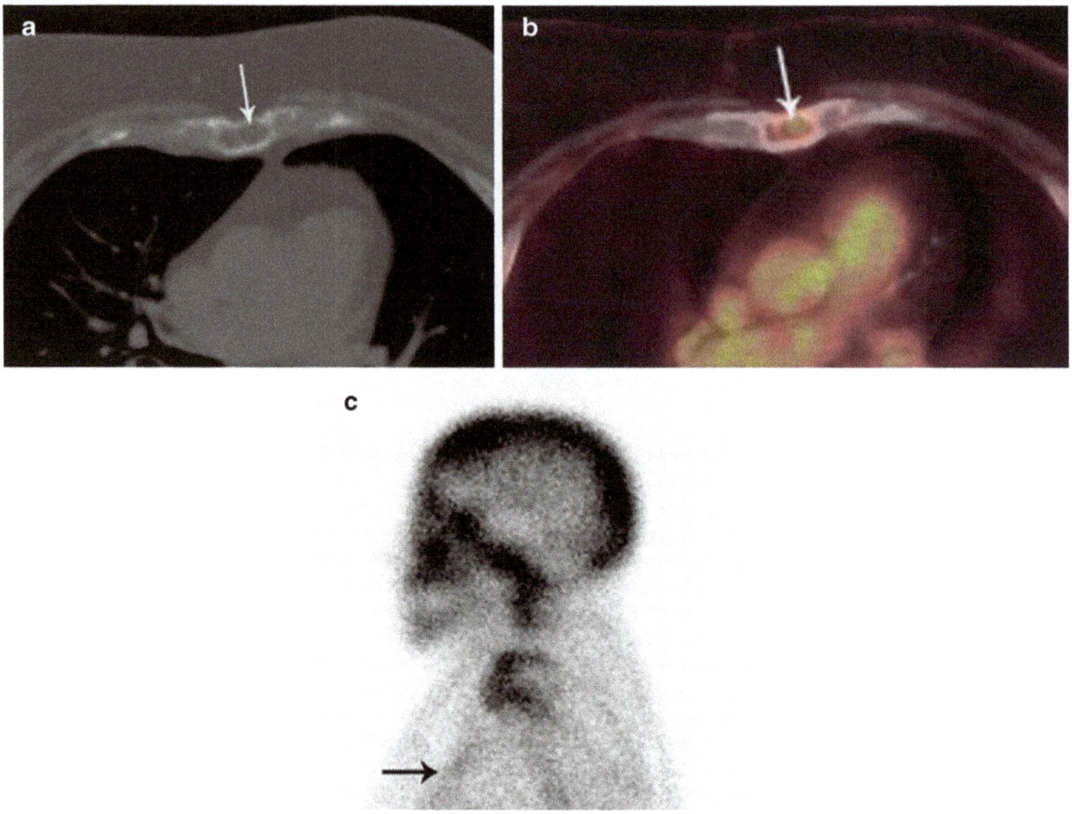

Fig. 8.13 Renal cell metastasis without uptake on bone scintigraphy but with uptake on ^{18}FDG-PET. There is lytic lesion (*arrow*) in the sternum on the axial CT image (**a**). The lesion (*arrow*) has radiotracer uptake (SUVmax 4.2) on the corresponding ^{18}FDG-PET image (**b**). On the bone scintigraphy exam (**c**), there is no uptake in the sternum at the expected location of the lesion (*arrow*). (Images courtesy of Dr. Phillip Kuo, Tucson, AZ)

Thyroid

- Most metastases are lytic
- Most bone metastases are seen in the papillary subtype
- Can be expansile and contain calcifications
- Can have a tendency to cross the joint space
- Rare to have osteoblastic metastases
- Radioiodine therapy can be used to treat patients with thyroid cancer and systemic disease, except for anaplastic/poorly differentiated (typically not radioiodine-avid)

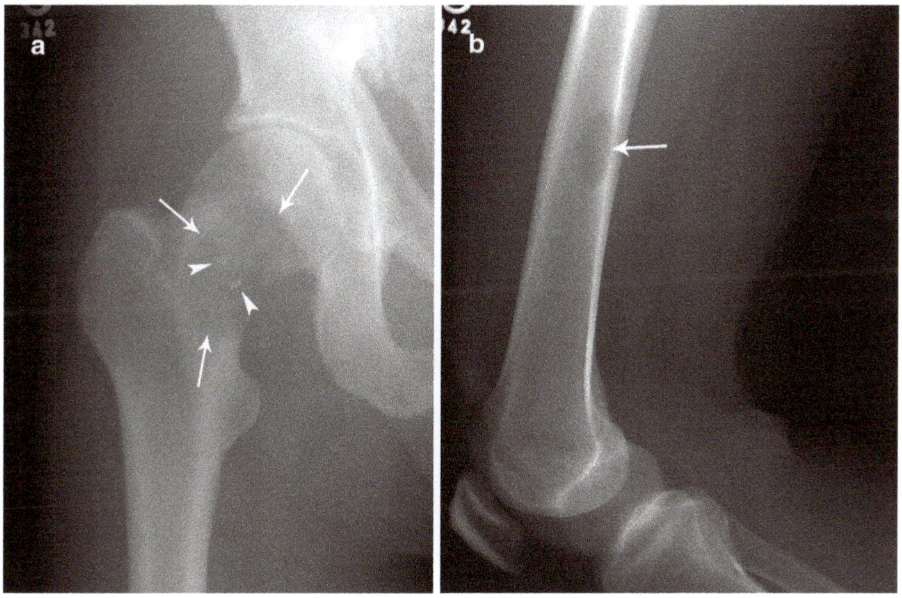

Fig. 8.14 Lytic metastases (*arrows*) in the proximal (**a**) and distal (**b**) femur from thyroid cancer. Note the punctate calcifications (*arrowheads*) in the femoral neck metastasis

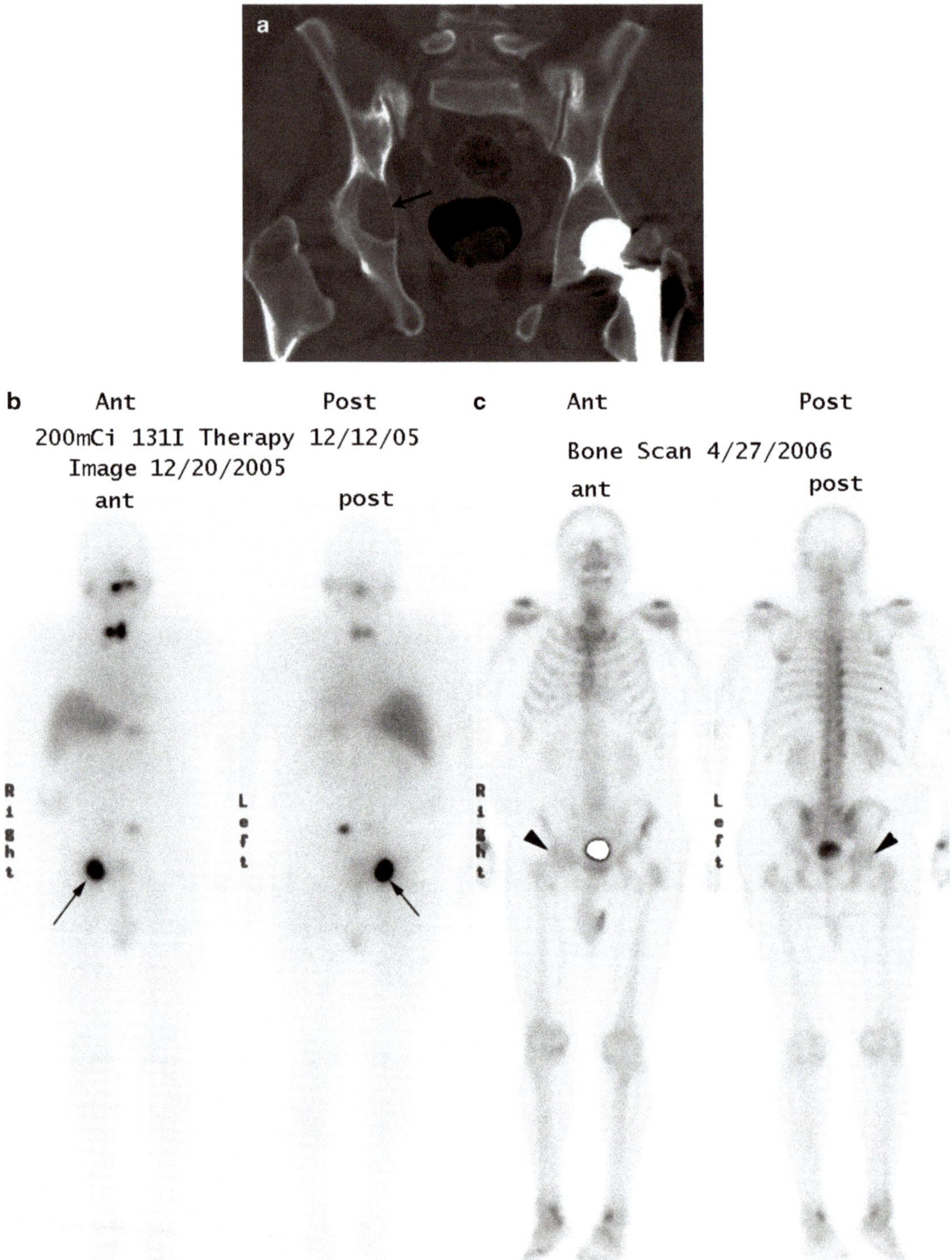

Fig. 8.15 Thyroid cancer metastasis. There is a lytic lesion (*arrow*) in the right posterior acetabulum on the coronal CT image (**a**). The lesion (*arrows*) has avid uptake on the whole body ^{131}I scan (**b**) performed for treatment of papillary thyroid carcinoma. Note the relative lack of radiotracer uptake in the right acetabulum (*arrowheads*) on the bone scintigraphy study (**c**). Cold spot in the left femoral neck is due to the hip prothesis. (Images courtesy of Dr. Phillip Kuo, Tucson, AZ)

Additional Bone Metastases

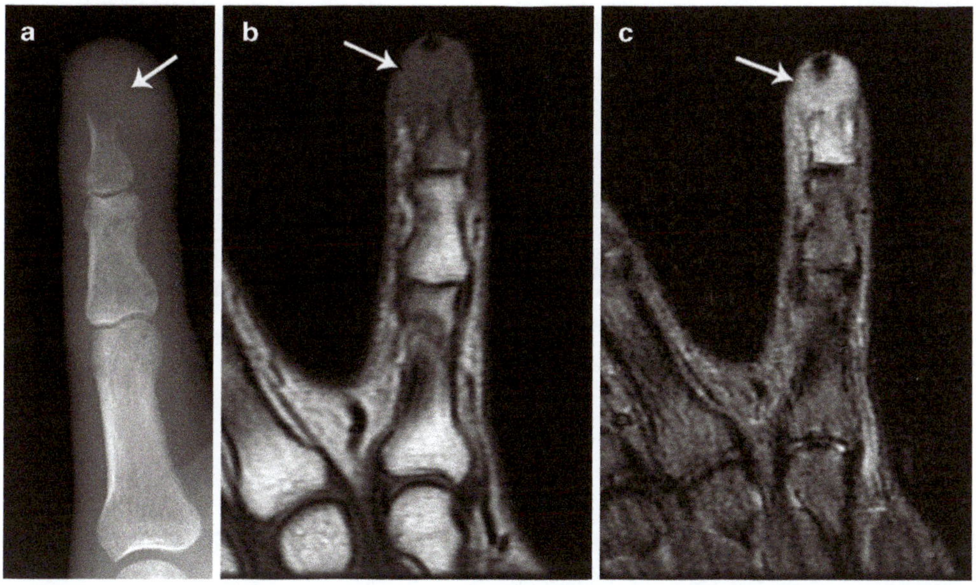

Fig. 8.16 Digital metastasis from squamous cell carcinoma of lung. On the radiograph (**a**), there is a lytic lesion (*arrow*) causing destruction of the distal tuft of the small finger. The metastasis (*arrow*) is dark on the T1-weighted (**b**) and bright on the T2-weighted (**c**) MR images. In general, metastases distal to the knee or elbow joint are rare; however, they can occur in lung, renal, and breast cancer. Lung cancer metastases in the hands and feet are believed to be due to shedding of tumor cells into the pulmonary veins

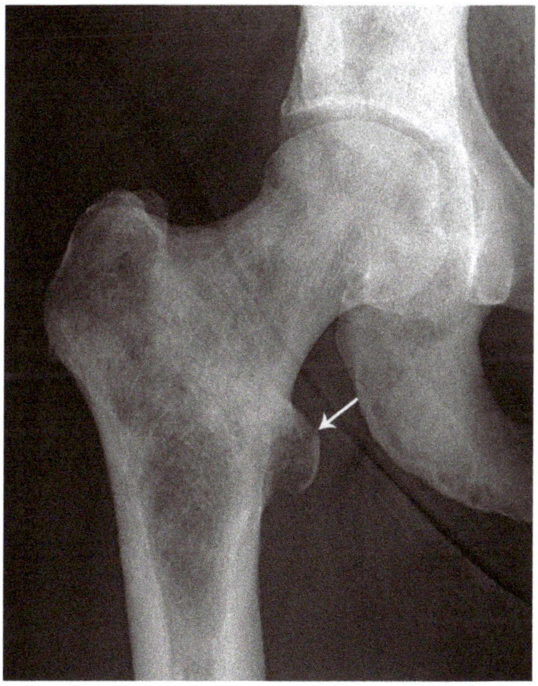

Fig. 8.17 Lesser trochanter metastasis. There are mixed lytic and sclerotic lesions in the proximal femur and acetabulum from breast cancer metastases. There is a nondisplaced fracture (*arrow*) at the lesser trochanter. Isolated lesser trochanter avulsion fractures should raise concern for metastases or other causes of pathologic fracture

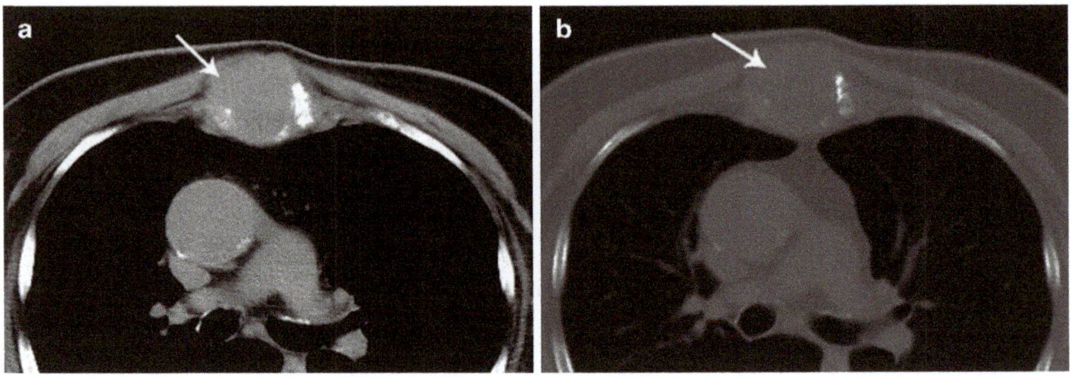

Fig. 8.18 Sternal breast cancer metastasis. Axial CT images using soft tissue (**a**) and bone (**b**) windows show a destructive lesion with a large soft tissue component (*arrows*) in the manubrium. In patients with malignancy, 80% of lesions in the sternum are due to metastatic disease

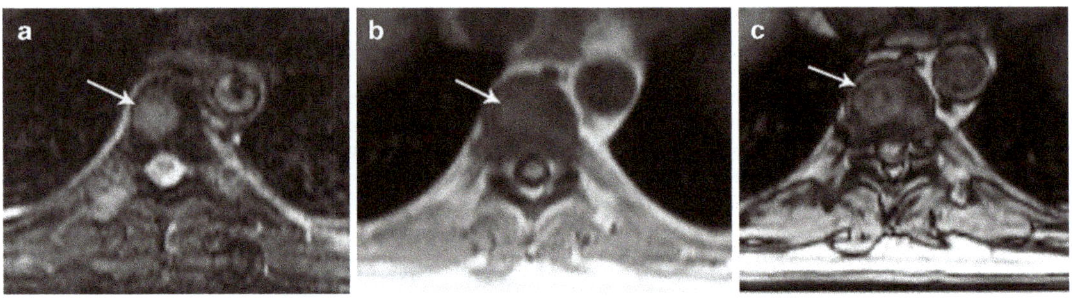

Fig. 8.19 Carcinoid metastasis on in- and out-of-phase MR imaging. There is a bright lesion (*arrow*) in a thoracic vertebral body on the axial fat-saturated T2-weighted MR image (**a**). On the T1-weighted MR images, the lesion (*arrow*) is isointense to slightly hyperintense to the vertebral body on the in-phase MR image (**b**). At this point, the differential would include both metastasis and intraosseous hemangioma, both of which can be hyperintense on T2-weighted images and iso- to hyperintense on in-phase T1-weighted images. However, the lesion remains hyperintense (does not lose signal) compared to the surrounding vertebral body on the out-of-phase MR image (**c**), supporting a diagnosis of metastasis. By contrast, red marrow and fat-containing hemangiomas would be expected to lose signal (become darker than the adjacent vertebral body) on the out-of-phase image, due to the presence of admixed microscopic fat and water. (Images courtesy of Dr. Suzanne Long, Philadelphia, PA)

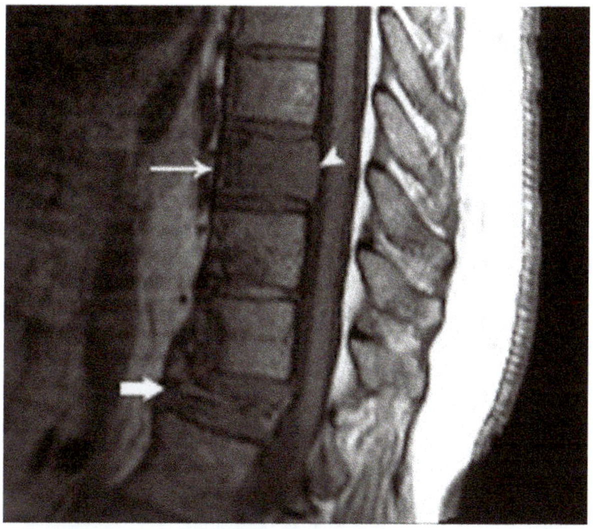

Fig. 8.20 Breast metastases. Sagittal T1-weighted MR image shows a slightly expansile T8 vertebral body (*arrow*) with a convex posterior margin (*arrowhead*). The T8 vertebral body has low signal compared to the neighboring vertebral bodies. There is a "vertebra plana" appearance of the T11 vertebra due to pathologic fracture (*thick arrow*)

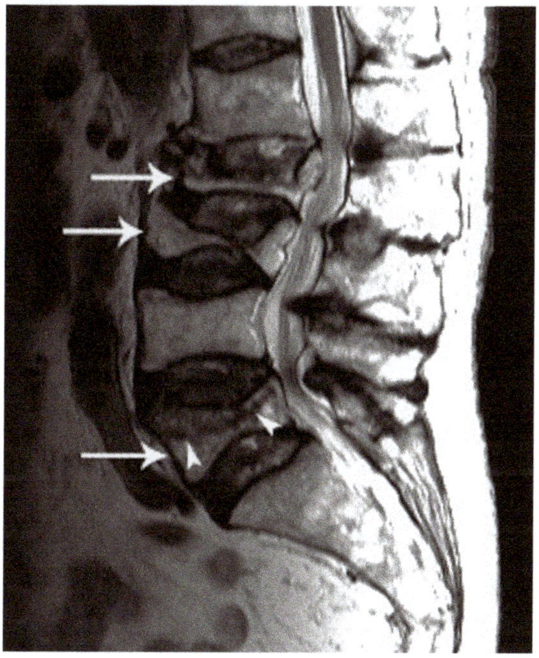

Fig. 8.21 T2-weighted MR image shows multiple osteoporotic fractures (*arrows*) in the lumbar spine. Note the linear fracture line (*arrowheads*) through the L5 vertebral body, which can help distinguish this benign fracture from a pathologic fracture

Features Favoring Metastatic Vertebral Compression Fracture Versus Osteoporotic Fractures

- Convex posterior border of the vertebral body
- Abnormal signal in pedicle or posterior elements
- Epidural mass
- Lack of low signal horizontal fracture line on T1- and T2-weighted MR images
- Retropulsion of posterior bone fragments
- Multiple noncontiguous fractures
- Normal adjacent discs
- Increased signal on diffusion weighted MR images and lower ADC values than normal vertebral bodies

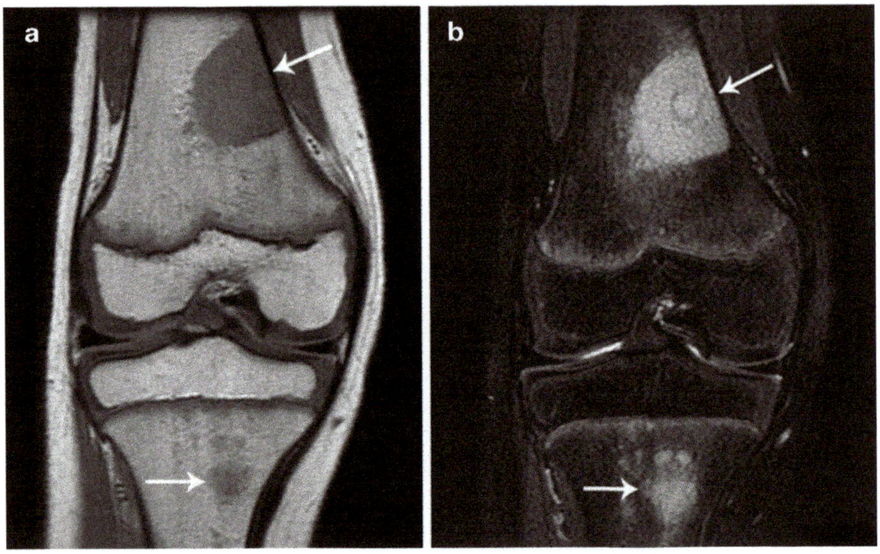

Fig. 8.22 Neuroblastoma metastases. The metastases (*arrows*) in the distal femur and proximal tibia are dark on the T1-weighted (**a**) and bright on the T2-weighted (**b**) fat-saturated MR images. Neuroblastoma is a common cause of pediatric osseous metastases

Most Common Bone Metastases in Children

- Neuroblastoma
- Rhabdomyosarcoma
- Clear cell sarcoma of kidney
- Ewing sarcoma
- Osteosarcoma
- Leukemia
- Metastases from soft tissue sarcomas

Acknowledgment We thank Drs. Mark Schweitzer and Phillip Kuo for helpful discussions related to this chapter.

Suggested Reading

1. Fidler M. Incidence of fracture through metastases in long bones. Acta Orthop Scand. 1981;52:623–7.
2. Fidler IJ, Yano S, Zhang RD, Fujimaki T, Bucana CD. The seed and soil hypothesis: vascularisation and brain metastases. Lancet Oncol. 2002;3:53–7.
3. Fogelman I, Cook G, Israel O, Van der Wall H. Positron emission tomography and bone metastases. Semin Nucl Med. 2005;35:135–42.
4. Graham TS. The ivory vertebra sign. Radiology. 2005;235:614–5.
5. Greenspan A, Jundt G, Remagen W. Differential diagnosis in orthopaedic oncology. 2nd ed. Philadelphia, PA: Lippincott Williams & Wilkins; 2007.
6. Kakonen SM, Mundy GR. Mechanisms of osteolytic bone metastases in breast carcinoma. Cancer. 2003;97:834–9.
7. Mirels H. Metastatic disease in long bones. A proposed scoring system for diagnosing impending pathologic fractures. Clin Orthop Relat Res. 1989;249:256–264.
8. Mundy GR. Mechanisms of bone metastasis. Cancer. 1997;80:1546–56.
9. Rodan GA. The development and function of the skeleton and bone metastases. Cancer. 2003;97:726–32.
10. Resnick D, editor. Diagnosis of bone and joint disorders. 4th ed. Philadelphia, PA: W.B. Saunders; 2002.
11. Rosenthal DI. Radiologic diagnosis of bone metastases. Cancer. 1997;80:1595–607.
12. Taira AV, Herfkens RJ, Gambhir SS, Quon A. Detection of bone metastases: assessment of integrated FDG PET/CT imaging. Radiology. 2007;243:204–11.
13. Tanaka Y, Nakayamada S, Okada Y. Osteoblasts and osteoclasts in bone remodeling and inflammation. Curr Drug Targets Inflamm Allergy. 2005;4:325–8.

9 Bone Tumor Mimickers

The previous chapters have been organized by the composition and tissue of differentiation for each tumor. However, many lesions that occur in bone are not true tumors and may be mistaken for a neoplasm, leading to the wrong diagnosis and inappropriate treatment. Therefore, this book would be incomplete without a section on common lesions and artifacts that can mimic tumors in bone. The lesions included here encompass several etiologies, including normal variants, congenital anomalies, posttraumatic lesions, metabolic and arthritic processes, infection, iatrogenic lesions, and pseudolesions created by technical artifacts. In this section, we present the common "mimickers" that one can expect to encounter in everyday practice. In most instances, the clinical history will be important in determining the true nature of the lesion.

Normal variants
- Red marrow
- Humeral pseudocyst
- Ward's triangle in the femur
- Calcaneal pseudocyst

Congenital/developmental anomalies
- Dorsal defect (patella)
- Synovial herniation of femoral neck (Pitt's pit)
- Avulsive cortical irregularity or cortical desmoid (posterior femur)
- Supracondylar process (humerus)
- Soleal line (tibia)

Trauma
- Subperiosteal hematoma
- Stress fracture
- Myositis ossificans

Metabolic/arthritic processes
- Brown tumor of hyperparathyroidism
- Melorheostosis
- Osteonecrosis
- Paget disease
- Calcific tendinitis (resorptive phase)
- Subchondral cyst (geode)

Osteomyelitis
- Brodie's abscess

Iatrogenic
- Biceps tenodesis
- Bone marrow biopsy
- Particle disease
- Radiation changes
- Contrast infiltration

Technical artifacts
- Humeral head (internal rotation view)
- Radial tuberosity (lateral view)
- MRI wrap-around (aliasing) artifact
- MRI pulsation artifact
- External objects

J.S. Wu and M.G. Hochman, *Bone Tumors: A Practical Guide to Imaging*,
DOI 10.1007/978-1-4419-0808-7_9,

Normal Variants

Red Marrow

Erythropoietic (red) marrow can be mistaken for a focal tumor, especially if it appears mass-like. Normal bone marrow typically transitions from red to yellow (fatty) marrow with increasing age. However, islands of red marrow can remain, especially in the metaphysis of long bones. Red marrow should be brighter than skeletal muscle on T1 weighted images. Moreover, red marrow should not extend into the epiphysis; rather, it should stop at the physeal scar. In and out of phase T1 imaging can be helpful for distinguishing red marrow from bone lesions, in difficult cases. Normal red marrow should lose signal (become darker) on out-of-phase imaging, because it invariably has some intermixed microscopic fat. By contrast, a focal bone lesion replaces normal marrow and should not contain internal fat (unless an intraosseous lipoma), so it would not be expected to lose signal on out-of-phase imaging.

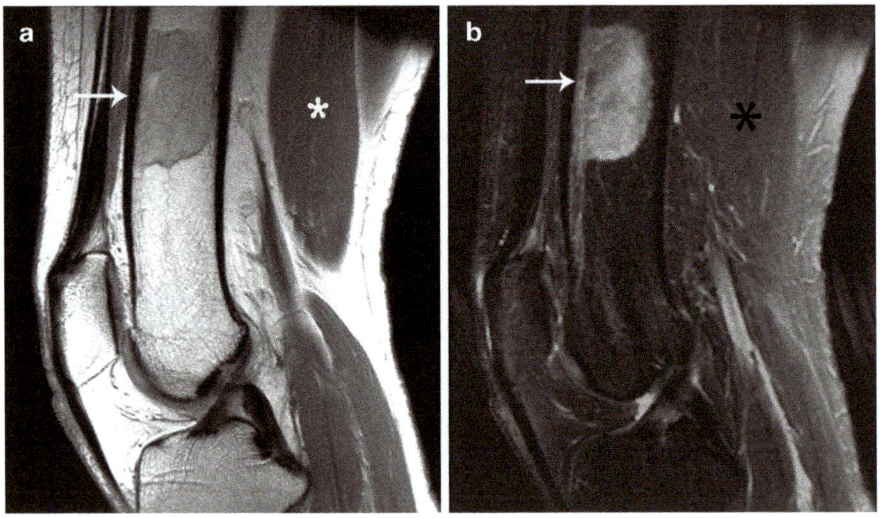

Fig. 9.1 Large island of red marrow in the distal femur. Note that the lesion (*arrows*) is hyperintense to skeletal muscle (*asterisk*) on both the T1- (**a**) and fat-saturated T2- (**b**) weighted MR images. Given the suspicion for metastatic breast cancer, a core needle biopsy was performed which confirmed erythropoietic (red) marrow

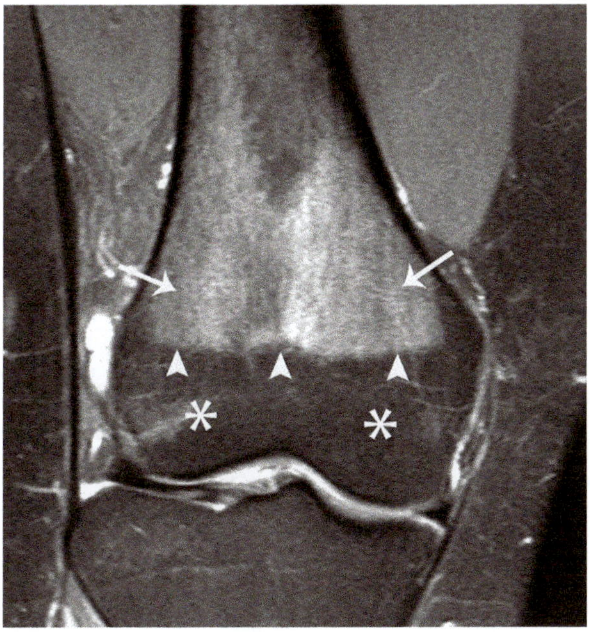

Fig. 9.2 Fat-saturated PD-weighted MR image shows hyperintense red marrow (*arrows*) ending abruptly at the physeal scar (*arrowheads*) of the distal femur, without crossing into the epiphysis (*asterisk*)

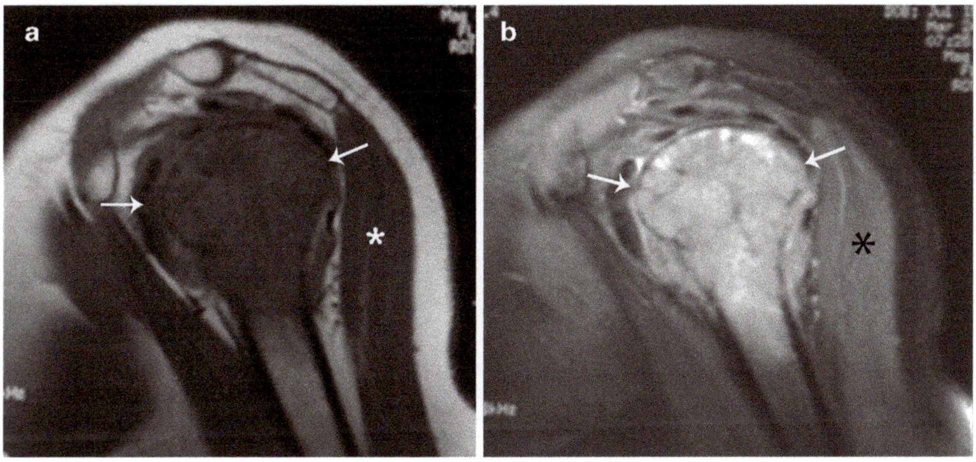

Fig. 9.3 On the T1-weighted MR image (**a**) there is a large lesion (*arrows*) replacing the humeral head which has signal intensity that is isointense to the adjacent muscle (*asterisk*). Erythropoietic marrow would be brighter than muscle. The tumor (*arrows*) is hyperintense to muscle (*asterisk*) on the fat-saturated T2-weighted MR image (**b**) extends into the epiphysis, and has a soft tissue component with cortical breakthrough

Humeral Pseudocyst

A lucent area can be seen in the superolateral aspect of the humeral head and mistaken for a chondroblastoma, giant cell tumor, Langerhans cell histiocytosis (EG), or lytic metastasis. This appearance is caused by a normal decrease in the amount of trabecular lines and often contains more fat than the rest of the humeral head, a difference that is well seen on MRI. The pseudolesion is best seen on external rotation views, and there is typically a sharp transition at the inferior margin of the pseudolesion formed by the fusion line of the greater tuberosity and the humeral shaft.

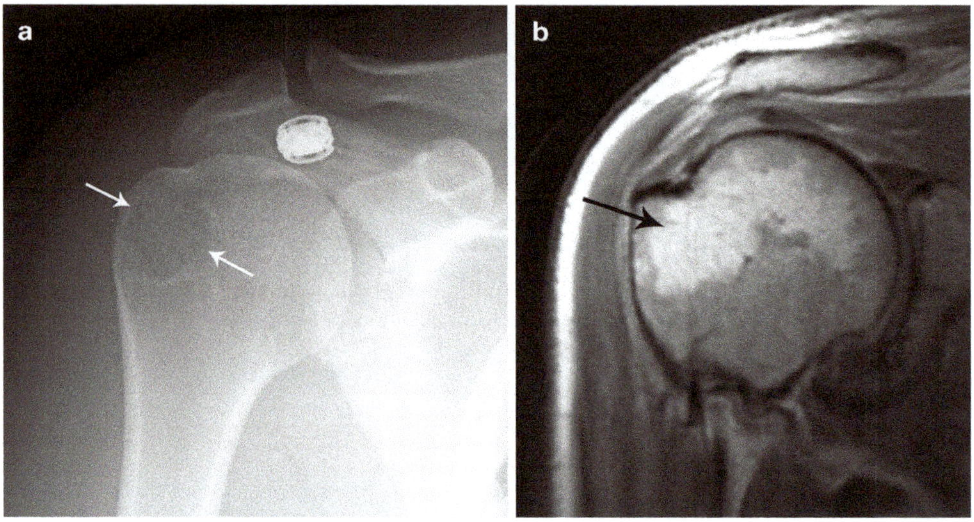

Fig. 9.4 Lucency in the greater tuberosity (*arrows*) on the external rotation shoulder radiograph (**a**) corresponds to normal fatty marrow (*arrow*) on the T1-weighted MR image (**b**)

Ward's Triangle

Ward's triangle refers to the triangular area of relative lucency in the femoral neck that is outlined by the compressive and tensile trabecular lines. This area is usually less apparent in osteoporotic patients due to decreased conspicuity of the trabecular lines.

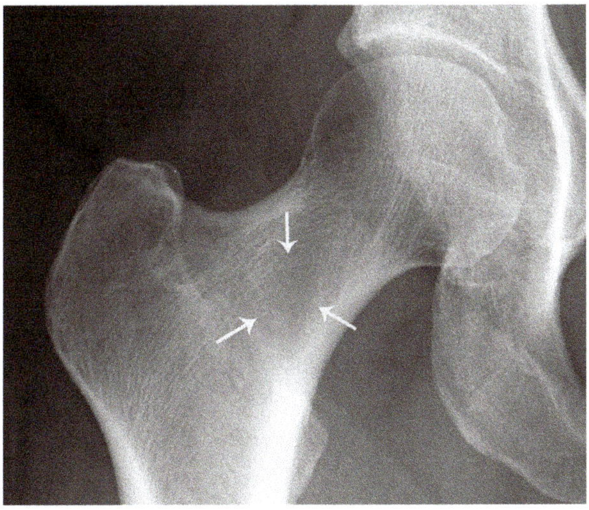

Fig. 9.5 Ward's triangle is seen as a lucency (*arrows*) in the femoral neck due to a decrease in trabecular lines

Calcaneal Pseudocyst

Similar to Ward's triangle in the proximal femur, a lucency in the body/anterior aspect of the calcaneus can appear in an area between major trabecular groups. This lucency can mimic an osteolytic tumor. However, several lesions can also occur in this location, including simple bone cysts, chondroblastomas, giant cell tumors, and intraosseous lipomas (which often contain central dystrophic calcification from fat necrosis).

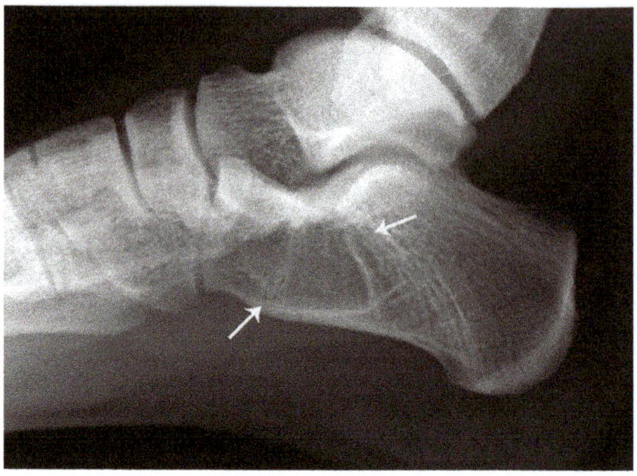

Fig. 9.6 There is a lucency (*arrows*) in the anterior calcaneus due to the decrease in trabeculae in this area

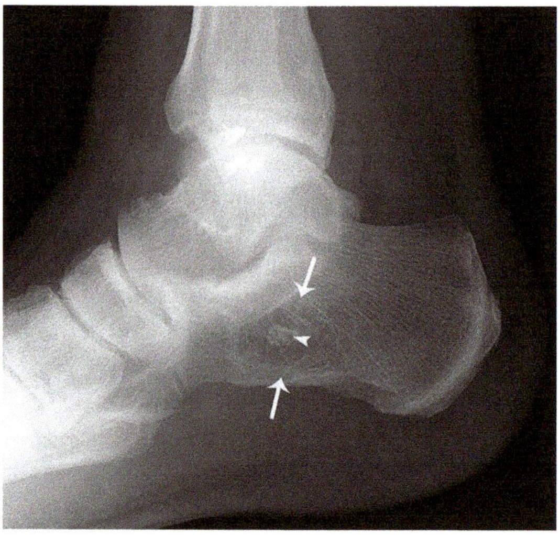

Fig. 9.7 An intraosseous lipoma (*arrows*) can also occur in the anterior calcaneus and often has a central calcification (*arrowhead*) from fat necrosis

Congenital/Developmental Anomalies

Dorsal Defect of the Patella

The dorsal defect of the patella is a well-marginated cortical defect in the superolateral patella (same location as a bipartite patella) and lies along the deep surface of the patella (the articular or dorsal surface). It is present in about 1% of people and can be bilateral. The defect contains fibrous material, with intact overlying cartilage. Although the cause is uncertain, hypotheses include incomplete fusion of multiple patellar ossification centers or, possibly, an acquired lesion related to traction at the insertion site of the vastus lateralis muscle. Rarely, this lesion can be associated with pain.

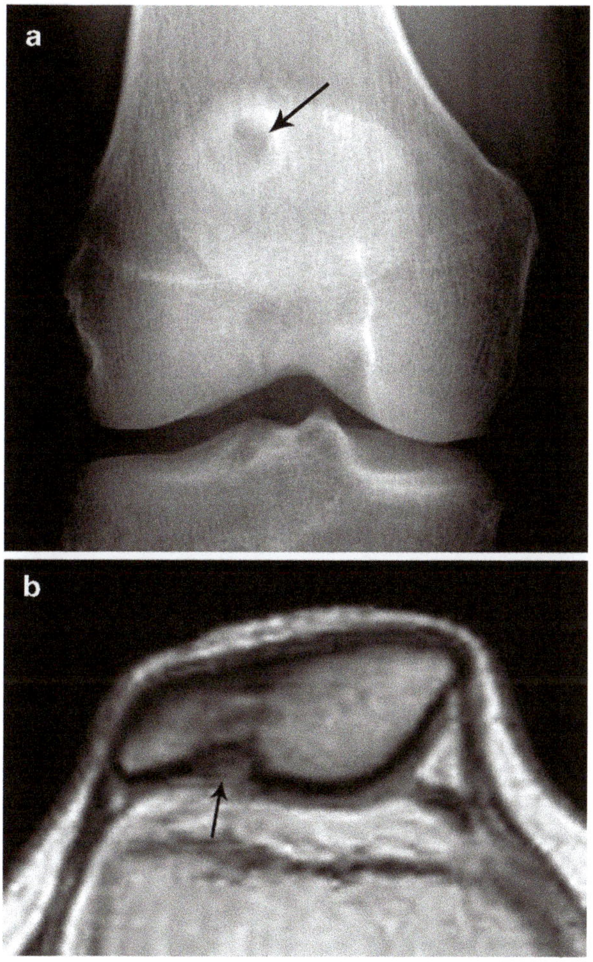

Fig. 9.8 Dorsal defect of patella. There is a small rounded lucency (*arrow*) in the superolateral aspect of the patella on the AP radiograph (**a**). On the axial PD-weighted MR image (**b**), intact overlying hyaline cartilage (*arrow*) is seen, which can help distinguish the dorsal defect of the patella from a cartilage defect

Synovial Herniation Pit in Proximal Femur (Pitt's Pit)

Synovial herniation pits of the proximal femur are common. Described by Dr. Michael Pitt in 1982, they are usually found in the anterosuperior aspect of the femoral neck and characteristically seen as a rounded lucent lesion with a thin sclerotic rim. They are typically less than 1 cm; however, can grow to 2–3 cm in size and can be lobulated. It is unclear whether these lesions are normal variants or the result of mechanical abrasion of the hip capsule against the femoral neck. Although herniation pits were thought for many years to be asymptomatic and incidental, more recently, an association between synovial herniation pits and femoral acetabular impingement (FAI) syndrome has been suggested. The presence of a sclerotic rim can help distinguish a synovial herniation pit from a metastasis.

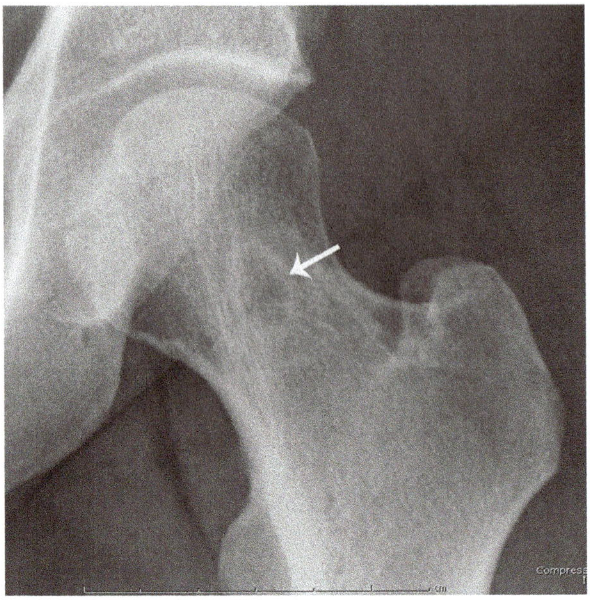

Fig. 9.9 Synovial herniation pit (*arrow*) with central lucency and thin sclerotic rim in the femoral neck

Avulsive Cortical Irregularity of the Posterior Femur

Avulsive cortical irregularity (formerly known as cortical desmoid) appears as an area of cortical irregularity arising from the posteromedial aspect of the distal femoral metaphysis in children and should not be mistaken for a surface osteosarcoma or osteomyelitis. The lesion is thought to arise from stresses exerted by the adductor magnus or the medial head of the gastrocnemius muscles. The lesion should resolve with skeletal maturity.

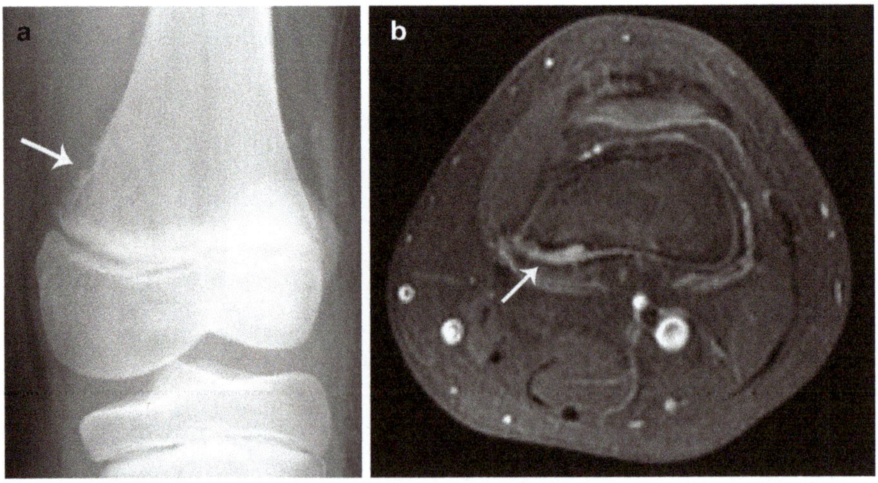

Fig. 9.10 On the AP radiograph (**a**), there is an area of cortical irregularity (*arrow*) at the medial aspect of the distal femoral metaphysis. The axial T2-weighted fat-saturated MR image (**b**) shows an area of cortical irregularity and mild edema (*arrow*) at the posteromedial aspect of the femoral metaphysis. (Images courtesy of Dr. Susan Connolly, Boston, MA)

Supracondylar Process of the Humerus

A bony spur can arise from the anteromedial aspect of the humerus in about 1–3% of the population. It is believed to represent a phylogenetic vestige of the supracondyloid foramen seen in some reptiles and mammals. Typically, it occurs as an incidental finding and should not be mistaken for an osteochondroma or surface osteosarcoma. Osteochondromas should point away from the elbow joint, whereas the supracondylar process points toward the elbow joint. Occasionally, the ligament of Struthers extends from the supracondylar process to the medial epicondyle, forming a tunnel that can entrap the median nerve and, occasionally, the brachial artery or one of its branches, leading to symptoms.

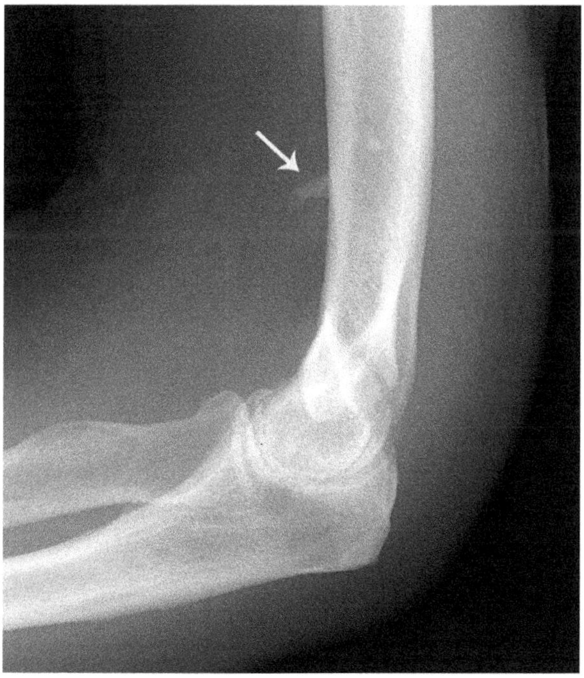

Fig. 9.11 Supracondylar process (*arrow*) arising from the distal humerus

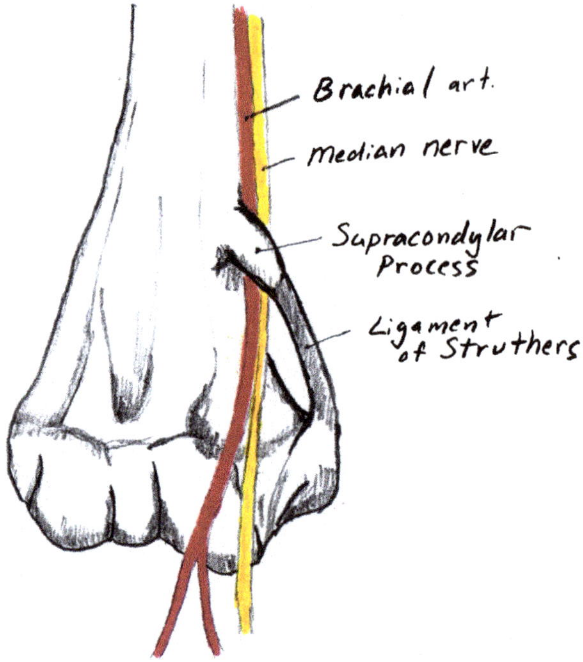

Fig. 9.12 Drawing illustrating how the ligament of Struthers and supracondylar process of the humerus can form a tunnel that can compress the median nerve and brachial artery

Soleal Line

The soleal line is a bony "tug lesion" that can form on the tibia at the attachment of the soleus muscle and mimic periostitis from a tumor or infection. When arising from the tibial head of the soleus, the cortical thickening extends lateral to medial along the posterior upper one-third of the tibia. Similar bony changes can be seen at the fibular attachment of the soleus.

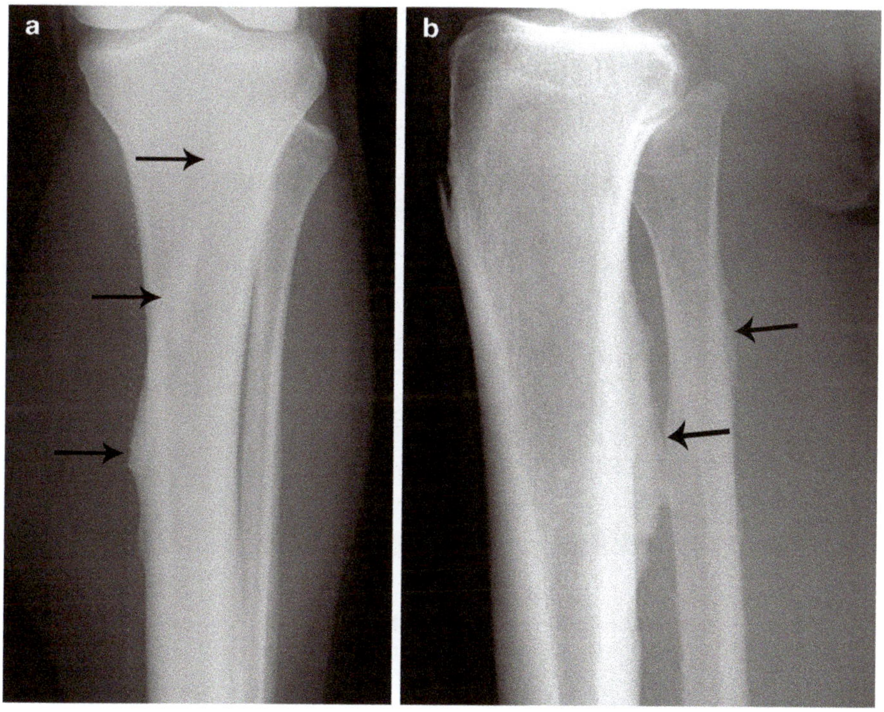

Fig. 9.13 Soleal line—"tug lesion" of the soleus attachment to the proximal tibia appears as a sclerotic line (*arrows*) extending lateral to medial along the proximal tibia shaft on the AP radiograph (**a**). The irregular cortical thickening (*arrows*) is well seen on the lateral radiograph along the tibia and fibula (**b**)

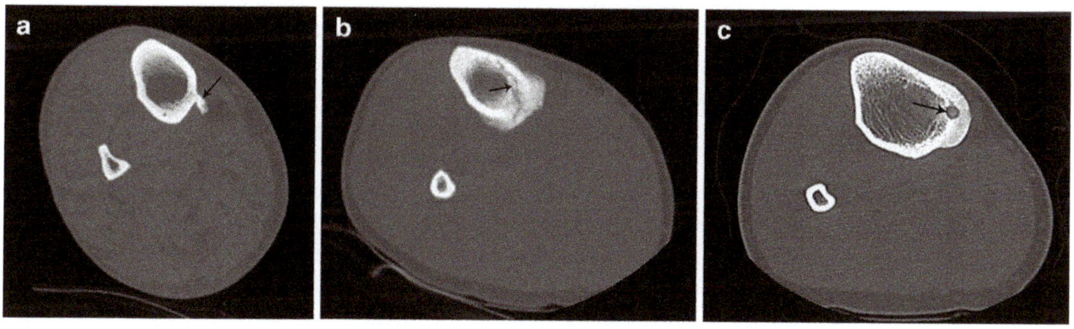

Fig. 9.14 CT scan can be helpful in distinguishing the soleal line (**a**) from a stress fracture (**b**) or osteoid osteoma (**c**) indicated by the *arrows*

Trauma

Subperiosteal Hematoma

Traumatic injury to the periosteum can lead to a focal mass, mimicking a surface bone lesion. The periosteum is a thick fibrous membrane on the surface of bone that nourishes the bone and provides a framework for bone healing when injury occurs. The periosteum is also highly vascular and closely adherent to the bone. Injury to the periosteum can result in a subperiosteal hematoma that lifts the periosteum off the bone surface, forming a focal mass. Often, these lesions will resolve without sequela; however, subperiosteal hematomas that persist can ossify. The lesions can be recognized by their nonaggressive appearance, subperiosteal location, and the fact that they contain fatty marrow when they ossify.

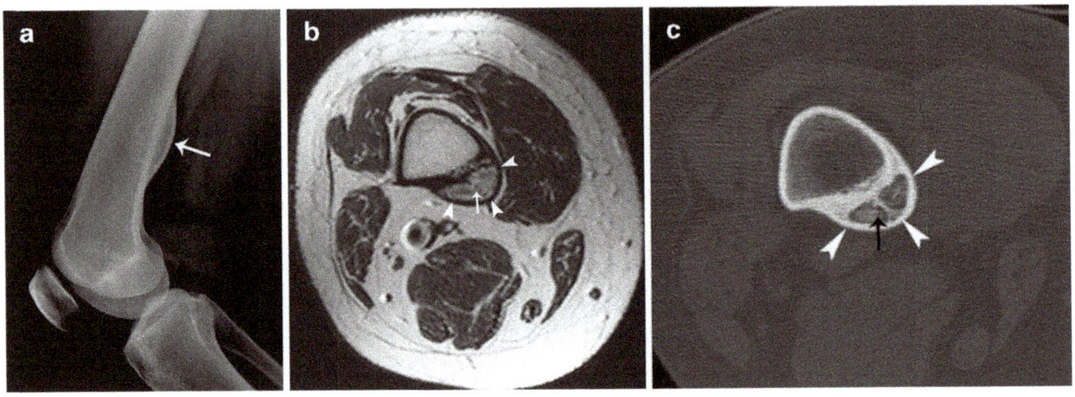

Fig. 9.15 Subperiosteal hematoma along the posterior femoral cortex. On the lateral radiograph (**a**), the lesion (*arrow*) has a smooth nonaggressive posterior border. T1-weighted MR (**b**) and axial CT (**c**) images demonstrate that the chronic subperiosteal hematoma contains fatty marrow signal (*arrow*) and cortical bone (*arrowheads*)

Stress Fracture

Stress fractures are overuse injuries that occur in the setting of unusual or repeated stress to bone. Stress fractures can be divided into (1) fatigue fractures, which occur when excessive repetitive force is applied to normal bone, as with a military recruit during "boot camp" training, and (2) insufficiency fractures, which occur when normal stress is applied to pathologically weakened bone, such as in osteoporotic bone, Paget disease or fibrous dysplasia. The most common sites for stress fractures are in the metatarsals, tarsals, and tibia (posterior aspect of proximal tibia). There is often a history of a recent increase in physical activity. The appearance of a stress fracture depends on the stage of healing. Early on, a stress fracture may not be visible radiographically but can be seen on bone scan or MRI. Later in its development, a stress fracture can show periosteal reaction and cortical resorption on radiographs. A lucent fracture line maybe present and is often perpendicular to the cortex. The fracture line is well seen with CT. The periosteal reaction can be aggressive, mimicking infection, osteoid osteoma, osteosarcoma, or Ewing sarcoma. The presence of a fracture line, lack of a soft tissue mass, and evidence of healing on follow-up studies should help distinguish stress fractures from other entities. Moreover, stress fractures may involve multiple contiguous bones, whereas primary bone neoplasms are unlikely to involve contiguous bones unless there is widespread metastatic disease.

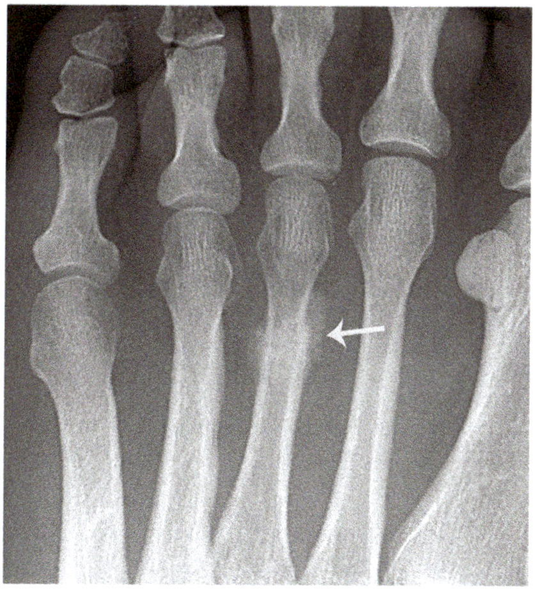

Fig. 9.16 Stress fracture in the third metatarsal of a 35-year-old man training for the Boston marathon. There is aggressive periosteal reaction (*arrow*) without a discernable fracture line

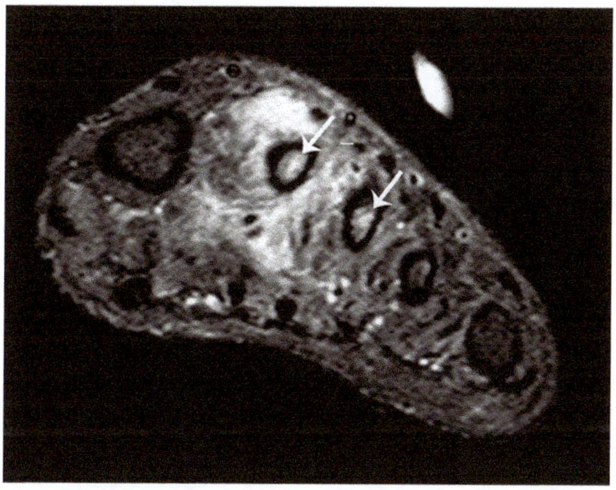

Fig. 9.17 STIR MR image shows edema (*arrows*) in the second and third metatarsal shafts (different patient than Fig. 9.16). Abnormality is seen in contiguous bones making primary bone neoplasm unlikely

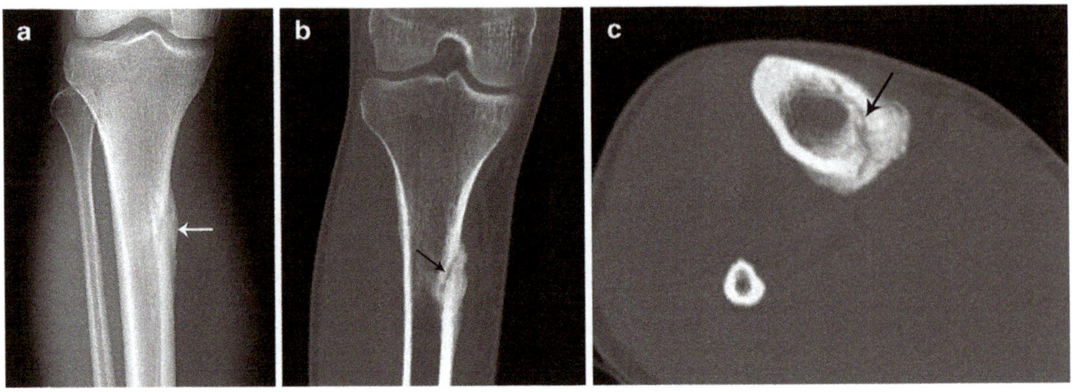

Fig. 9.18 A 22-year-old karate instructor with tibial stress fracture. There is cortical thickening (*arrows*) in the medial tibial shaft on the radiograph (**a**). The linear configuration of the fracture line (*arrows*) on the coronal (**b**) and axial (**c**) CT images is different than the rounded lucency of an osteoid osteoma

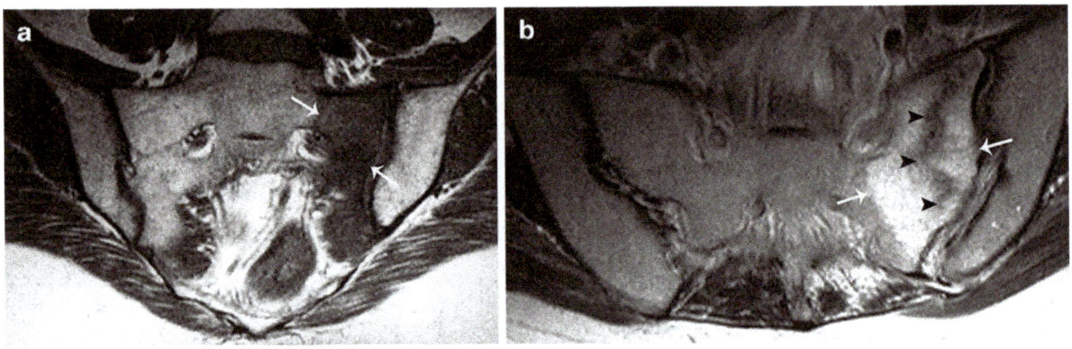

Fig. 9.19 Stress fracture (with fracture line). The T1-weighted MR image (**a**) shows an area of dark signal (*arrows*) in the left sacral ala which is nonspecific. The T2-weighted MR image (**b**) shows a low signal fracture (*arrows*) surrounded by marrow edema (*arrowheads*)

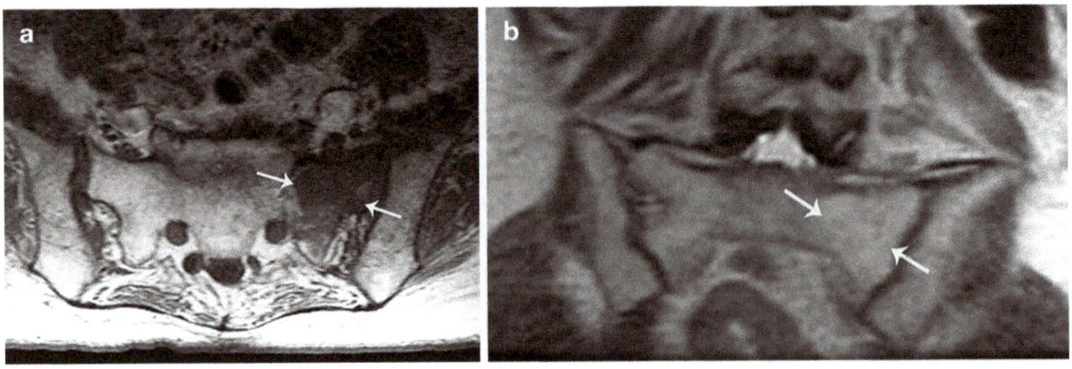

Fig. 9.20 Stress fracture (healing). T1-weighted MR image (**a**) shows an area of dark signal (*arrows*) in the left sacral ala, which is nonspecific but may represent a focal tumor. Six months later, the left sacral area (*arrows*) has normal fatty signal on the T1-weighted MR image (**b**) consistent with healing of a stress fracture

Myositis Ossificans

Myositis ossificans refers to heterotopic ossification occurring in muscle and often forms, to varying degrees, following trauma. Other predisposing factors have been reported, including burns, paraplegia, surgery, traumatic brain injury, hemophilia, ankylosing spondylitis, and diffuse idiopathic skeletal hyperostosis (DISH). Although myositis ossificans is believed to arise following trauma, patients often cannot recall any antecedent trauma. Patients may be asymptomatic or may present with pain, swelling, and, occasionally, an elevated erythrocyte sedimentation rate. Most lesions arise in the large muscles of the extremities. The appearance of myositis ossificans varies depending on its stage of development. Calcification is rarely seen on radiographs in the first few weeks, but can become apparent 3–8 weeks after onset, starting peripherally and progressing centrally, in a "zonal" pattern. Mineralization in the mass evolves from faint, irregular, floccular densities to dense calcifications and, ultimately, to a rim of mature lamellar bone with central osteoid matrix. The MR appearance also varies, reflecting the histologic changes. Early lesions are poorly defined; are isointense on T1-weighted images and heterogeneously hyperintense on T2-weighted images; and have diffuse surrounding soft-tissue edema. As peripheral calcification develops, peripheral low signal intensity may become visible on MR images. Mature lesions appear as well-defined masses that are isointense to fat centrally and have low signal intensity peripherally (on both T1- and T2-weighted images), without surrounding soft-tissue edema. Early-stage myositis ossificans can enhance and can be mistaken for a soft tissue sarcoma, as the characteristic zonal ossification pattern is not present. Moreover, some lesions may be closely adherent to the cortical surface, occasionally "wrapping" around the entire circumference of the bone, mimicking an osteochondroma or parosteal osteosarcoma. In these instances, CT is extremely helpful in demonstrating a plane of soft tissue between the ossified mass and the bone cortex. Unlike osteochondromas, myositis ossificans adherent to bone should not demonstrate contiguity of the lesion marrow cavity with that of the host bone.

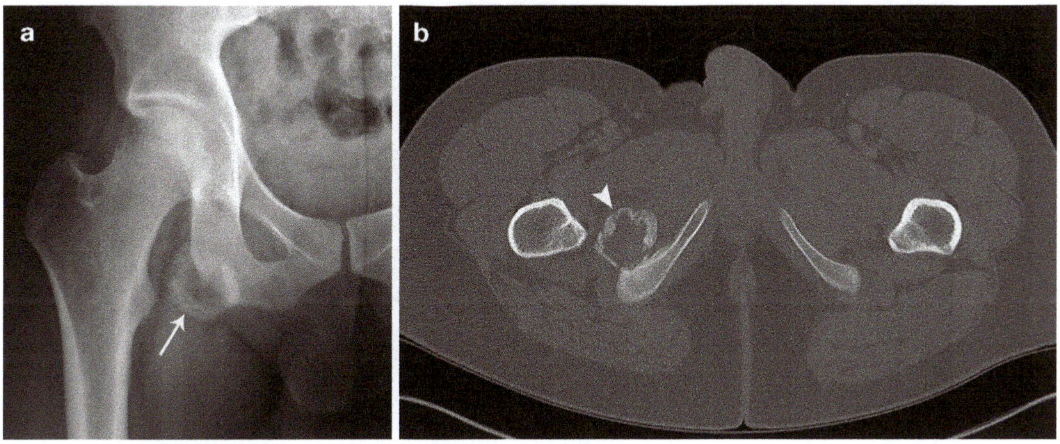

Fig. 9.21 A 25-year-old soccer player with maturing myositis ossificans in the right adductor muscles. There is a round peripherally dense lesion (*arrow*) at the right inferior pubic ramus on the AP radiograph (**a**). The lesion has peripheral zonal calcification (*arrowhead*) characteristic of myositis ossificans on the axial CT image (**b**)

Metabolic/Arthritic Processes

Brown Tumor of Hyperparathyroidism

Osteolytic lesions can develop in patients with longstanding untreated hyperparathyroidism and are called brown tumors or osteoclastomas. They can be seen in patients with primary hyperparathyroidism and in patients with secondary hyperparathyroidism due to renal failure. These lesions represent accumulation of fibrous tissue and giant cells related to microfracture and hemorrhage. Brownish blood products within the lesions give rise to the name. Brown tumors are reportedly seen in 5% of patients with hyperparathyroidism, but their occurrence has decreased with improved early diagnosis of hyperparathyroidism. A history of generalized weakness, paresthesias, abdominal pain, and mental status changes, as well as abnormal levels of serum calcium, phosphorous, alkaline phosphatase, and parathyroid hormone (PTH), can aid in the diagnosis of hyperparathyroidism. Brown tumors appear as well-defined lytic lesions with or without septations, can expand the bone, and can sometimes appear quite aggressive. They are found in the long bones, ribs, pelvis, and facial bones. With treatment, e.g., removal of the parathyroid adenoma, the lesions can become sclerotic. Lack of a change in the appearance of the lesion, with adequate treatment for hyperparathyroidism, should raise suspicion for an alternative diagnosis.

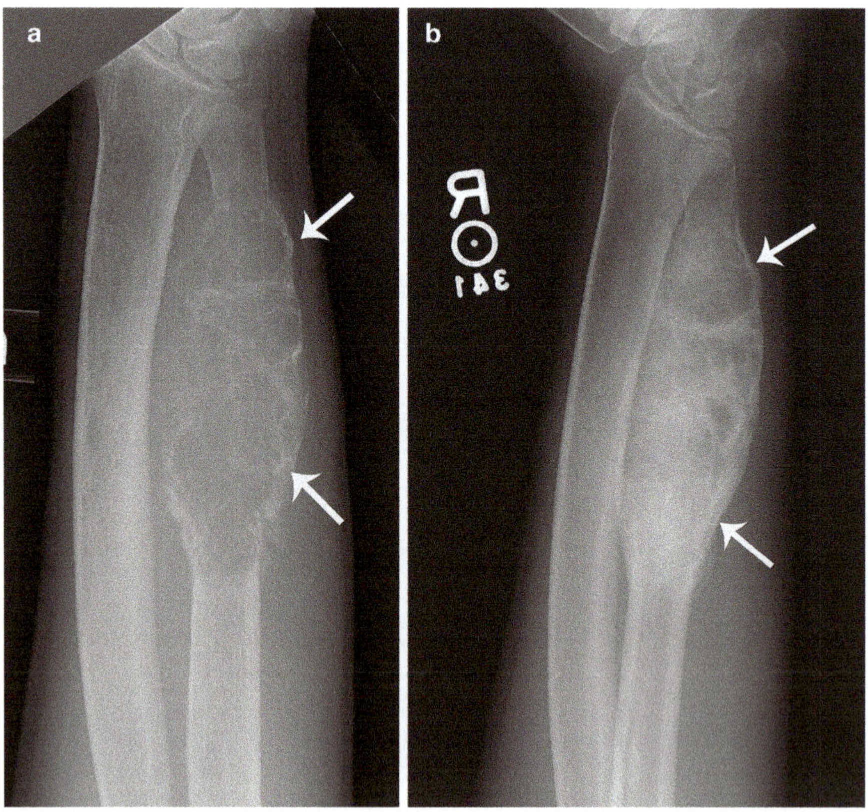

Fig. 9.22 Destructive expansile brown tumor (*arrows*) in the distal ulna before (**a**) and after (**b**) removal of a parathyroid adenoma. Note the increased sclerosis of the lesion following treatment

Melorheostosis

Melorheostosis is a benign bone dysplasia characterized by sclerotic bone lesions, often involving several bones along a single limb, in the distribution of a sclerotome. The appearance has been compared to "dripping candle wax" along the side of a candle. It is a nonhereditary disorder and 50% of patients will exhibit signs of the disease by age 20. Melorheostosis can be asymptomatic; however, when symptomatic, clinical problems include pain, limb deformities and contractures related to muscle and tendon shortening, skin disorders, and poor circulation. Melorheostosis can be associated with soft tissue hemangiomas and neurofibromas and is believed to be related to osteopathia striata and osteopoikilosis. On imaging, the lesions can be mistaken for a surface osteosarcoma or osteochondroma. Radiographs demonstrate characteristic flowing cortical hyperostosis and seeing this appearance in multiple contiguous bones in a sclerotomal distribution can help with the diagnosis. The lesions are low signal on all MR pulse sequences, but can have edema in the surrounding soft tissue. Moreover, the lesions can be active on bone scan, distinguishing them from bone islands or osteopathia striata.

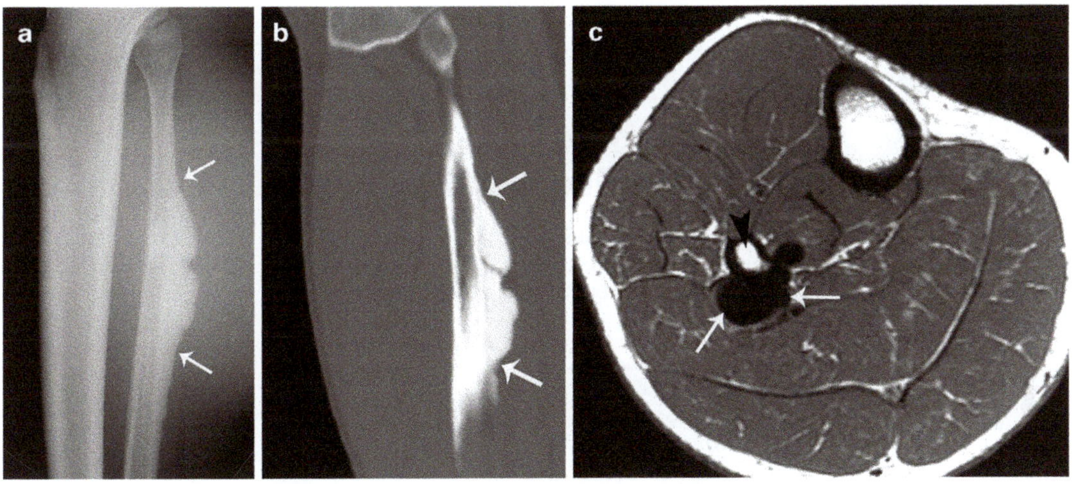

Fig. 9.23 Melorheostosis along the posterior shaft of the fibula. The cortical thickening (*arrows*) along the fibula is well seen on the lateral radiograph (**a**) and sagittal CT image (**b**). The axial T1-weighted MR image (**c**) shows dense low signal cortical thickening (*arrows*) with normal bright marrow (*arrowhead*) in the fibula

Osteonecrosis

Osteonecrosis refers to ischemic necrosis of the bone and marrow and has many causes, including: trauma, steroids, hemoglobinopathies (such as sickle cell anemia), alcoholism, pancreatitis, systemic lupus erythematosus, Gaucher's disease, irradiation, chemotherapy, and Caisson's disease. Osteonecrosis can be subdivided into (1) intramedullary bone infarcts, occurring in the metaphysis and diaphysis and (2) epiphyseal bone infarcts (avascular necrosis) that involve the subchondral bone and that can lead to collapse of the articular surface. Early on, bone infarcts are occult and quite subtle on radiographs. More advanced bone infarcts will appear as a focal lesion comprised of a central lucency and serpentine sclerotic border on radiographs. Bone infarcts can have a similar appearance to enchondromas on radiographs; however, enchondromas typically have central calcifications, with peripheral lucency. Even when they are occult on radiographs, bone infarcts can be seen (even in the early stage) on MRI. Early bone infarcts demonstrate nonspecific marrow edema. Later lesions can develop more characteristic features, such as subchondral signal changes or a "double line sign," i.e., an outer band of low signal associated with an inner band of high signal on non-fat-saturated T2-weighted images. Bone infarcts can have variable appearances on bone scintigraphy.

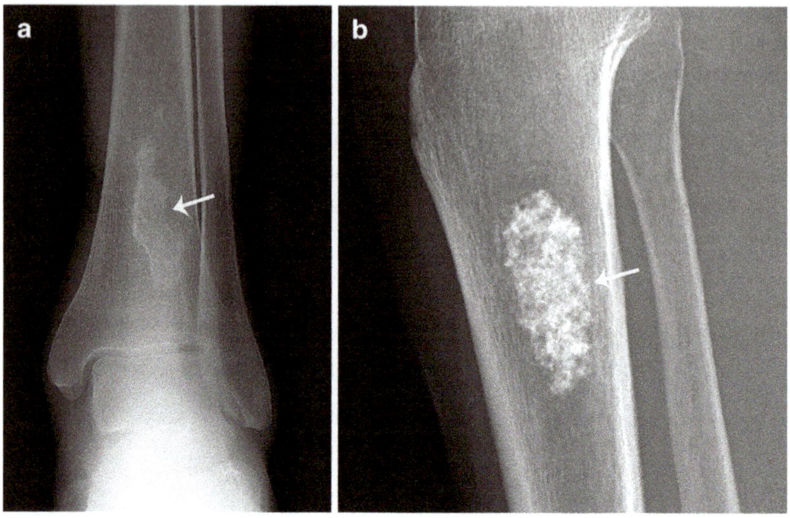

Fig. 9.24 Bone infarct versus enchondroma. Note pattern of peripheral density and smoother borders (*arrows*) on the AP ankle radiograph (**a**), which helps distinguish the bone infarct from the central calcification and more lobulated borders of an enchondroma (*arrow*) on the lateral tibia radiograph (**b**)

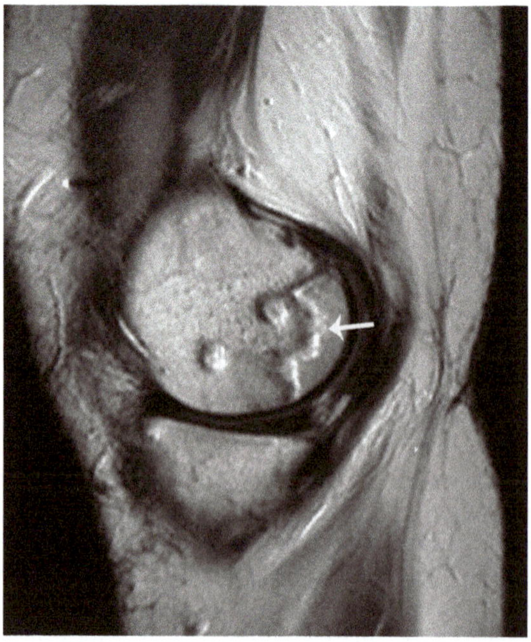

Fig. 9.25 Avascular necrosis of the distal femur. Note the "double line" of low and high signal (*arrow*) on the T2-weighted MR image

Paget Disease

Paget disease (osteitis deformans) is a chronic condition of abnormal bone remodeling that leads to osseous expansion and deformity. The condition is rare under the age of 55 and present in 10% of patients over age 80. There is a higher occurrence of Paget disease in individuals from Australia, Great Britain, and Europe, and the entity is rare in individuals of Chinese origin. The cause of Paget disease is unknown; however, it has been linked to viral infection from paramyxoviruses. Patients may be asymptomatic, with incidental findings of Paget disease on imaging studies, or may present with unexplained elevated alkaline phosphatase, bone pain, fractures, arthritis, hearing loss from involvement of the auditory ossicles, increasing head size, renal stones, loose teeth, and high output cardiac failure from hypervascular pagetic bone. Rarely (<1%) malignant transformation to a sarcoma, typically osteosarcoma, can occur. The active phase of Paget disease is characterized by bone resorption. In long bones, the osteolytic form of Paget begins at the end of a long bone and the leading edge of the lesion extends toward the mid-diaphysis, in a pointed-edge "blade of grass" or "flame" pattern. The tibia is an exception, in that the lucent area may be centered in the diaphysis, without involvement of the ends of the bone. The quiescent phase of Paget disease is characterized by bone deposition, with thickening of the medullary trabeculae and bone cortex and with overall bony enlargement. The pelvis is the most commonly involved site and involvement there is often unilateral. The skull, vertebral bodies, and long bones (femur, tibia, and humerus) can also be involved.

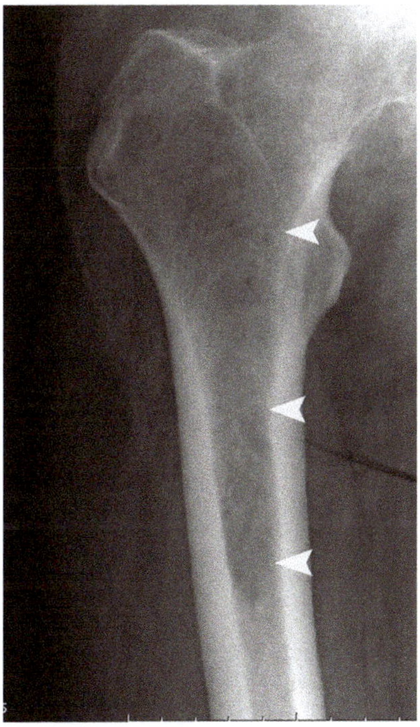

Fig. 9.26 Paget disease (active phase)—osteolytic "blade of grass" lucency (*arrowheads*) extending towards the mid-diaphysis of the femur

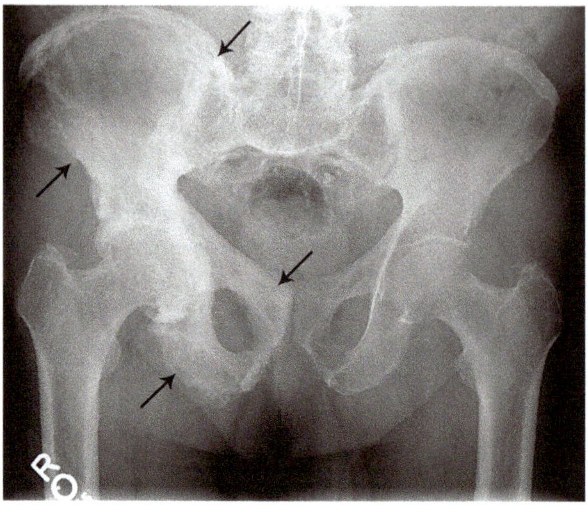

Fig. 9.27 Paget disease (quiescent phase) in right hemipelvis. Note both cortical and medullary expansion and trabecular thickening (*arrows*) of the right pelvic bones

Calcific Tendinitis

Calcific tendinitis, a form of hydroxyapatite deposition disease (HADD), is caused by the deposition of calcium hydroxyapatite crystals in the tendons and is a common cause of joint pain and stiffness. Calcific tendinitis is most common in the tendons of the rotator cuff and the hip; however, it can involve any tendon. At times, during the resorptive phase, calcific tendinitis can mimic an aggressive process such as infection or neoplasm. In some instances, calcific tendinitis can be associated with erosion of the adjoining bone, mimicking a destructive bone lesion. This aggressive pattern is common at the gluteus maximus insertion along the posterior proximal femoral diaphysis. The disease is typically self-limiting, but percutaneous needle aspiration and steroid injection can provide relief.

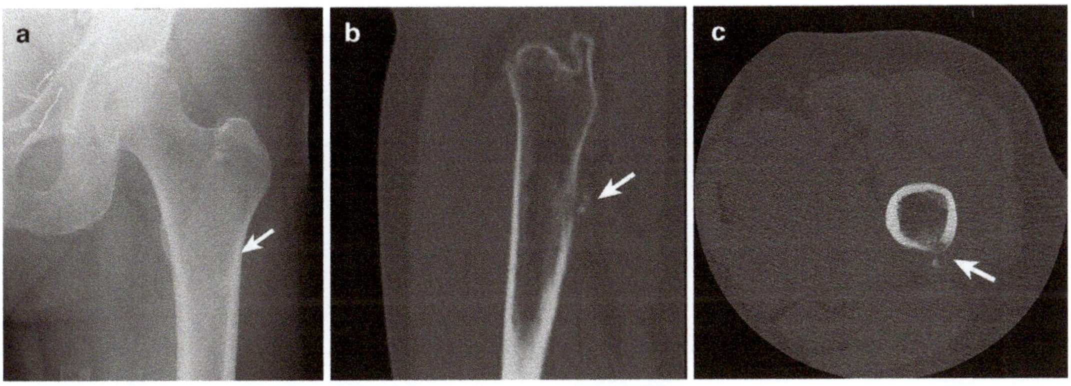

Fig. 9.28 Calcific tendinitis (resorptive phase)—hip radiograph (**a**) shows faint sclerosis in the proximal femur (*arrow*). Sagittal (**b**) and axial (**c**) CT images show hazy amorphous densities with cortical erosion (*arrows*) at the insertion site of the gluteus maximus tendon to the femur

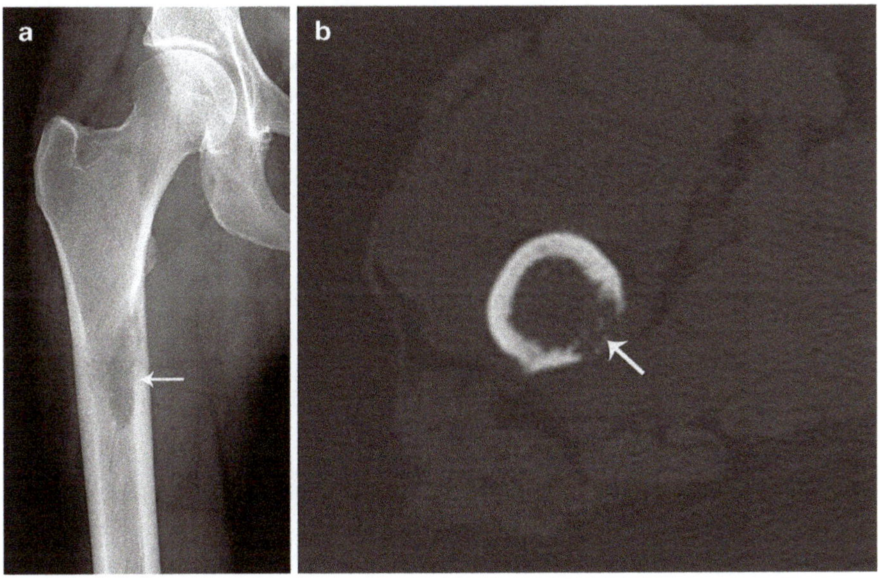

Fig. 9.29 Breast cancer metastasis—there is a lytic lesion (*arrows*) with ill-defined margins in the proximal femoral shaft on the radiograph (**a**). Note the cortical erosion/destruction (*arrow*) on the axial CT image (**b**), similar to Fig. 9.28 showing calcific tendinitis of the gluteus maximus tendon. Knowing that the gluteus maximus tendon attaches to the posterolateral and not the posteromedial femur can help distinguish the two processes

Subchondral Cyst

Subchondral cysts or geodes are extremely common and are seen in the setting of osteoarthritis. They form as synovium and joint fluid enters the subchondral bone via defects in the overlying articular cartilage, due to increased joint pressure. They are typically small in size, abut the joint surface, and have a sclerotic margin. However, they can grow to large sizes and even extend down the shaft of a long bone. Because the incidence of osteoarthritis increases with age, these lesions are commonly seen in the older population. CT can be helpful to demonstrate the sclerotic margin. On MRI, the lesion is usually iso- or hyperintense to muscle on T1-weighted images and high signal on T2-weighted images, with peripheral enhancement. However, high T1 signal or internal enhancement may occur in lesions that contain proteinaceous material or fibrous material, respectively. The presence of osteoarthritis in the joint should help distinguish a subchondral cyst from other epiphyseal lesions such as chondroblastoma, giant cell tumor, clear cell chondrosarcoma, Langerhans cell histiocytosis, and lytic metastases (which typically do not have a sclerotic border).

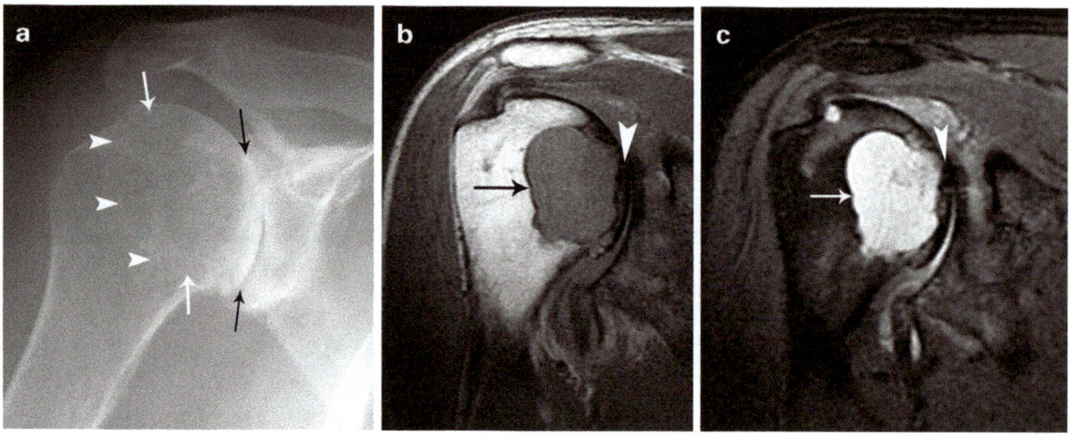

Fig. 9.30 Large subchondral cyst (geode)—radiograph (**a**) shows a subarticular lucency (*arrows*) with a faint sclerotic rim (*arrowheads*) in the humeral head. There is narrowing of the joint space, osteophytes, and subchondral sclerosis (*black arrows*) from severe glenohumeral osteoarthritis. The T1-weighted (**b**) and fat-saturated T2-weighted (**b**) MR images show a well demarcated cystic lesion (*arrows*) abutting the narrowed joint space (*arrowheads*)

Osteomyelitis

Brodie's Abscess

Osteomyelitis can have a varied imaging appearance depending on its clinical stage. In the acute stage, radiographs can reveal areas of aggressive periostitis, cortical destruction, endosteal scalloping, and intracortical tunneling. There can be associated soft tissue swelling, abscess, and gas formation. However, it is important realize that radiographic findings of osteomyelitis may not be present for 1–2 weeks following initial infection. MRI and bone scintigraphy are more sensitive in the detection of early osseous signs of osteomyelitis. Subacute or chronic osteomyelitis can result in a radiolucent intraosseous abscess called a Brodie's abscess, often in the metaphysis of long bones. These lesions were first described by Sir Benjamin Collins Brodie in 1832 and appear on radiographs as a single or multilobulated lucent lesion with surrounding sclerosis that fades towards the periphery. Depending on the amount of sclerosis, these lesions can mimic an osteoid osteoma or osteosarcoma. Lesions without significant sclerosis can mimic Langerhans cell histiocytosis, chondroblastoma, giant cell tumor, and Ewing sarcoma. A sinus tract extending away from the central abscess can be nicely depicted by CT and can help to distinguish a Brodie's abscess from other lesions, especially an osteoid osteoma. Systemic signs of infection can be helpful; however, several of the lesions listed in the differential can also present with fever, pain, and other clinical signs of infection. Bone biopsy is often necessary for diagnosis and sampling of the fluid and soft tissue components can lead to a higher diagnostic yield than only the sclerotic bone. Moreover, sending additional specimens for microbiologic culture is helpful to guide antibiotic therapy.

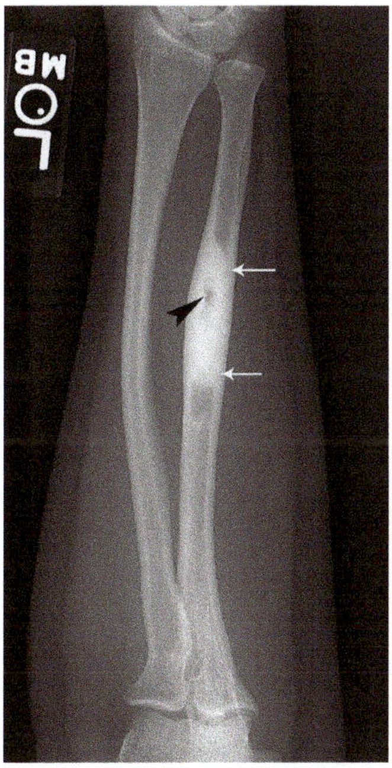

Fig. 9.31 Brodie's abscess. There is an area of sclerosis (*arrows*) with a small central lucency (*arrowhead*) in the mid shaft of the ulna in a patient with chronic osteomyelitis

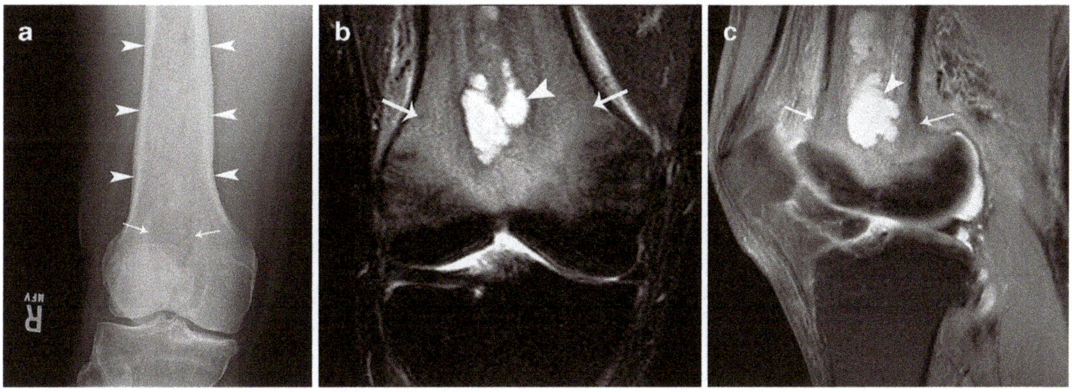

Fig. 9.32 Acute on chronic osteomyelitis with Brodie's abscess. Radiograph (**a**) demonstrates an area of lucency (*arrows*) in the distal femoral metaphysis. The distal femur has a mottled appearance with cortical thickening (*arrowheads*) from chronic osteomyelitis. Coronal (**b**) and sagittal (**c**) STIR MRI images nicely show the bright intraosseous abscess (*arrowhead*) with surrounding marrow edema (*arrows*). Purulent fluid was aspirated at the time of biopsy and cultures of the bone specimens grew *Staphylococcus aureus*

Iatrogenic Causes

Biceps Tenodesis

In patients with tears or inflammation of the long head of the biceps tendon, biceps tenodesis may be performed. The intra-articular portion of the long head of the biceps tendon is cut and the remaining portion of the tendon is attached to the proximal humeral diaphysis. This postoperative appearance can produce a lucent lesion with a sclerotic border. Checking the patient's surgical history and awareness of this procedure is the key to mistaking this finding for a neoplasm.

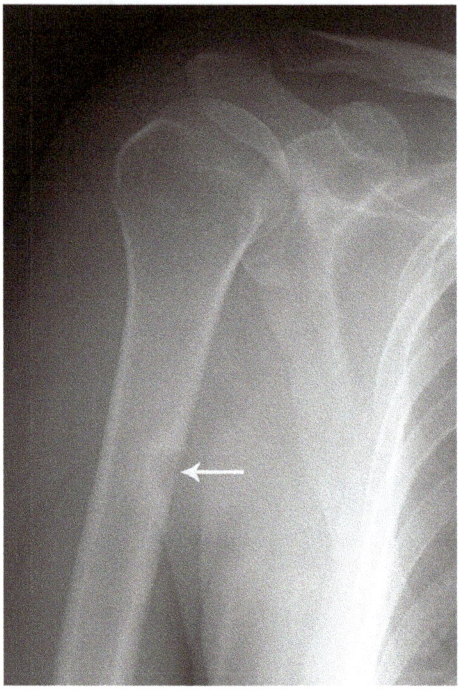

Fig. 9.33 Lucent lesion (*arrow*) in the proximal humeral shaft from a biceps tenodesis

Bone Marrow Biopsy

A bone marrow aspirate is commonly obtained from the iliac bone from a posterior approach. If there is a history of recent bone marrow biopsy, then edema in the marrow should not be mistaken for a focal lesion. Confirming the history of bone marrow biopsy is central to making this diagnosis.

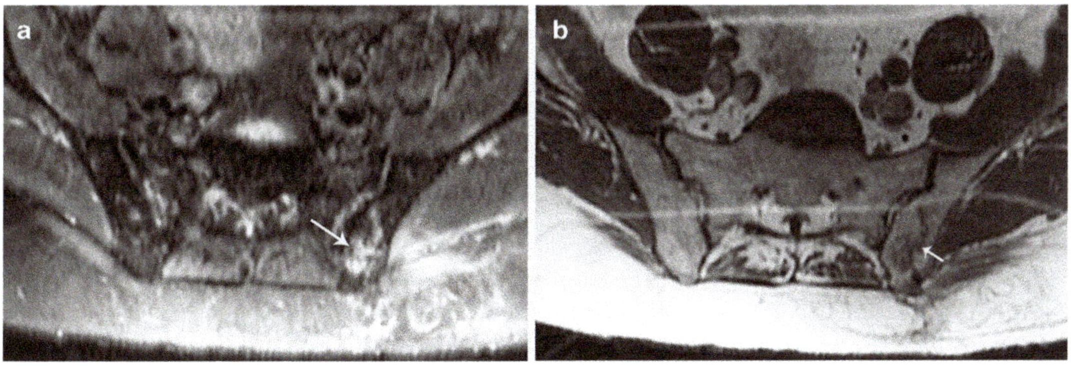

Fig. 9.34 Bone marrow biopsy changes. There are linear areas of low T1 and high T2 signal (*arrows*) on the T1-weighted (**a**) and T2-weighted (**b**) MR images at the site of a bone marrow biopsy

Particle Disease

Particle disease is one of the most common causes of hardware failure, especially in hip arthroplasty. The polymethylmethacrylate cement, polyethylene, or metal in the arthroplasty components can incite a macrophage-mediated granulomatous response, which can stimulate osteoclast activity. The process will create areas of lucency surrounding the hardware components. However, unlike mechanical loosening, the lytic areas seen with particle disease typically do not follow the outline of the prosthesis. The lucencies are often larger and less linear than the periprosthetic lucencies seen with mechanical loosening. Particle disease can mimic osteolytic tumors or infection. The key features distinguishing particle disease from neoplasm are the presence of hardware and that fact that particle disease often creates abnormal lucencies on both sides of the joint.

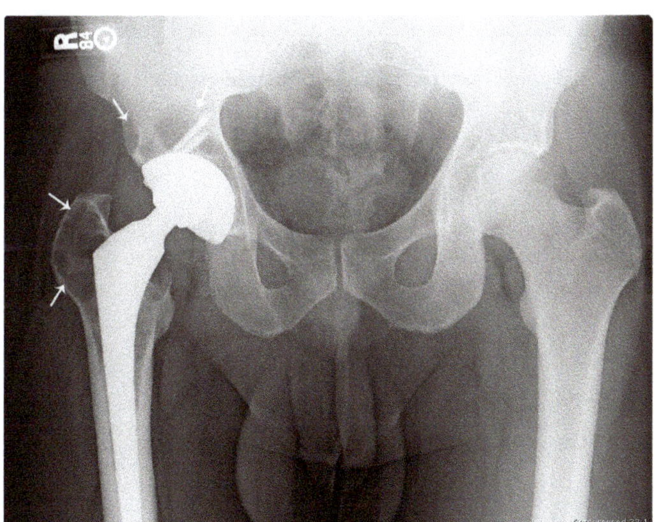

Fig. 9.35 Particle disease. There are multiple lucent lesions (*arrows*) on both sides of the right hip joint abutting both the femoral and acetabular components

Radiation Changes

Radiation is commonly used in the treatment of certain malignancies. In the early stages (hours to days), radiation causes vascular congestion, edema, and hypocellularity in the bone marrow. This will appear as low signal on T1-weighted MR images and high signal on T2-weighted images. Later (weeks to months), the bone marrow will be replaced with fat and occasionally with fibrosis, with high signal on T1- and mixed signal on T2-weighted images. Often, one can see a clear line of demarcation between the irradiated and nonirradiated tissue, corresponding anatomically to the borders of the radiation field. The affect on the bone marrow can depend on the timing and dose of radiation. Fatty conversion can be reversible at doses less than 30–40 Gy. Irradiated bone is at increased risk for insufficiency fractures, osteonecrosis, and radiation-induced sarcomas.

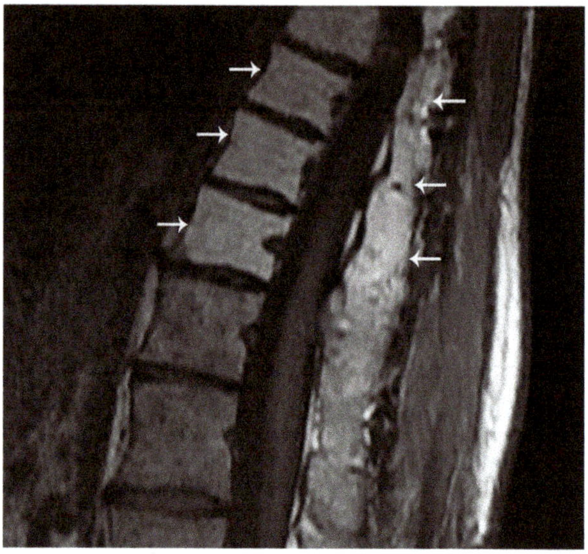

Fig. 9.36 T1-weighted MR image shows fatty marrow replacement in several upper thoracic vertebral bodies (*arrows*) with a sharp demarcation from the lower thoracic vertebral bodies (*arrowheads*) indicating the edge of the radiation field in a patient treated for lung cancer

Contrast Infiltration

Iodinated contrast used for CT imaging can extravasate into the soft tissues if a venous access catheter is displaced. This is especially problematic when using power injection and in unresponsive patients who cannot alert the technologist about pain at the injection site. The increased density at the injection site can persist for several days and, if not treated, can lead to tissue necrosis. Prompt treatment is necessary to minimize tissue necrosis.

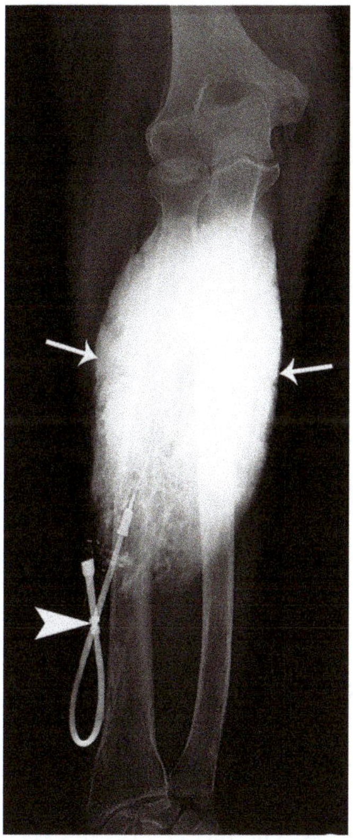

Fig. 9.37 There is a large oval density in the forearm (arrows) mimicking an osseous lesion in a patient who experienced extravasation of iodinated contrast from a power injection due to a displaced IV catheter (arrowhead) during a CT scan

Technical Artifacts

Humeral Head Pseudolesion on Internal Rotation View

A pseudolesion with a sclerotic border and lucent center can appear in the humeral head on the internal rotation view. The sharp sclerotic border forms at the humeral neck as the diameter of the bone changes abruptly. The pseudolesion should disappear on the external rotation view and should not be mistaken for an osteolytic lesion.

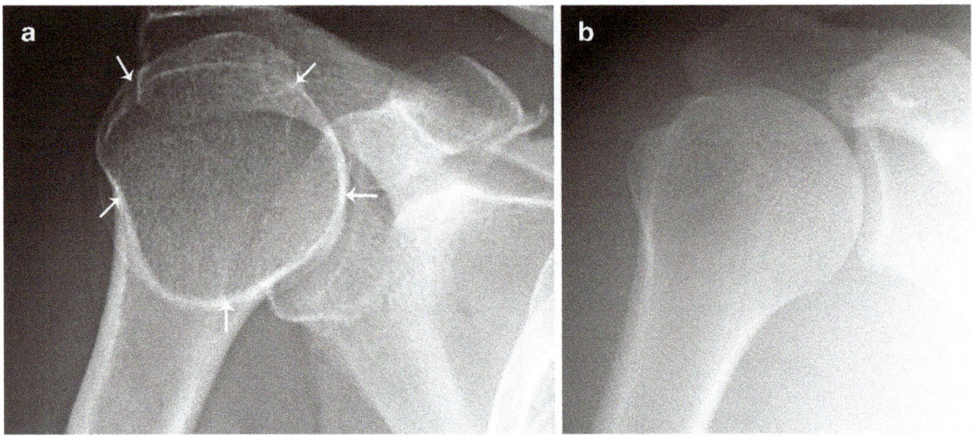

Fig. 9.38 A lucent pseudolesion with a sclerotic border (arrows) appears on the internal rotation view (**a**) of the humeral head and disappears on the external rotation view (**b**)

Radial Tuberosity Pseudolesion on Lateral View

On lateral views of the proximal radius, the normal radial tuberosity is imaged en face and can appear as an ovoid lucent lesion. On AP and oblique views, the tuberosity becomes visible and the artifactual intramedullary lucency disappears. The lucency occurs because the density of trabeculae in the tuberosity is decreased compared with the normal medullary bone of the diaphysis. This artifact is analogous to the pseudolesion seen on internal rotation views of the humeral head described previously. The same effect can be seen when looking "down the barrel" of any bony protruberance and it explains why osteochondromas used to be called "diaphyseal aclasia." The bony protuberance of an osteochondroma can mimic a lucent lesion when seen en face. To avoid this pitfall, it is important to check an orthogonal image of the same bone.

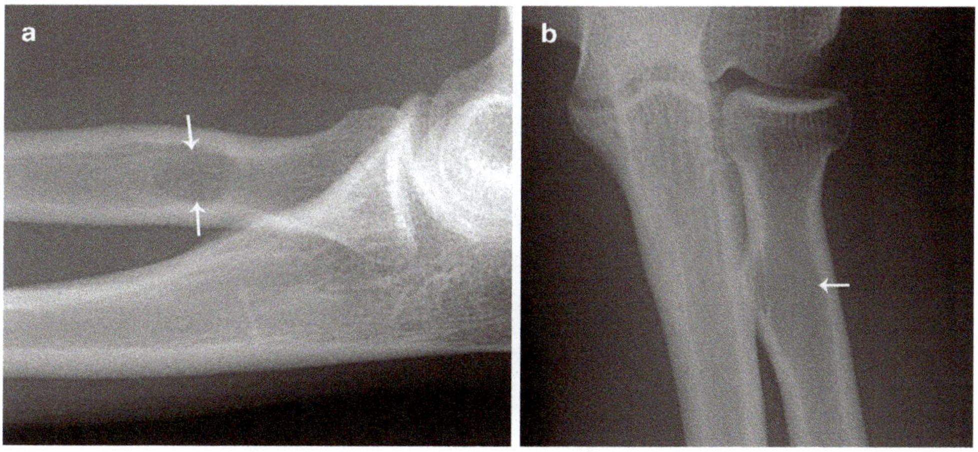

Fig. 9.39 There is an apparent lucent lesion (*arrows*) in the radial tuberosity on the lateral view (**a**) that disappears on the AP view (**b**)

MRI Wrap-Around (Aliasing) Artifact

Wrap-around or aliasing artifacts on MR imaging can occur if the field of view (FOV) is smaller than the body part being imaged. This can lead to image data that is outside the FOV being "wrapped-around" and artifactually included within the image. This artifact is a more common problem in the phase encoding direction, but can also occur in the frequency encoding direction. Wrap-around artifact can be corrected by employing a large enough FOV in the phase-encoding direction such that the entire body part is included in the image or by using phase oversampling techniques during imaging. Swapping phase and frequency can help determine whether the apparent lesion is artifact or a real lesion. Awareness of this technical artifact can prevent mistaking wrap-around artifact for focal lesions.

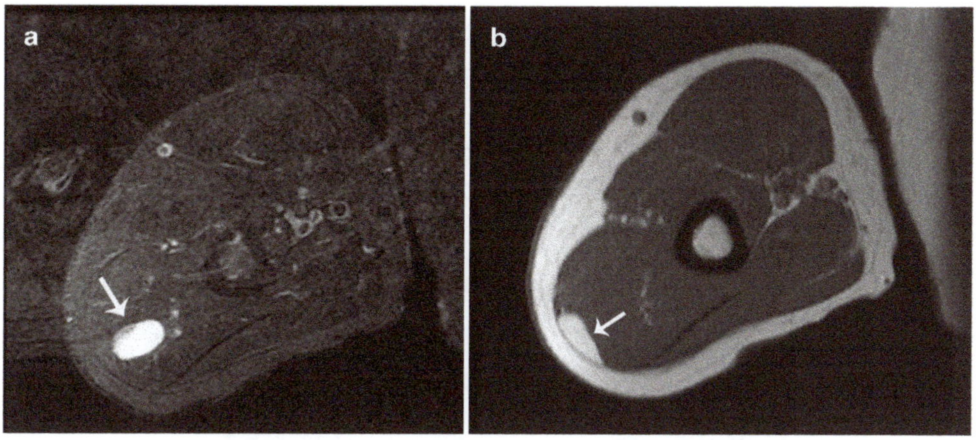

Fig. 9.40 On the STIR MR image (**a**) there is wrap-around (aliasing) artifact from a bright sebaceous cyst (*arrow*) in the posterior chest wall (not included in the imaging FOV) which is erroneously registering onto the triceps muscle, mimicking a soft tissue tumor. The study was performed to evaluate a lipoma (*arrow*) in the upper arm which is well seen on the T1-weighted MR image (**b**) (Images courtesy of Dr. Colm McMahon, Dublin, Ireland)

MRI Pulsation Artifact

Ghosting artifact from pulsatile arterial or venous flow can mimic lesions, as artifactual image data from the vessels is superimposed onto bone or soft tissue. Repeating the imaging sequence after swapping the phase and frequency encoding directions can help to determine whether or not the lesions are real.

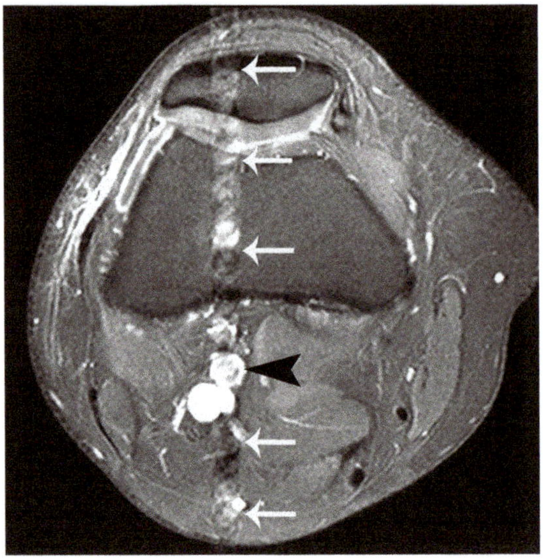

Fig. 9.41 On the T2-weighted fat-saturated MR image, there is extensive pulsation artifact (*arrows*) related to the popliteal artery (*black arrowhead*)

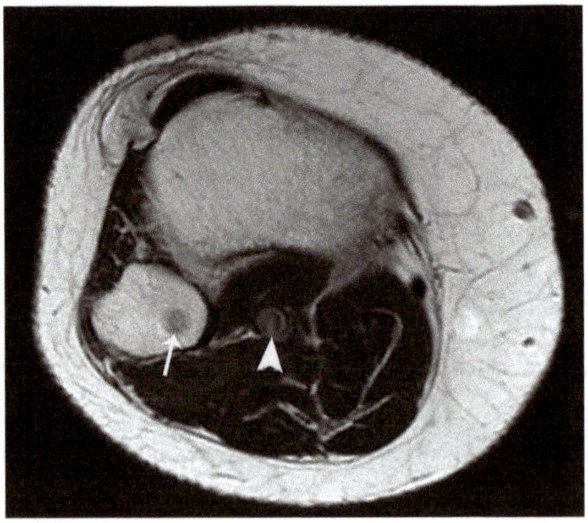

Fig. 9.42 Subtle pulsation artifact causes a low signal rounded focus (*arrow*) in the fibula from the popliteal artery (*arrowhead*) which mimics a tumor (different patient than Fig. 9.41)

External Object Artifact

Objects lying over or under the patient during imaging can mimic a bone lesion. This is especially problematic in cases of acute trauma where the studies need to be performed quickly and imaging technique may not be optimal.

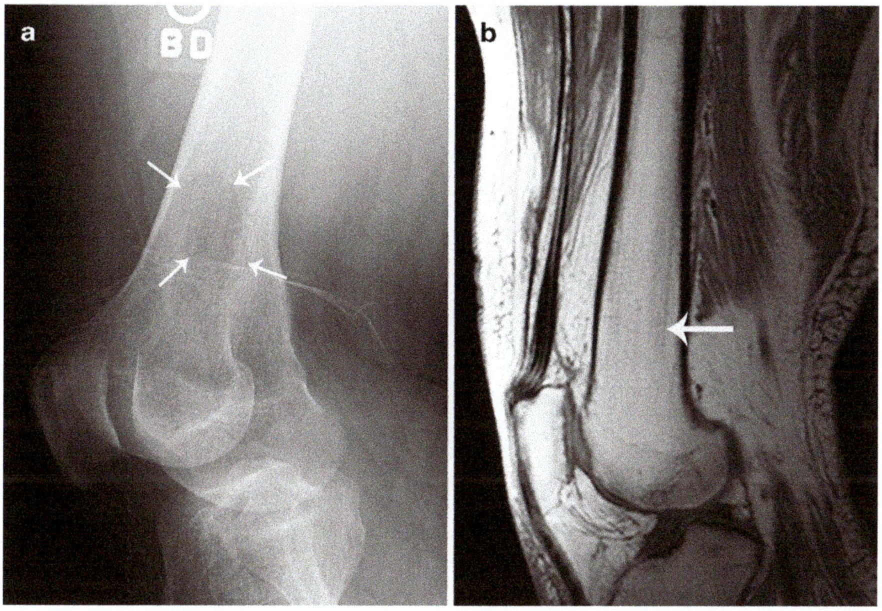

Fig. 9.43 On the lateral radiograph (**a**) there is an oval lucency (*arrows*) in the distal femur mimicking a lytic lesion. Subsequent T1-weighted MRI image (**b**) shows a normal distal femur (*arrow*), confirming the artifactual nature of the lesion. The lucency was caused by handle holes in the trauma board lying underneath the patient

Suggested Reading

1. Anderson SE, Johnston JO, Steinbach LS. Pseudotumors of the shoulder invited review. Eur J Radiol. 2008;68:147–58.
2. Daldrup-Link HE, Henning T, Link TM. MR imaging of therapy-induced changes of bone marrow. Eur Radiol. 2007;17:743–61.
3. Davies AM, Evans N, Mangham DC, Grimer RJ. MR imaging of brown tumour with fluid-fluid levels: a report of three cases. Eur Radiol. 2001;11:1445–9.
4. De Wilde V, De Maeseneer M, Lenchik L, Van Roy P, Beeckman P, Osteaux M. Normal osseous variants presenting as cystic or lucent areas on radiography and CT imaging: a pictorial overview. Eur J Radiol. 2004;51:77–84.
5. Gould CF, Ly JQ, Lattin Jr GE, Beall DP, Sutcliffe 3rd JB. Bone tumor mimics: avoiding misdiagnosis. Curr Probl Diagn Radiol. 2007;36:124–41.
6. Johnson JF, Brogdon BG. Dorsal effect of the patella: incidence and distribution. AJR Am J Roentgenol. 1982;139:339–40.
7. Kransdorf MJ, Meis JM, Jelinek JS. Myositis ossificans: MR appearance with radiologic-pathologic correlation. AJR Am J Roentgenol. 1991;157:1243–8.
8. Levine AH, Pais MJ, Berinson H, Amenta PS. The soleal line: a cause of tibial pseudoperiostitis. Radiology. 1976;119:79–81.
9. Mitchell MJ, Logan PM. Radiation-induced changes in bone. Radiographics. 1998;18:1125–136.
10. Natsis K. Supracondylar process of the humerus: study on 375 Caucasian subjects in Cologne, Germany. Clin Anat. 2008;21:138–41.
11. Pitt MJ, Graham AR, Shipman JH, Birkby W. Herniation pit of the femoral neck. AJR Am J Roentgenol. 1982;138:1115–21.
12. Resnick D, editor. Diagnosis of bone and joint disorders. 4th ed. Philadelphia, PA: W.B. Saunders; 2002.

10 Cases

In this chapter, we have selected cases that highlight teaching points discussed in the previous nine chapters. Also included here are some uncommon entities that were only briefly mentioned in prior chapters due to space constraints, but that can be important in the differential diagnosis for certain lesions. Each case has a brief history followed by a description of the imaging findings. Next, we provide a "Best 3" differential diagnosis list, based on the belief that giving an exceedingly long list is usually not practical in everyday clinical practice. The discussion for each case focuses on the distinguishing features among the "Best 3" and provides a rationale for why the final diagnosis is the most logical one. Lastly, we provide some "Key Points" which briefly highlight important facts about the disease entity or the specific teaching point.

J.S. Wu and M.G. Hochman, *Bone Tumors: A Practical Guide to Imaging*,
DOI 10.1007/978-1-4419-0808-7_10, © Springer Science+Business Media, LLC 2012

Case 1

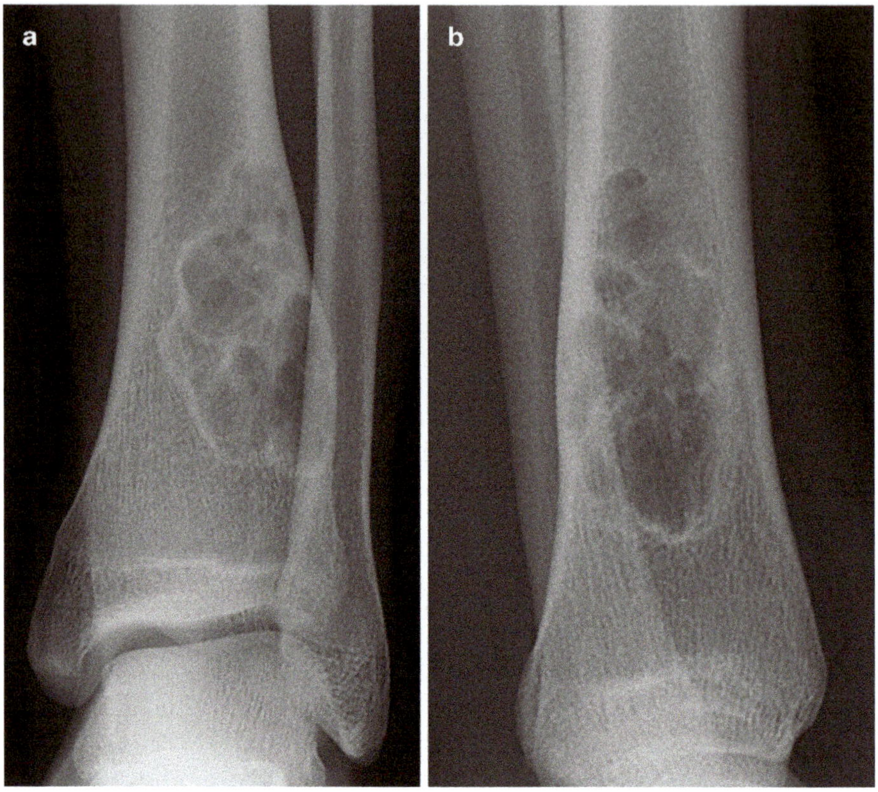

Fig. 10.1

History

A 19-year-old female with continued ankle pain after sports injury.

Imaging Findings

AP (a) and lateral (b) radiographs show an ovoid, bubbly, mixed lucent and sclerotic lesion, located eccentrically in the distal tibial metadiaphysis and abutting the posterior cortex. The lesion has a sclerotic rim, expands the bone slightly, and thins the overlying cortex. There is no periosteal new bone formation.

Differential Diagnosis (Best 3)

Non-ossifying fibroma (NOF)
Fibrous dysplasia
Aneurysmal bone cyst (ABC)

Discussion

The location (metadiaphyseal, intramedullary, eccentric, and abutting cortex) and appearance are highly suggestive of NOF. Fibrous dysplasia (FD) can have a similar appearance and can occur in the metaphysis, but it is usually located centrally and favors the diaphysis. Both NOF and monostotic FD are usually incidental, asymptomatic findings. ABC is also eccentrically located, but is more expansile and, unlike NOF, often demonstrates fluid levels on MRI. ABCs typically present with pain and swelling, whereas NOFs are usually asymptomatic, unless there is a pathologic fracture. Like NOFs, fibrous cortical defects are also fibrous xanthomas, but are smaller (usually <3 cm) than NOFs and centered in the cortex.

Diagnosis

Non-ossifying fibroma

Key Points

- Common incidental finding—seen in 30% of normal individuals in first two decades.
- Classic "don't touch" lesion—imaging is usually diagnostic.
- Most (55%) occur around knee, less common in distal tibia and fibula, rare in upper extremity.
- Occurs in the metaphysis of long bones; usually posterior and medial.
- Migrates toward diaphysis as bone lengthens.
- Asymptomatic, except for large lesions, where stress and pathologic fractures can occur.
- Fracture more likely in lesions >3 cm, >50% diameter, and in weight-bearing bones.
- No treatment, unless atypical clinical or radiologic features or risk for pathologic fracture.

Suggested Reading

Betsy M, Kupersmith LM, Springfield DS. Metaphyseal fibrous defects. J Am Acad Orthop Surg. 2004;12:89–95.

Case 2

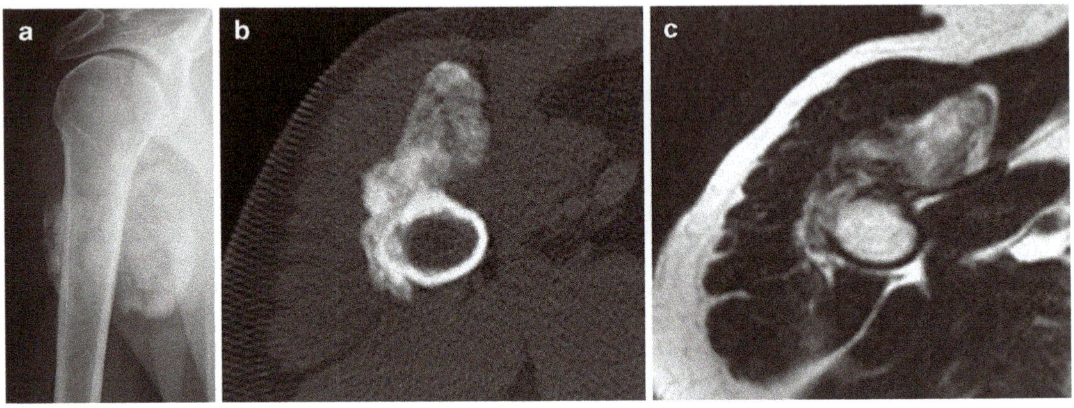

Fig. 10.2

History

A 47-year-old man with arm pain.

Imaging Findings

The radiograph (a) shows a dense lesion with ossification adjacent to (or arising from) the proximal humeral shaft, extending into the adjacent soft tissues. The axial CT (b) and T2-weighted MR image (c) confirm that the lesion is arising from the cortical surface and that there is a lack of medullary/cortical continuity between the lesion and the humerus.

Differential Diagnosis (Best 3)

Myositis ossificans
Parosteal osteosarcoma
Osteochondroma

Discussion

From the radiograph, it is difficult to determine whether the lesion is arising from the humerus or from the soft tissues. If localized to the soft tissues, then myositis ossificans will be most likely. The CT and MR clearly show that the lesion is arising from the bone and that there is no connection between the medullary cavities of the humerus and the lesion. Thus, the mass is most likely a parosteal osteosarcoma rather than an osteochondroma. Myositis ossificans is usually separate from bone, but rarely can be adherent to the cortical surface.

Diagnosis

Parosteal osteosarcoma

Key Points

- Most common surface osteosarcoma subtype.
- Tumor arises from the outer layer of periosteum.
- Most commonly found in the distal femur and proximal humerus.
- Can have symptoms due to exophytic mass injuring adjacent soft tissue structures.
- CT and MRI are helpful in showing that the tumor arises from the bone surface and that the medullary cavities are not continuous, in order to distinguish it from an osteochondroma.
- Slightly better prognosis than conventional osteosarcoma subtype and occurs 1–2 decades older (30–50 years old).

Suggested Reading

Dönmez FY, Tüzün U, Başaran C. MRI findings in parosteal osteosarcoma: correlation with histopathology. Diagn Interv Radiol. 2008;14(3):142–52.
Okada K, Frassica FJ, Sim FH, Beabout JW, Bond JR, Unni KK. Parosteal osteosarcoma. A clinicopathological study. J Bone Joint Surg Am. 1994;76:366–78.
Jelinek JS, Murphey MD, Kransdorf MJ, Shmookler BM, Malawer MM, Hur RC. Parosteal osteosarcoma: value of MR imaging and CT in the prediction of histologic grade. Radiology. 1996;201:837–42.

Case 3

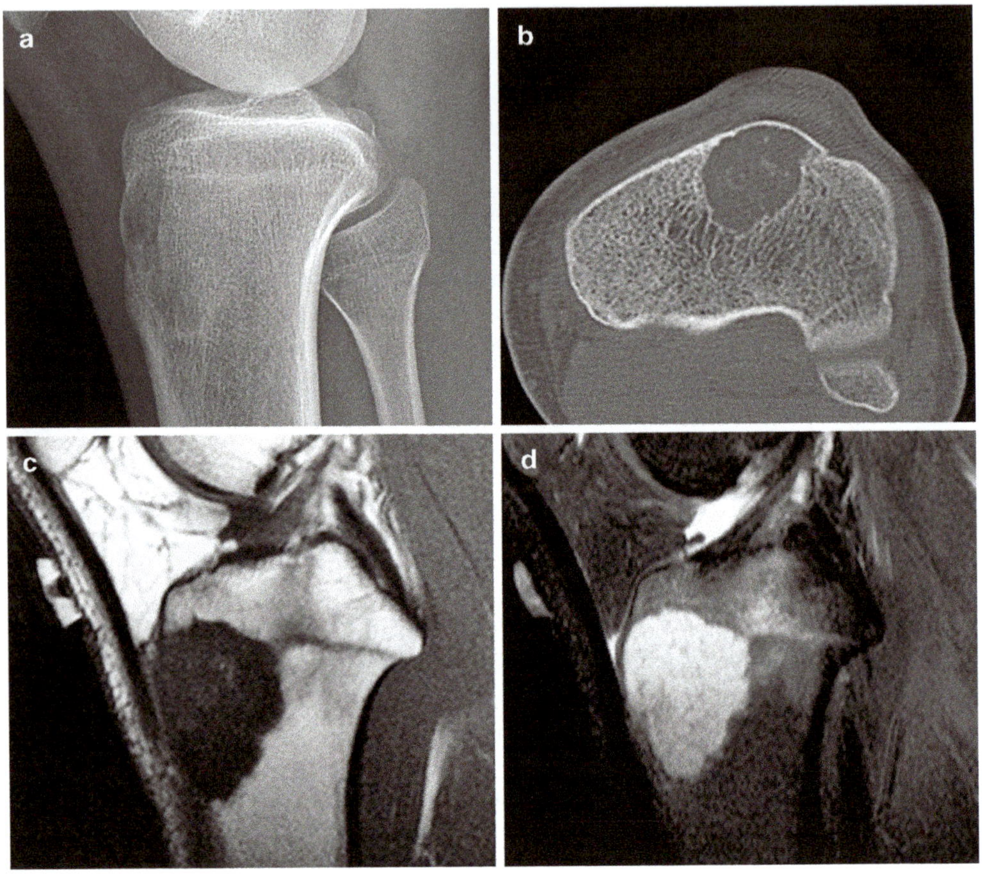

Fig. 10.3

History

A 20-year-old man with knee pain.

Imaging Findings

Lateral knee radiograph (a) shows a lucent lesion with faint sclerotic rim in the tibial tubercle (an apophysis). The axial CT (b) shows that the lytic lesion is geographic with a thin, sclerotic, well-circumscribed border and faint internal chondroid matrix. The MR images show a low T1 lesion (c) with prominent marrow edema adjacent to the posterosuperior aspect of the lesion, best seen on the fat-saturated T2-weighted MR image (d).

Differential Diagnosis (Best 3)

Giant cell tumor
Chondroblastoma
Clear cell chondrosarcoma

Discussion

The radiograph is fairly nonspecific and numerous lucent lesions can be included in the differential diagnosis including: giant cell tumor, chondroblastoma, chondromyxoid fibroma, Langerhans cell histiocytosis, and osteomyelitis. On the CT, chondroid matrix is seen in the lesion, making LCH and GCT unlikely. Clear cell chondrosarcoma is possible but typically occurs in an older population, is larger in size, has aggressive features, and is more likely to extend beyond the epiphysis into the soft tissues or metaphysis.

Diagnosis

Chondroblastoma

Key Points

- Rare benign cartilage tumor of bone.
- Occurs in the skeletally immature.
- Epiphyseal and apophyseal locations.
- Minimal to no internal cartilaginous matrix.
- Can have an aggressive appearance with periosteal reaction and marrow edema.
- High percentage have secondary aneurysmal bone cysts.

Suggested Reading

Kim J, Kumar R, Raymond AK, Ayala AG. Non-epiphyseal chondroblastoma arising in the iliac bone, and complicated by an aneurysmal bone cyst: a case report and review of the literature. Skeletal Radiol. 2010;39:583–7.

Kaim AH, Hugli R, Bonel HM, Jundt G. Chondroblastoma and clear cell chondrosarcoma: radiological and MRI characteristics with histopathological correlation. Skeletal Radiol. 2002;31:88–95.

Case 4

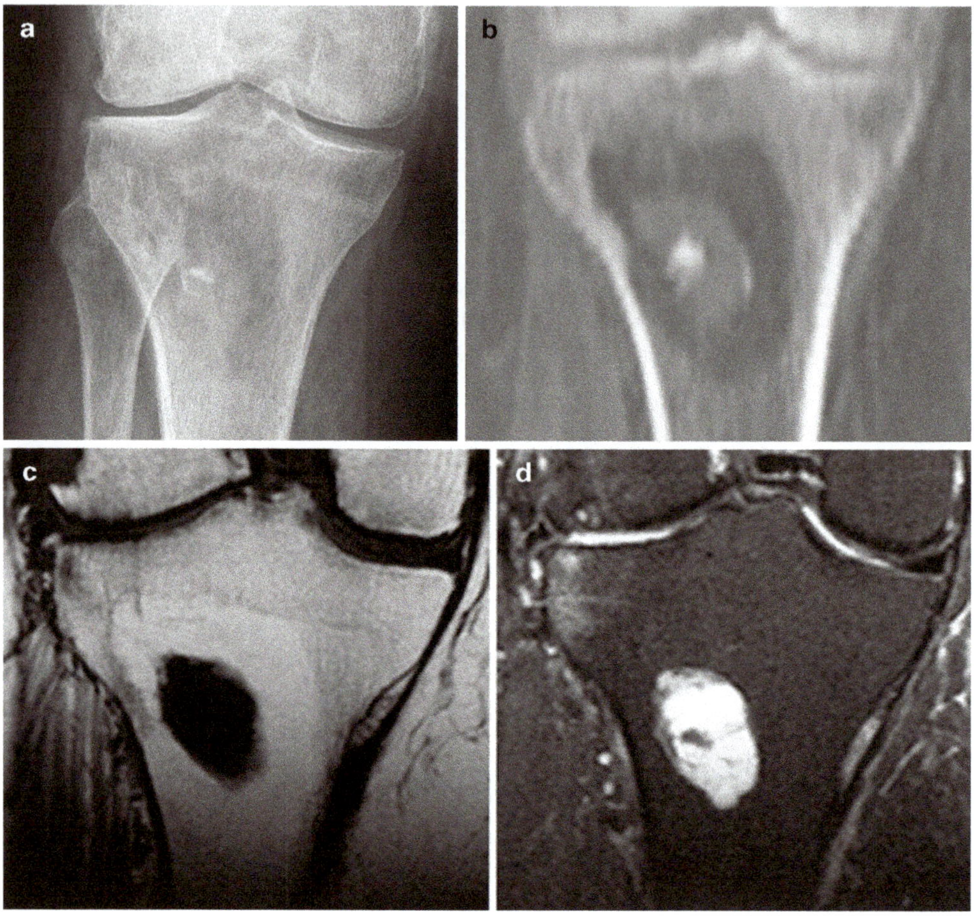

Fig. 10.4

History

A 51-year-old woman with knee pain.

Imaging Findings

Radiograph (a) —There is a lesion in the proximal tibia with a central calcification and peripheral zone of lucency. Moderate osteoarthritis of the lateral compartment of the knee is seen.
CT (b) —The lesion has a central focus of calcification, middle layer of fluid density, and outer layer of fatty density.
MRI—T1-weighted MR image (c) shows a low signal lesion surrounded by a peripheral zone of fat density. The central calcification is obscured by the area of low signal. The fat-saturated T2-weighted MR image (d) confirms that the peripheral layer contains fat as it is no longer visible. The central dystrophic calcification is now visible as a focus of low signal surrounded by fluid density. Incidental note is made of marrow edema and cartilage loss in the lateral compartment from osteoarthritis.

Differential Diagnosis (Best 3)

Fibrous dysplasia
Osteomyelitis with abscess
Intraosseous lipoma

Discussion

Recognizing that the lesion is composed mostly of fat and that intraosseous lipomas can have internal fluid signal are the key features of this case. The MR images are very helpful, but, if read independent of the radiograph or CT, can be confusing. The dystrophic calcification is obscured by the central necrosis on the T1 image and the peripheral zone of fat disappears against the background of the normal fatty marrow on the fat suppressed MR image. Fibrous dysplasia would be unlikely to have central necrosis and dystrophic calcification. An intraosseous abscess could be considered based on the T2 MR image; however, the peripheral fatty component would not be expected with an abscess.

Diagnosis

Intraosseous lipoma

Key Points

- Rare benign fatty tumor of bone.
- Asymptomatic, occasionally dull pain.
- Most common in proximal femur, calcaneus, and tibia.
- Can undergo involution, necrosis, cyst formation, and central calcification (from fat necrosis).
- CT and MRI can be useful to show fatty content, cystic necrosis, and central calcification.
- Milgram classification (based on involutional changes):
  - *Stage 1*—lesions have viable fat cells with no necrosis.
  - *Stage 2*—lesions have viable fat cells and areas of necrosis and calcification.
  - *Stage 3*—lesions have complete or near-complete fat necrosis with calcification, cyst formation, and reactive new bone formation.
- Asymptomatic lesions without risk for fracture are followed; otherwise, treatment consists of curettage and bone grafting.

Suggested Reading

Mandl P, Mester A, Balint PV. A black hole in the bone – intraosseous lipoma. J Rheumatol. 2009;36(2):434–6.
Milgram JW. Intraosseous lipomas: radiologic and pathologic manifestations. Radiology. 1988; 167:155–60.

Case 5

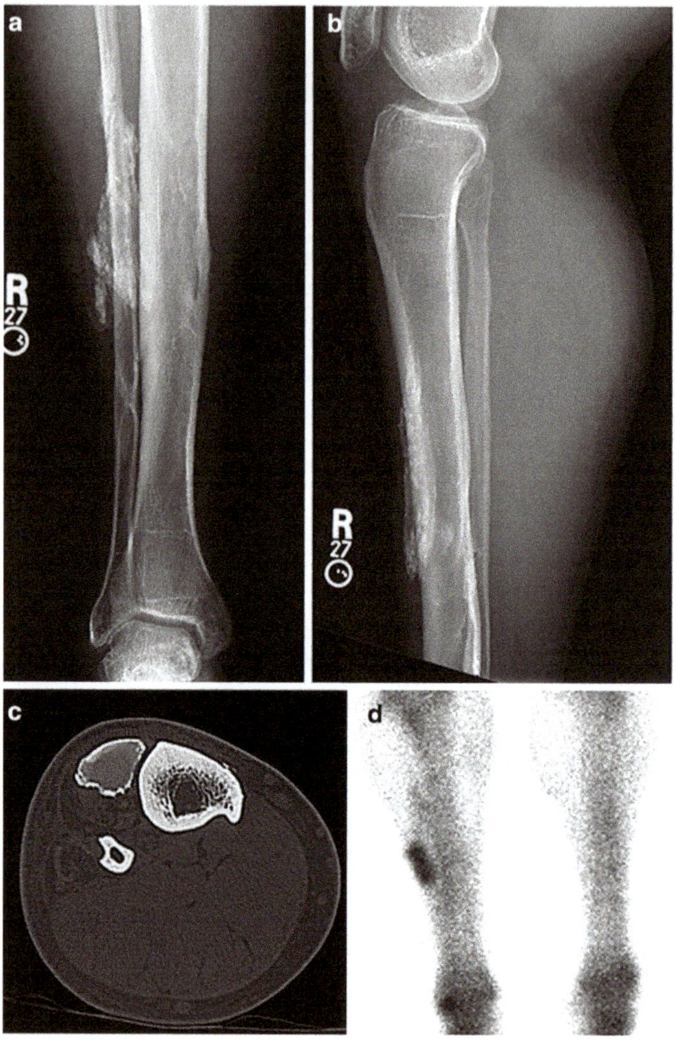

Fig. 10.5

History

A 65-year-old man with chronic mild lower leg pain.

Imaging Findings

The AP (a) and lateral (b) lower leg radiographs show dense mineralization adjacent to the tibia anterolaterally at its midportion. There is deformity of the fibula and tibia suggestive of old healed fractures. The axial CT image (c) shows a soft tissue mass with peripheral mineralization in the anterior muscle compartment of the lower leg separate from the tibial cortex. The tibia at this same level shows mild cortical thickening. The bone scintigraphy scan (d) shows moderate uptake in the calcified soft tissue mass, but no activity in the tibia.

Differential Diagnosis (Best 3)

Parosteal osteosarcoma
Myositis ossificans
Synovial sarcoma

Discussion

Based on the radiographs, it is unclear whether the calcifications are arising from the tibia or localized to the soft tissues. Cortically based lesions would include a surface osteosarcoma and osteochondroma. The CT image demonstrates that the lesion is clearly separate from the bone and the peripheral calcifications are more typical of maturing myositis ossificans than the irregular calcifications seen with a synovial sarcoma. Moreover, the healed fracture deformities confirm prior trauma at this site as a cause of the heterotopic ossification.

Diagnosis

Myositis ossificans

Key Points

- Abnormal formation of mature lamellar bone in the soft tissues.
- Can be posttraumatic, nontraumatic, or neurogenic in origin.
- Predisposing factors include burns, paraplegia, surgery, traumatic brain injury, hemophilia, polio, ankylosing spondylitis, and diffuse idiopathic skeletal hyperostosis (DISH).
- Due to metaplasia of the soft tissue elements into tissue capable of forming bone.
- Patients may be asymptomatic or have pain, swelling, and elevated erythrocyte sedimentation rate.
- Although the new bone formation can be contiguous with the adjacent bone, it is typically separate and does not involve the periosteum.
- Mineralization is rarely seen on radiographs in the first few weeks, but can become apparent 3–8 weeks after onset, starting peripherally and progressing centrally, in a "zonal" pattern.
- Bone scintigraphy is likely the best imaging modality to assess the maturity of the bone formation (decreased activity with maturation).
- Nonsurgical options using indomethacin, bisphosphonates (prophylaxis), and radiation are typically favored over surgical intervention.

Suggested Reading

Kransdorf MJ, Meis JM, Jelinek JS. Myositis ossificans: MR appearance with radiologic–pathologic correlation. AJR Am J Roentgenol. 1991;157:1243–8.
Mavrogenis AF, Soucacos PN, Papagelopoulos PJ. Heterotopic ossification revisited. Orthopedics. 2011;34(3):177.
Parikh J, Hyare H, Saifuddin A. The imaging features of post-traumatic myositis ossificans, with emphasis on MRI. Clin Radiol. 2002;57:1058–66.

Case 6

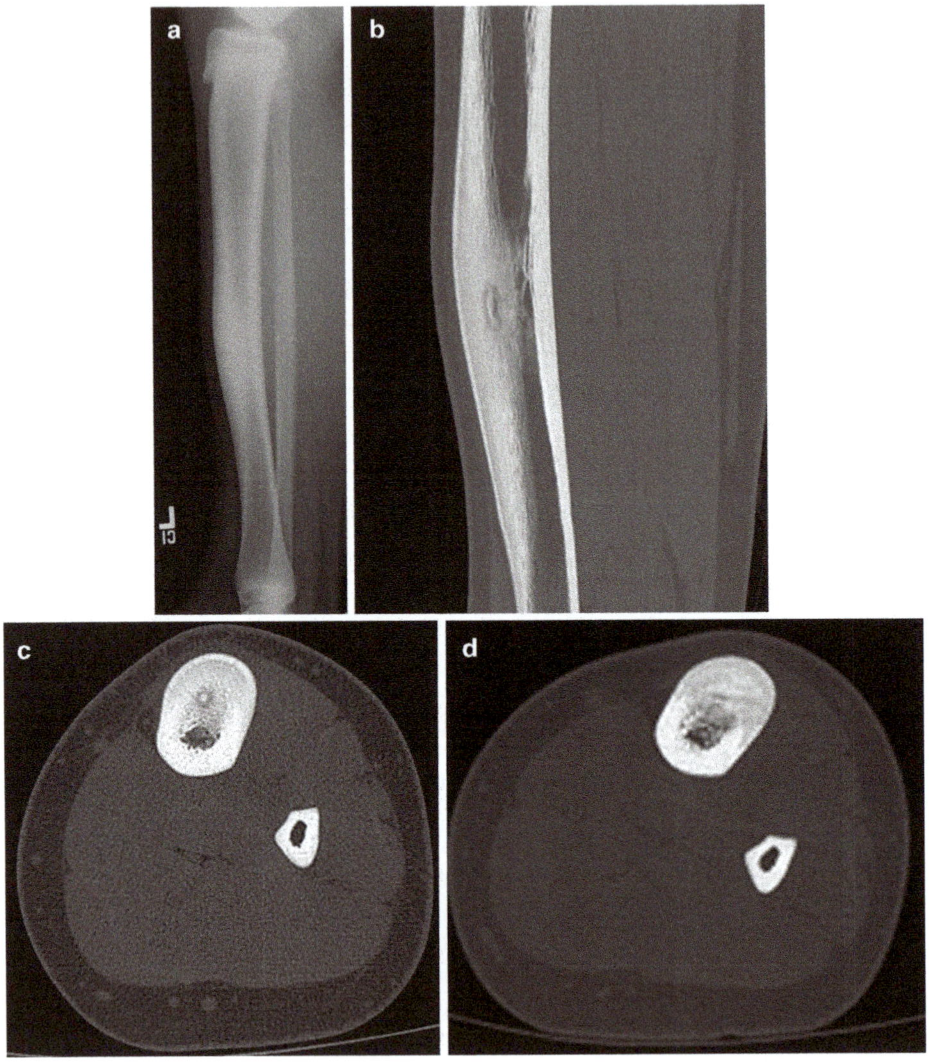

Fig. 10.6 (**d**) Six months after treatment. Images courtesy of Dr. Jennifer Son, Boston, MA

History

A 15-year-old girl with shin pain.

Imaging Findings

Lateral radiograph (a) of the lower leg shows an area of smooth nonaggressive periosteal thickening of the anterior tibial cortex. The sagittal (b) and axial (c) CT images show a small lucency with central calcification in the anterior cortex, with surrounding cortical thickening in the anterior tibial cortex. Axial CT image (d), 6 months after treatment, shows resolution of the lucency.

Differential Diagnosis (Best 3)

Osteoid osteoma
Osteomyelitis (Brodie's abscess)
Stress fracture

Discussion

From the radiograph alone, any diagnosis in the "Best 3" would be equally appropriate without additional clinical history. From the CT images, an osteoid osteoma is most likely given the small nidus and cortical location, which would be less typical of a Brodie's abscess. The lucency seen in stress fractures is typically more linear. The follow-up CT image after radiofrequency ablation (RFA) shows resolution of the central nidus.

Diagnosis

Osteoid osteoma

Key Points

- Common bone tumor in the young.
- The lucent nidus, which contains highly vascularized connective tissue, is the actual tumor.
- The sclerosis or periosteal reaction is a sequela of the tumor acting on the host bone.
- Almost always painful and although "pain relieved by aspirin" can occur with many bone tumors, this feature is very common with osteoid osteomas.
- The lucent nidus may not be visible on radiographs (as in this case) and is better seen with CT.
- No malignant potential. Can spontaneously resolve.
- Treated with pain management, excision, or radiofrequency ablation.

Suggested Reading

Chai JW, Hong SH, Choi JY, et al. Radiologic diagnosis of osteoid osteoma: from simple to challenging findings. Radiographics. 2010;30:737–49.

Case 7

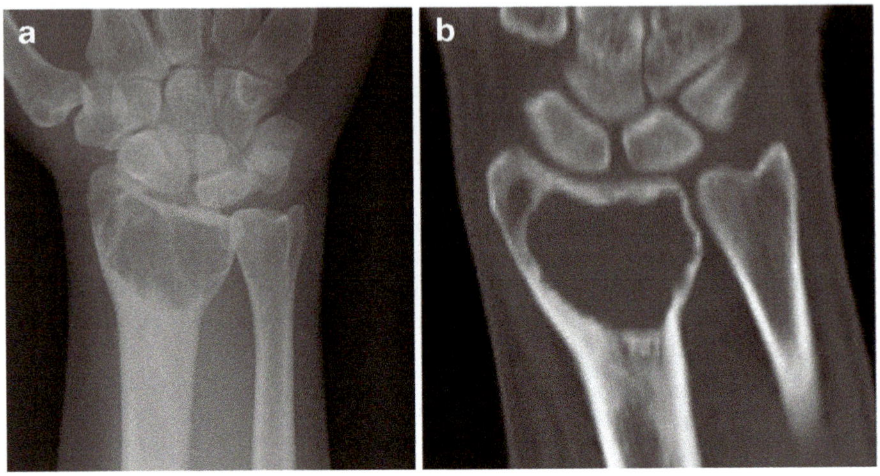

Fig. 10.7

History

A 32-year-old woman with wrist pain.

Imaging Findings

There is a well-circumscribed, geographic, lucent lesion in the distal radius, extending from the metaphysis to the subarticular surface, with negligible surrounding sclerosis and no internal matrix. The cortex is thinned and expanded, without periosteal new bone formation. A few pseudotrabeculae are noted on the radiograph (a), but no true septations are seen on the CT (b).

Differential Diagnosis (Best 3)

Aneurysmal bone cyst (ABC)
Simple bone cyst (SBC)
Giant cell tumor (GCT)

Discussion

Extension from the metaphysis to the epiphysis is very typical for GCT, as is the Type IB (well-defined, without sclerotic rim) pattern of bone destruction. ABCs are classically more expansile, with more pronounced cortical thinning. Both lesions are eccentric. SBC is unlikely in this case, because, when in long bones, it usually occurs in individuals less than 20 years old, and only a small percentage of SBCs occur outside the proximal humerus, femur, or tibia. Moreover, SBCs can extend up to the metaphyseal plate, but usually do not extend beyond it. Diagnosis notwithstanding, this lesion is at high risk for pathologic fracture and warrants treatment.

Diagnosis

Giant cell tumor

Key Points

- Relatively common, almost exclusively in skeletally mature patients, peak 20–45 years old.
- Majority occur in the long bones about the knee.
- GCTs originate in metaphysis and extend into epiphysis.
- Cortical thinning is common, with cortical expansion and penetration in 50%.
- Sclerotic rim is unusual.
- Benign GCTs can be locally aggressive, with soft tissue extension, and can recur locally.
- Many GCTs are treated due to fracture risk; may be packed with methylmethacrylate cement.
- Benign "metastasizing" GCT in 2–3%, with benign metastases (or perhaps implants) to lungs.
- Malignant transformation can occur after multiple resections for recurrence or after radiation.

Suggested Reading

Murphey MD, Nomikos GC, Flemming DJ, et al. From the Archives of the AFIP: imaging of giant cell tumor and giant cell reparative granuloma of bone: radiologic pathologic correlation. Radiographics. 2001;21:1283–309.
Turcotte RE. Giant cell tumor of bone. Orthop Clin N Am. 2006;37:35–51.
Siebenrock KA, Unnni KK, Rock MG. Giant-cell tumour of bone metastasizing to the lungs. JBJS (Br). 1998;80B:43–7.

Case 8

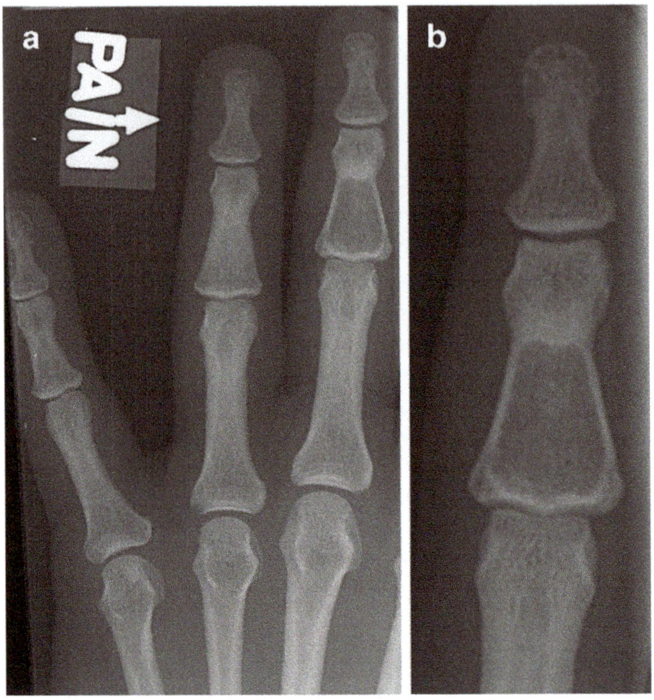

Fig. 10.8

History

A 26-year-old woman with pain in the tip of the ring finger after trauma.

Imaging Findings

AP radiographs (a, b) of the hand shows a geographic well-circumscribed nonaggressive lesion in the middle phalanx of the long finger (away from the site of pain). There is no appreciable matrix mineralization and there is slight bony expansion with thinning of the cortex.

Differential Diagnosis (Best 3)

Enchondroma
Giant cell tumor (GCT)
Aneursymal bone cyst (ABC)

Discussion

Statistically, enchondroma would be the most likely lesion, based its common occurrence in the hands. Benign giant cell tumors and aneursymal bone cysts could have an identical radiographic appearance, but are less common. A metastasis would be unlikely in the digits, especially in someone under 40 years of age without known disease. An important consideration in this case is the degree of cortical thinning, which can predispose to pathologic fracture following minor trauma. Prophylactic treatment with curettage and cancellous bone grafting should be considered.

Diagnosis

Enchondroma

Key Points

- Most common bone tumor in the hand.
- Enchondromas in the hands and feet often lack cartilaginous matrix when compared to enchondromas in larger long bones (femur, humerus, and tibia).
- Bony expansion, cortical endosteal scalloping, and pathologic fracture are more likely to occur in the small tubular bones of the hands and feet and do not necessarily indicate malignant transformation.
- Enchondromas in the hands very rarely undergo malignant transformation to chondrosarcomas.
- Recurrence rate is relatively high with curettage and bone grafting, thus radiographic follow-up is important.

Suggested Reading

Gaulke R, Suppelna G. Solitary enchondroma at the hand. Long-term follow-up study after operative treatment. J Hand Surg. 2004;29(1):64–6.

Case 9

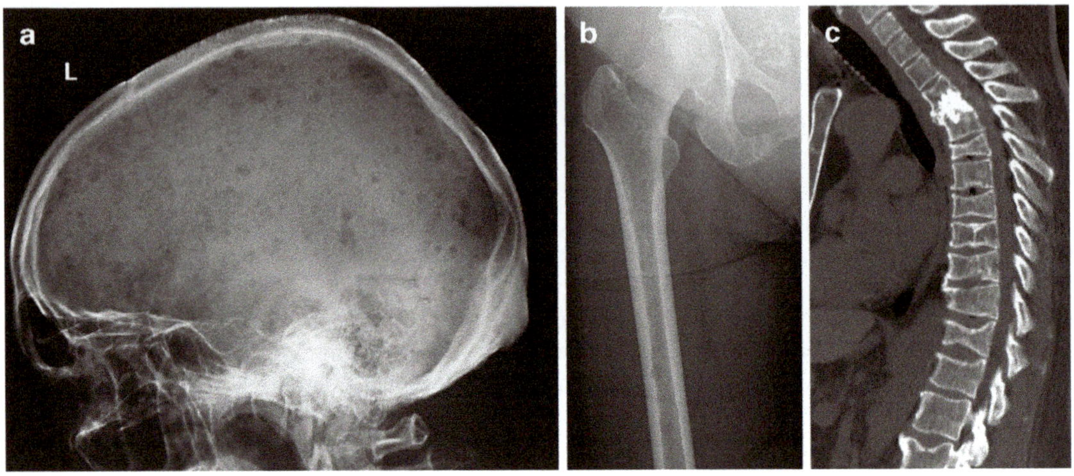

Fig. 10.9

History

A 58-year-old man with back pain.

Imaging Findings

Radiographs (a, b) demonstrate innumerable small rounded lytic lesions in the skull and right femur. The lesions are mostly similar in size (<1 cm), have a "punched out" appearance, and lack a sclerotic rim. Pathologic superior and inferior pubic ramus fractures are also noted. The sagittal CT image (c) demonstrates diffuse osteopenia and multiple vertebral body compression fractures.

Differential Diagnosis (Best 3)

Multiple myeloma
Lytic metastases
Langerhans cell histiocytosis (LCH)

Discussion

Multiple "punched out" round lytic lesions in the skull are highly suggestive of myeloma, particularly when similar in size. The diagnosis is supported by diffuse osteopenia and vertebral body compression fractures. Lytic metastases are less likely to be discrete and uniform in size or to create discrete endosteal scalloping. LCH can cause multiple lytic lesions and vertebral body compressions in children, but, in adults, it usually presents with only one to a few bone lesions.

Diagnosis

Multiple myeloma

Key Facts

- Most common primary malignant tumor of bone.
- Can occur in any bone, but axial skeleton is the most common site (follows sites of adult hematopoietic marrow).
- At presentation, 12–25% have diffuse osteopenia, without detectable focal lesion.
- Monoclonal M component spike is present in serum or urine protein electrophoresis in 99%, Bence Jones proteins (monoclonal light chain) in serum in 75%.
- Workup and follow-up is performed with skeletal survey rather than bone scan, because only a small percentage of lesions will show activity on bone scans; some sites use PET scans or "whole body" MRI.
- Small percentage (<3%) of lesions are purely sclerotic and some of these are associated with POEMS syndrome.

Suggested Reading

Angtuaco EJ, Fassas AB, Walker R, et al. Multiple myeloma: clinical review and diagnostic imaging. Radiology. 2004;231:11–23.
Susanne Lütje S, & de Rooy, JWJ, Sandra Croockewit S, et al., Role of radiography, MRI and FDG-PET/CT in diagnosing, staging and therapeutical evaluation of patients with multiple myeloma. Ann Hematol. 2009;88:1161–8.
Meletios A, Dimopoulos LA, Moulopoulos ID, et al. Imaging of myeloma bone disease. Acta Oncol. 2000;39(7):823–7.

Case 10

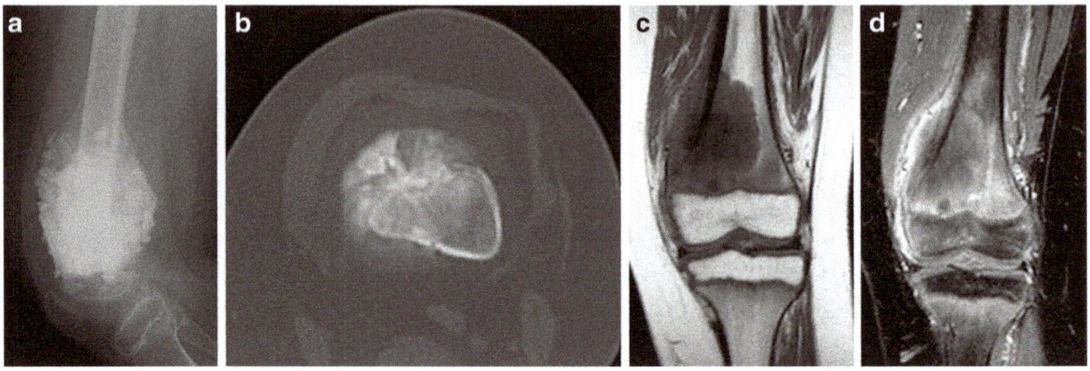

Fig. 10.10 Images courtesy of Dr. Jennifer Son, Boston, MA

History

A 16-year-old girl with knee pain and swelling.

Imaging Findings

The radiograph (a) shows a large mass in the distal femur containing dense mineralization, irregular borders, and cortical breakthrough anteriorly and posteriorly. The axial CT image (b) shows osteoid matrix extending into the adjacent soft tissues. The T1 (c) and fat-saturated T2-weighted (d) MR images show that the lesion involves that majority of the medial medullary cavity and contains areas of low signal due to osteoid matrix. The lesion does not extend into the joint space and ends near the physis.

Differential Diagnosis (Best 3)

Chondrosarcoma
Fracture (hypertrophic nonunion)
Osteosarcoma (conventional)

Discussion

The lesion is aggressive, based on the cortical breakthrough and extensive new bone formation. The appearance of osteosarcomas can depend on the amount of osteoid matrix, varying from very dense lesions (as in this case) to lytic lesions containing minimal osteoid matrix. The calcifications in chondrosarcomas tend to be more delicate, ranging from punctate to "arcs and rings" patterns. However, the type of matrix mineralization can be difficult to classify at times. Poorly healing fractures can sometimes present with exuberant, aggressive-appearing callus, but the fracture line should be discernable on CT. Nonetheless, the aggressiveness of this lesion should lead to biopsy.

Diagnosis

Osteosarcoma (conventional)

Key Points

- Second most common primary tumor of bone (#1 is myeloma), 20% of all bone malignancies.
- Distal femur is the most common site (40%); typically metaphyseal (90%).
- Variable appearance on radiographs, depending on the amount of osseous matrix and lesion aggressiveness.
- May contain chondroblastic or fibroblastic elements (i.e., chondroblastic osteosarcoma). Even if only 1% of the lesion is osseous, it is still classified as an osteosarcoma.
- Many reactive processes that produce reparative bone can mimic osteosarcoma. These include infection, trauma, and myositis ossificans.

Suggested Reading

Federman N, Bernthal N, Eilber FC, Tap WD. The multidisciplinary management of osteosarcoma. Curr Treat Options Oncol. 2009;10:82–93.
Suresh S, Saifuddin A. Radiological appearances of appendicular osteosarcoma: a comprehensive pictorial review. Clin Radiol. 2007;62:314–23.
Picci P. Osteosarcoma (osteogenic sarcoma). Orphanet J Rare Dis. 2007;2:6.

Case 11

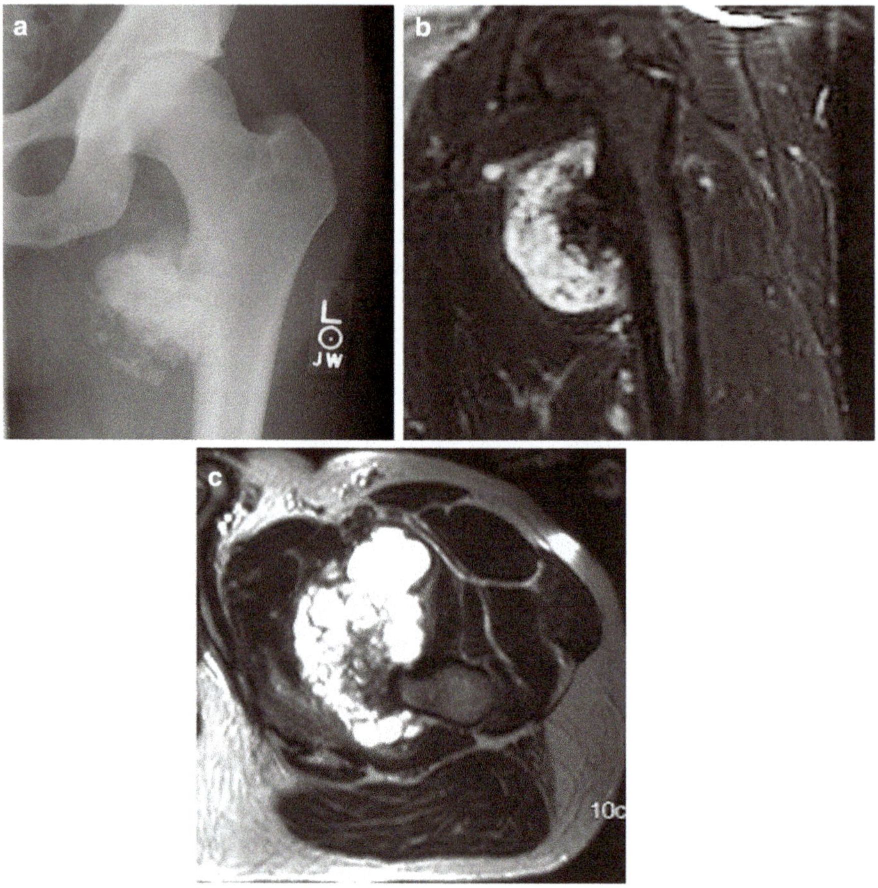

Fig. 10.11

History

A 39-year-old man with groin pain.

Imaging Findings

The AP hip radiograph (a) shows a surface-based lesion arising from the medial aspect of the proximal femur just below the lesser trochanter. There is dense mineralization centrally with suggestion of chondroid matrix at the periphery. The MRI images (b and c) show a C-shaped cap (maximum 8 cm thick), which is high signal on T2-weighted images. Note the continuity between the medullary cavities of the lesion and the host bone on the axial T2-weighted image (c).

Differential Diagnosis (Best 3)

Osteochondroma
Chondrosarcoma
Surface osteosarcoma (parosteal)

Discussion

The key to this lesion is determining whether there is continuity with the host bone or not. If so, then an osteochondroma should be highest on the differential. In this case, the medullary cavities are connected (best seen on the axial MR image instead of the radiographs), thus a surface chondrosarcoma or osteosarcoma is less likely and this lesion is most likely an osteochondroma. The cartilage cap is abnormally enlarged (>1.5 cm) and malignant transformation should be suspected. Biopsy and surgical resection revealed an osteochondroma with malignant transformation of the cartilage cap into a chondrosarcoma.

Diagnosis

Chondrosarcoma (malignant degeneration of cartilage cap in an osteochondroma)

Key Points

- Osteochondroma is the most common benign tumor of bone.
- Complications are related to local mass effect (bursitis and aneurysms), fractures, and malignant transformation of the cartilaginous cap into chondrosarcoma (1% of lesions).
- The cartilage cap decreases with age and should not grow after skeletal maturity.
- Although cartilage caps greater than 1.5 cm in thickness should raise suspicion for malignant transformation, the cap usually measures >5 cm in proven cases of malignant transformation.
- Changes in the orientation of the chondroid mineralization in the cap on radiographs can be a subtle sign of malignant transformation.

Suggested Reading

Woertler K, Lindner N, Gosheger G, Brinkschmidt C, Heindel W. Osteochondroma: MR imaging of tumor-related complications. Eur Radiol. 2000;10:832–40.
Lee KC, Davies AM, Cassar-Pullicino VN. Imaging the complications of osteochondromas. Clin Radiol. 2002;57:18–28.
Murphey MD, Choi JJ, Kransdorf MJ, Flemming DJ, Gannon FH. Imaging of osteochondroma: variants and complications with radiologic–pathologic correlation. Radiographics. 2000;20:1407–34.

Case 12

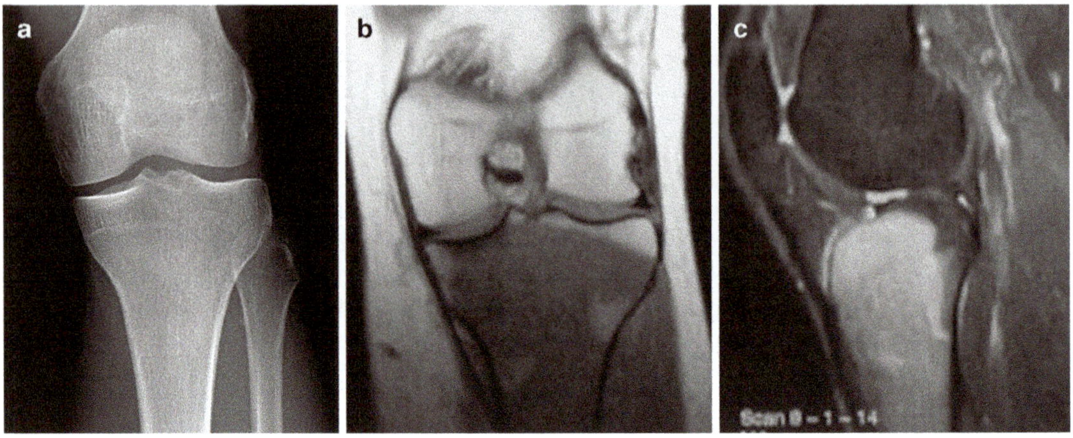

Fig. 10.12

History

A 24-year-old woman with knee pain.

Imaging Findings

The AP knee radiograph (a) is normal. The T1-weighted MR image (b) shows low signal in the proximal tibia which is isointense to muscle and extends to the articular surface, traversing the expected location of the physeal scar (seen as a thin line of sclerosis on the radiograph). The lesion is hyperintense on the fat-saturated T2-weighted MR image (c).

Differential Diagnosis (Best 3)

Hematopoietic (red marrow)
Primary non-Hodgkin lymphoma (B cell) of bone
Stress fracture

Discussion

It is important not to dismiss the signal abnormality in the tibia as hematopoietic marrow. Hematopoietic marrow typically has low signal on T1 weighted images; however, the signal should be brighter than the adjacent skeletal muscle. Moreover, hematopoietic marrow typically ends at the physeal scar and should not extend across into the epiphysis (except in the femoral and humeral heads, where it can be subarticular). These findings in this case suggest a marrow-replacing process, which includes lymphoma. Edema related to a stress fracture is possible; however, the signal abnormality in this case is quite diffuse and there is a sharp interface between the tumor and the adjacent normal marrow. Moreover, although not necessary to diagnose a stress fracture, no fracture line is identified. Note that the marrow abnormalities are occult on the radiograph and only seen on the MRI.

Diagnosis

Primary non-Hodgkin lymphoma (B cell) of bone

Key Points

- Primary lymphoma of bone is defined as lymphoma occurring only in bone, without disease in the lymph nodes or other tissue.
- Bony metastases from systemic Hodgkin or non-Hodgkin lymphoma (NHL) is much more common than primary lymphoma of bone.
- Primary lymphoma of bone is almost always due to NHL (usually diffuse B cell) instead of Hodgkin's (only few case reports).
- Can have a varied appearance with osteolytic and sclerotic lesions. There is marrow replacement and the lesions can have a large soft tissue component.
- The femur, pelvis, tibia, and humerus are the most commonly affected sites.
- Has a favorable cure rate (80–90%) using radiotherapy and chemotherapy.

Suggested Reading

Singh T, Satheesh CT, Lakshmaiah KC, Suresh TM, Babu GK. Primary bone lymphoma: a report of two cases and review of the literature. J Can Res Therap. 2010;6(3):296–8.
Bhagavathi S, Fu K. Primary bone lymphoma. Arch Pathol Lab Med. 2009;133:1868–71.
Krishnan A, Shirkhoda A, Tehranzadeh J, Armin AR, Irwin R, Les K. Primary bone lymphoma: radiographic-MR imaging correlation. Radiographics. 2003;23:1371–87.

Case 13

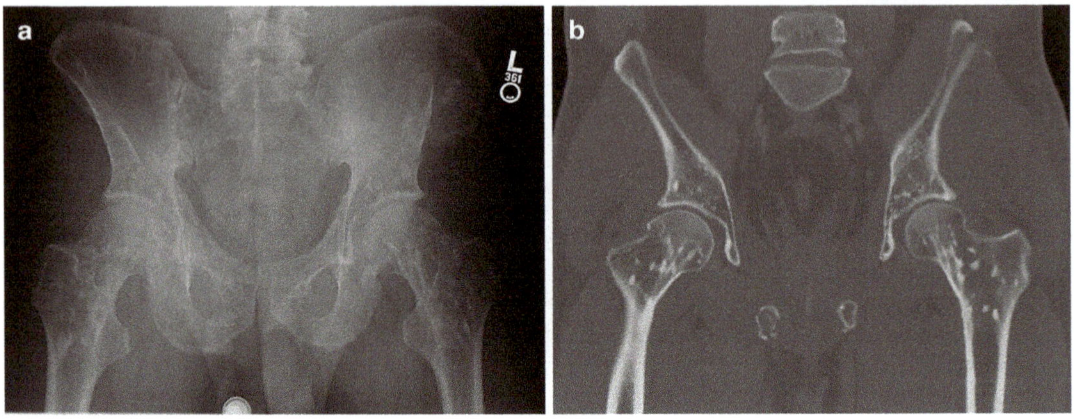

Fig. 10.13

History

A 58-year-old man with left sided pelvic pain following car accident.

Imaging Findings

There are numerous small round sclerotic foci in the femurs and pelvic bones. Fracture of the left upper iliac wing is seen on both the radiograph (a) and CT image (b).

Differential Diagnosis (Best 3)

Osteopoikilosis
Osteoblastic metastases
Tuberous sclerosis

Discussion

The sclerotic foci in osteopoikilosis are typically smaller that those seen with diffuse osteoblastic metastases or tuberous sclerosis. Patients with tuberous sclerosis often have other clinical findings (renal masses, subependymal tubers, nail and skin abnormalities, and seizures). Prostate cancer is the most common malignancy to cause sclerotic metastases and patients usually have a PSA level >10 ng/mL.

Diagnosis

Osteopoikilosis

Key Points

- Aka "spotted bones" disease.
- Sclerosing bone dysplasia characterized by numerous small sclerotic foci (bone islands) in periarticular osseous regions.
- Pelvic bones are the most common site of involvement.
- Cause is unknown.
- Typically no uptake in bone scinitigraphy.
- Usually asymptomatic, but occasionally associated with joint pain (15–20%).
- Can have scleroderma-like skin lesions, dwarfism, dystocia (difficult childbirth), and spinal stenosis.
- Association with other sclerosing bone dysplasias (osteopathia striata and melorheostosis).

Suggested Reading

Ellanti P, Clarke B, Gray J. Osteopoikilosis. Ir J Med Sci. 2010;179:615–6.
Lagier R, Mbakop A, Bigler A. Osteopoikilosis: a radiological and pathological study. Skeletal Radiol. 1984;11(3):161–8.

Case 14

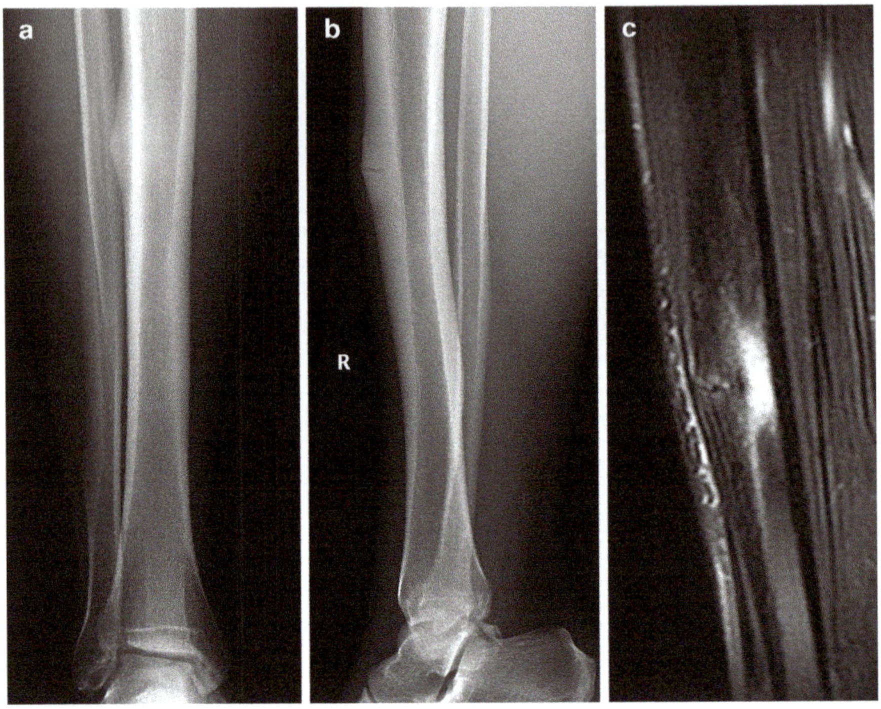

Fig. 10.14

History

A 23-year-old long distance runner with pain in the anterior tibia.

Imaging Findings

AP (a) and lateral (b) radiographs of the lower leg shows an area of thick periosteal reaction in the anterolateral tibial shaft. Centered in the periosteal reaction, there is a linear lucency which is perpendicular to the long axis of the tibia. The fat-saturated T2-weighted MR image (c) demonstrates edema in and adjacent to the linear defect.

Differential Diagnosis (Best 3)

Osteoid osteoma
Brodie's abscess
Stress facture

Discussion

Periosteal reaction and marrow edema can be seen in any of the three entities listed above. The linear lucent fracture line is the most helpful feature, as the nidus in an osteoid osteoma or Brodie's abscess is round in most cases. However, a linear cloaca can be seen with a Brodie's abscess. Based on the history, stress fracture is the most likely of the three. Additional considerations in this case would include osteosarcoma and Ewing sarcoma; however, both of these tumors typically have a more aggressive appearance and can have a soft tissue component. Lastly, stress fracture, in contrast to many of the other processes, can show healing on subsequent exams.

Diagnosis

Stress fracture

Key Points

- Stress fractures are overuse injuries that occur in the setting of unusual or repeated stress to normal bone (fatigue fracture) or normal stress to abnormally weakened bone (insufficiency fracture).
- The most common sites for stress fractures are in the femoral neck, metatarsals, tarsals, and tibia (posterior medial or anterolateral aspect).
- Mechanism is partly due to poor response of the bone to tensile instead of compressive forces.
- The appearance of a stress fracture depends on the stage of healing and is often not visible on early radiographs.
- MRI and bone scan can help detect stress fractures and stress response earlier than radiographs.
- The lucent fracture line is often perpendicular to the cortex.

Suggested Reading

Spitz DJ, Newberg AH. Imaging of stress fractures in the athlete. Radiol Clin N Am. 2002;40: 313–31.

Bergman AG, Fredericson M, Ho C, Matheson GO. Asymptomatic tibial stress reactions: MRI detection and clinical follow-up in distance runners. AJR. 2004;183:635–8.

Case 15

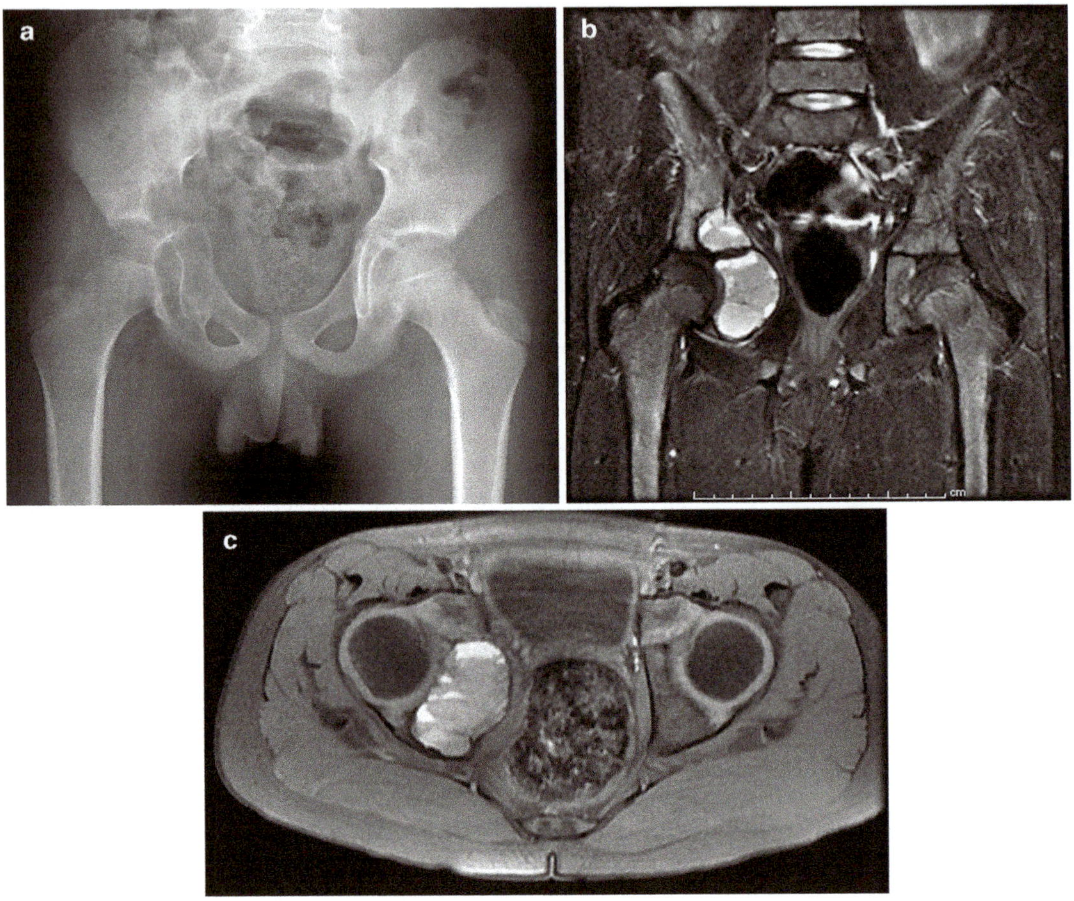

Fig. 10.15 Images courtesy of Dr. Jennifer Son, Boston MA

History

A 13-year-old boy with right hip pain.

Imaging Findings

The patient is skeletally immature, with a large, expansile lytic lesion in the right acetabulum. A segment of cortex along the medial iliac bone appears indistinct on the radiograph (a), but thinly intact on the MRI. Fat-saturated coronal T2 (b) and axial T1 (c) MR images show a geographic lesion, with multiple fluid–fluid levels.

Differential Diagnosis (Best 3)

Simple bone cyst (SBC)
Telangiectatic osteosarcoma
Aneurysmal bone cyst (ABC)

Discussion

All three lesions could have this appearance and could occur in a skeletally immature person. MRI excludes SBC, which should be unilocular. Telangiectatic osteosarcoma can also occur in this age group and can mimic ABC, but, on MRI, 89% of telangiectatic osteosarcomas have cortical breakthrough, with a soft tissue component. Though osteoblastoma can look like ABC on MRI, with multiple fluid levels, osteoblastoma is a rare lesion, especially in the pelvis, and ABC-like osteoblastomas usually occur in the spine.

Diagnosis

Aneurysmal bone cyst

Key Points

- Not common; most patients are 5–20 years old.
- Seventy percent of ABCs are primary and benign, but 30% occur as secondary lesions and can be found in association with other benign or malignant tumors.
- Eccentric, metaphyseal, and markedly expansile, with severe cortical thinning, often with periosteal new bone (even when cortex intact).
- Most occur in long bones (femur, tibia, and humerus), also posterior elements of spine, pelvis and hands.
- Can cross disc into adjoining vertebral body.
- Multiple fluid–fluid levels are best seen on CT and MRI.

Suggested Reading

Mankin HJ, Hornicek FJ, Ortiz-Cruz E, et al. Aneurysmal bone cyst: a review of 150 patients. J Clin Oncol. 2005;23(27):6756–62.
Munk PL, Helms CA, Holt RG. MR imaging of aneurysmal bone cysts. AJR Am J Roentgenol. 1989;153:99–101.

Case 16

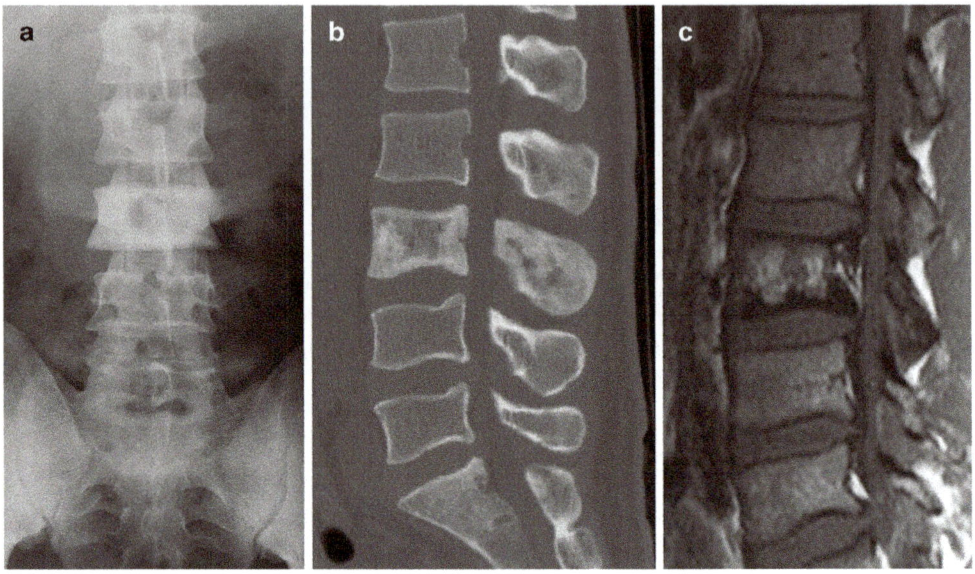

Fig. 10.16

History

Back pain.

Imaging Findings

AP radiograph (a) shows diffusely increased density in the L3 vertebral body, an "ivory vertebral body." CT (b) reveals that the bony sclerosis is somewhat patchy, the cortices of L3 are thickened, and the abnormality also involves the L3 spinous process, which appears larger than those at other levels. T1 weighted MRI image (c) shows high signal fat in the lesion, with low signal sclerosis.

Differential Diagnosis (Best 3)

Paget disease
Sclerotic metastasis
Lymphoma (rarer sclerotic form)

Discussion

Paget disease commonly affects lumbar vertebral bodies and results in thickened cortex, coarsened trabeculae, and enlargement of the bone. Bony enlargement is highly suggestive of Paget. Both metastases and lymphoma could produce patchy sclerosis in a vertebral body, but would not result in cortical thickening or bony enlargement, and sclerotic lymphoma is very rare. CT exams of hemangiomas typically demonstrate a "corduroy" or "polka dot" pattern of prominent vertical trabeculae and fatty marrow density.

Diagnosis

Paget disease

Key Facts

- Classic definition of ivory vertebral body: increased radiographic density, without change in the size or shape of the vertebra and without abnormalities of the adjacent disc spaces.
- Differential diagnosis: metastasis (breast, prostate, and less likely, carcinoid), lymphoma, Paget disease (though can cause enlarged vertebra), infection (often multiple vertebrae), and idiopathic segmental sclerosis (response to stress).
- In children, consider: Hodgkin lymphoma (most common), osteosarcoma, metastases (neuroblastoma and medulloblastoma), and osteoblastoma.
- Paget disease is due to excessive, abnormal bone remodeling, perhaps caused by paramyxovirus.
- Majority of cases involve the axial skeleton (pelvis) and/or proximal femur; often polyostotic, but asymmetric.
- Can be asymptomatic, incidental, with elevated alkaline phosphatase.
- Imaging appearance is varied and depends on the phase of the disease (lytic, mixed, and sclerotic).
- In the lytic phase, osteolysis begins at the epiphysis and advances towards the diaphysis (flame-shaped, blade of grass appearance), though in the tibia, changes can begin away from epiphysis.
- Sclerotic phase hallmarks are coarsened trabeculae, cortical thickening, and bony enlargement; may develop "cotton wool" appearance in skull.
- Patterns in spine: "picture frame", ivory vertebra.
- Usually diagnosed on radiograph but CT can be useful to show characteristic features.
- MRI appearance is variable, but normal marrow fat signal excludes sarcomatous degeneration.

Suggested Reading

Graham TS. The ivory vertebra sign. Radiology. 2005;235:614–5.
Theodorou DJ, Theodorou SJ, Kakitsubata Y. Imaging of Paget disease of bone and its musculoskeletal complications: review. Am J Roentgenol. 2011;196 (6):S64–75.
Silverman IE, Flynn JA. Images in clinical medicine. Ivory vertebra. N Engl J Med. 1998;338:100.

Case 17

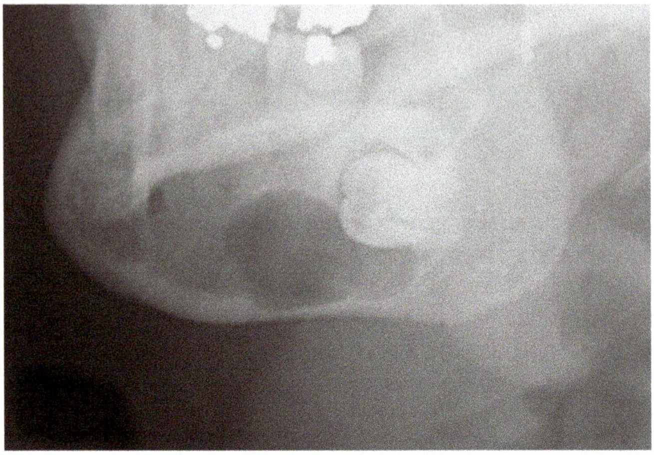

Fig. 10.17

History

A 51-year-old man with jaw pain.

Imaging Findings

There is a well-circumscribed lucent lesion in the mandibular ramus without appreciable internal matrix. There is scalloping of the cortex, but no cortical breakthrough or obvious soft tissue component. The lesion is adjacent to an unerupted molar tooth.

Differential Diagnosis (Best 3)

Dentigerous cyst
Ameloblastoma
Aneurysmal bone cyst (ABC)

Discussion

Cystic lesions in the mandible are quite common and are often odontogenic cysts (i.e., lesions related to tooth development). The dentigerous cyst is a common odontogenic cyst that develops in the normal dental follicle surrounding an unerupted tooth. It usually appears as a single lucent lesion with well-defined margins. Ameloblastoma is an epithelial tumor that arises from the dental lamina and can appear as an expansile multilocular radiolucency, often near the third lower molar. Aneursymal bone cysts are also multilocular and can have a honeycomb or soap bubble appearance, with eccentric expansion. Periosteal reaction may be present with ABCs but is not common with dentigerous cysts, unless fractured.

Diagnosis

Dentigerous cyst

Key Points

- A subtype of odontogenic cysts (not neoplastic).
- Overgrowth of a normal dental follicle surrounding an unerupted (often molar) tooth.
- Typically asymptomatic, but can distort adjacent teeth and cause pain.
- Often an incidental radiographic finding, but can grow to a large size, leading to pathologic fracture.
- Usually a single cystic lesion adjacent to an unerupted molar tooth, without bony expansion or periostitis.
- Can occasionally contain dystrophic calcifications.
- Multilocular and expansile lucent lesions in the mandible should raise suspicion for tumors such as an ameloblastoma or ABC.
- Tumors can arise from cells in the walls of the dentigerous cyst, including mucoepidermoid carcinoma, ameloblastoma, and squamous cell carcinoma.
- If small and asymptomatic, dentigerous cysts can be observed; large lesions should be biopsied and removed.

Suggested Reading

Avelar RL, Antunes AA, Carvalho RW, Bezerra PG. Odontogenic cysts; a clinicopathological study of 570 cases. J Oral Sci. 2009;51(4):581–6.
Núñez-Urrutia S, Figueiredo R, Gay-Escoda C. Retrospective clinicopathological study of 418 odontogenic cysts. Med Oral Patol Oral Cir Bucal. 2010;15(5):e767–73.

Case 18

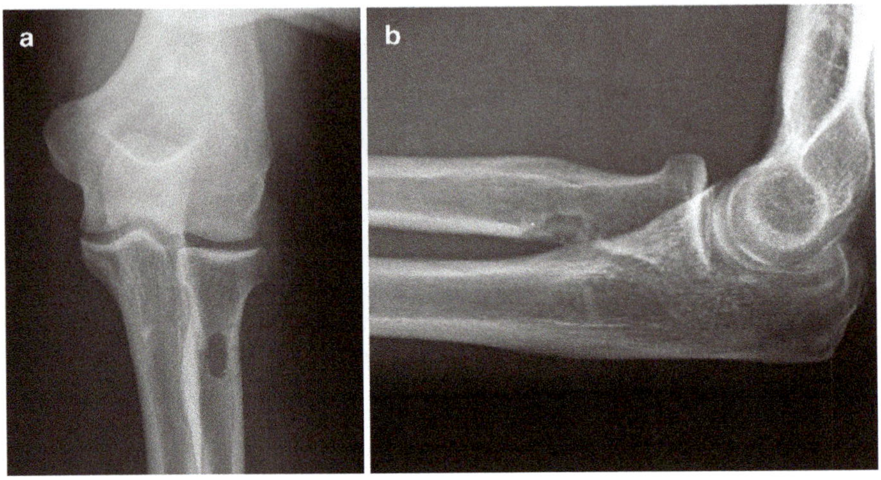

Fig. 10.18

History

A 48-year-old man with improved elbow pain.

Imaging Findings

There is lucent oval lesion in the radial tuberosity on both the AP (a) and lateral (b) views of the elbow. The lesion has a well-defined margin without sclerotic borders. It extends from the cortex into the medullary cavity on the lateral view and there is no associated periostitis or soft tissue component.

Differential Diagnosis (Best 3)

Radial tuberosity pseudolesion
Distal biceps tendon repair pseudolesion
Multiple myeloma

Discussion

The key to this case is the location of the lesion. The lesion is at the radial tuberosity, the distal biceps tendon attachment site. Although a lucent pseudolesion can be seen on a lateral view of the elbow due to a relative paucity of trabeculae, the lucent lesion in this case is well seen on both the AP and lateral views. The appearance is consistent with a distal biceps tendon repair. Coupled with the correct clinical/surgical history (which may require some detective work), the diagnosis should be relatively straightforward. If there has been no prior surgery, then both metastasis and myeloma should be considered as they are common bone tumors in adults.

Diagnosis

Distal biceps tendon repair pseudolesion

Key Points

- Iatrogenic causes can create focal osseous lesions leading to unnecessary workup/treatment, thus it is important to investigate all relevant clinical/surgical history thoroughly.
- Rupture of the distal biceps tendon typically occurs on the dominant side, in middle-aged men, during eccentric stress with the elbow in a flexed position.
- More common in males and increased risk with smokers and steroid users.
- Two predisposing factors for biceps tendon rupture are (1) poor vascular supply to the tendon near the radial attachment and (2) mechanical impingement during pronation and supination.
- The postoperative lucency is a trough created by a motorized burr, through which the biceps tendon is threaded and sutured down.
- Heterotopic ossification can occur at the site of repair, further confusing the picture, if one is not aware of the surgical history.

Suggested Reading

Chillemi C, Marinelli M, De Cupis V. Rupture of the distal biceps brachii tendon: conservative treatment versus anatomic reinsertion – clinical and radiological evaluation after 2 years. Arch Orthop Trauma Surg. 2007;127:705–8.

Case 19

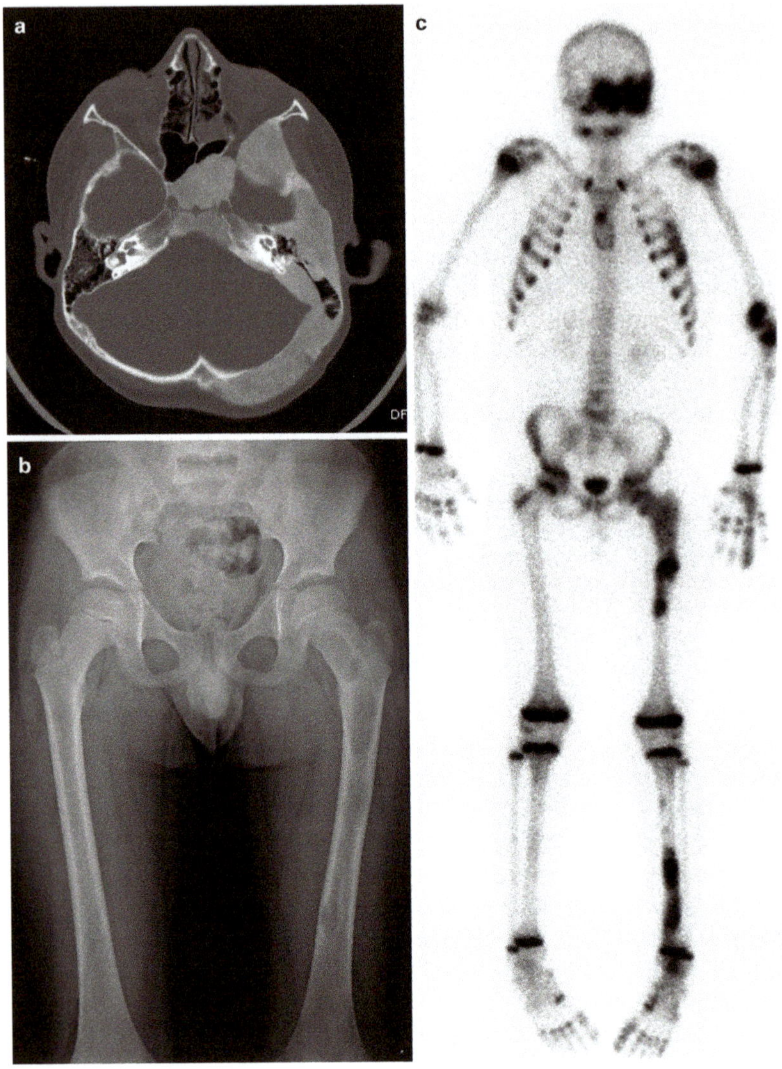

Fig. 10.19 Images courtesy of Dr. Jean-Marc Gauguet, Boston, MA

History

A 13-year-old boy with skull deformity.

Imaging Findings

Axial CT (a) shows expansion of the left cranial vault with ground glass density and absence of the usual corticomedullary differentiation. The radiograph (b) demonstrates multiple elongated, well-circumscribed, lucent lesions in the left femur, also with ground glass density. The radiouclide bone scan (c) shows multiple areas of increased activity in the skull, ribs, and left femur and tibia, corresponding to abnormalities on the CT and radiographs. Increased activity at the unfused physes is a normal finding.

Differential Diagnosis (Best 3)

Maffucci syndrome with multiple enchondromas
Jaffe–Campanacci syndrome (JC) with multiple non-ossifying fibromas
Polyostotic fibrous dysplasia

Discussion

Although all three diagnoses could account for multiple lucent lesions in an adolescent, the appearance of the skull, with enlargement of the bones and ground glass density, is pathognomonic for fibrous dysplasia. Enchondromas should demonstrate chondroid calcifications and are generally more rounded and lobulated, though, in Maffucci syndrome, the enchondromas often create more pronounced bone deformities. In any event, enchondromas are not associated with the intense bone scan activity seen here. JC syndrome is quite rare, has "coast of California" café au lait spots, and, like other non-ossifying fibromas, the lesions are metadiaphyseal and often eccentric.

Diagnosis

Polyostotic fibrous dysplasia

Key Points

- Polyostotic fibrous dysplasia can occur independently or as part of McCune–Albright syndrome.
- McCune–Albright consists of (1) polyostotic fibrous dysplasia, (2) cafe au lait spots, and (3) sexual precocity and/or other endocrine abnormalities and is more common in women. Need only two features to diagnose the syndrome.
- While monostotic FD is often asymptomatic, polyostotic fibrous dysplasia is more likely to be earlier-onset, have larger lesions, and be symptomatic: pain, swelling, limp, bowing of limbs, fractures, craniofacial deformity, and scoliosis.
- Common sites: femur, tibia, pelvis, foot, and craniofacial.
- Usually predominantly on one side of body.
- Skull findings: widening of diploic space, outer table convexity; deformity of orbits, sinuses and neural foramina.
- Leontiasis ossea (lion face)—refers to a rare form of craniofacial polyostotic fibrous dysplasia causing facial deformity and enlargement.
- Bone scans are helpful for demonstrating polyostotic disease—normal to marked activity.
- Most lesions cease or have slow growth at puberty, but deformities can continue.

Suggested Reading

Fitzpatrick KA, Taljanovic MS, Speer DP, et al. Imaging findings of fibrous dysplasia with histopathologic and intraoperative correlation. AJR Am J Roentgenol. 2004;182:1389–98.
Chapurlat RD, Orcel P. Fibrous dysplasia of bone and McCune–Albright syndrome. Best Pract Res Clin Rheumatol. 2008;22(1):55–69.
Theoret CM, Packota GV, Leswick DA. Case of the month #153. Leontiasis ossea. Can Assoc Radiol J. 2009;60(4):213–6.

Case 20

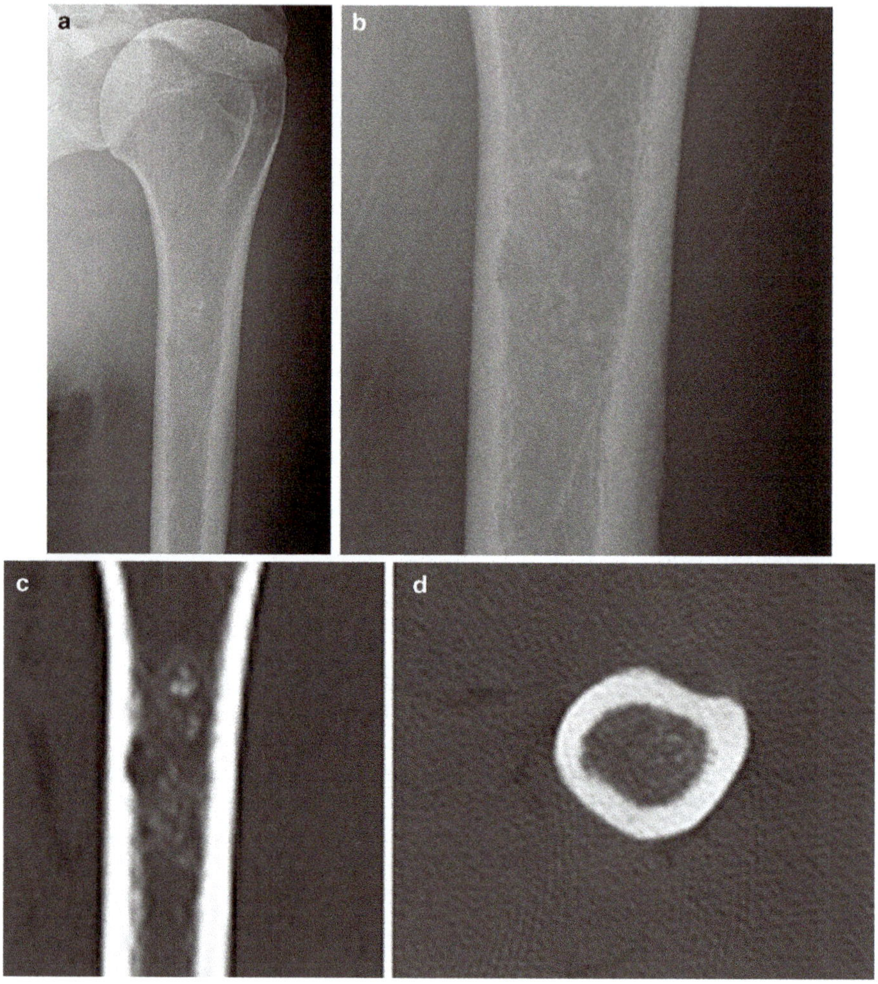

Fig. 10.20

History

A 43-year-old woman with asymptomatic lesion seen in humerus.

Imaging Findings

The radiograph (a) and magnified view (b) show a lesion in the proximal humeral diaphysis containing punctuate central calcifications. There is mild endosteal scalloping of the medial cortex involving <2/3 of the thickness. There is no associated periostitis or cortical breakthrough. The CT images (c and d) confirms the presence of a chondroid lesion with punctuate calcifications and mild endosteal scalloping of the medial humeral cortex.

Differential Diagnosis (Best 3)

Enchondroma
Bone infarct
Chondrosarcoma

Discussion

The first step in this case is determining whether chondroid matrix is present. Although this lesion has fewer calcifications than the typical enchondroma, the punctate morphology and central location of the calcifications suggests a chondroid lesion. Bone infarcts tend to have well-demarcated sclerotic borders. Next, the scalloping of the medial humeral cortex should raise some concern for a higher grade chondroid lesion. Endosteal scalloping of >2/3 of the cortical thickness is the best distinguishing feature between an enchondroma and a low grade chondrosarcoma. This lesion has roughly 25% cortical scalloping, thus is still within normal limits for an enchondroma.

Diagnosis

Enchondroma

Key Points

- Enchondromas are very common.
- Lesions typically have a lobulated appearance due to lobulated growth of hyaline cartilage (increased surface area allows better use of adjacent nutrients).
- Endosteal scalloping of the cortex (amongst other factors) can help distinguish an enchondroma from chondrosarcoma.
- CT is very useful in depicting the degree of endosteal scalloping.
- Other features, such as periosteal reaction, cortical breakthrough, soft tissue extension, and large lesion size (>5 cm), would raise concern for either a low grade chondrosarcoma or dedifferentiation into a higher grade chondrosarcoma.

Suggested Reading

Bui KL, Ilaslan H, Bauer TW, Lietman SA, Joyce MJ, Sundaram M. Cortical scalloping and cortical penetration by small eccentric chondroid lesions in the long tubular bones: not a sign of malignancy? Skeletal Radiol. 2009;38:791–6.

Case 21

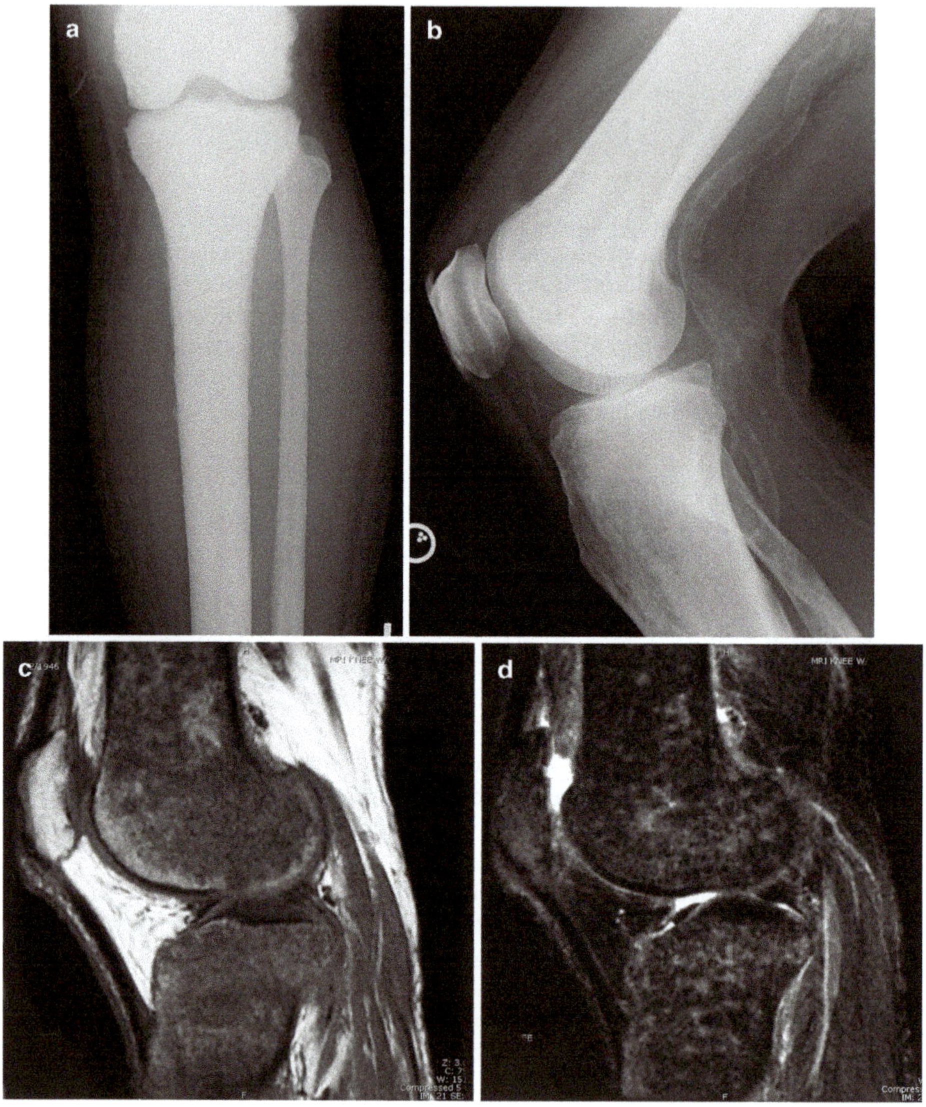

Fig. 10.21

History

A 55-year-old man with hepatosplenomegaly and weakness.

Imaging Findings

The radiographs of the lower leg (a) and knee (b) show diffuse sclerosis of the distal femur, proximal tibia, and to a lesser extent, the fibula. There is no cortical breakthrough or soft tissue component. There is diffuse low signal marrow on both the T1- (c) and T2-weighted (d) MR images extending to the articular surface, without much marrow edema.

Differential Diagnosis (Best 3)

Mastocytosis
Myelofibrosis
Osteoblastic metastases

Discussion

From the radiographs, one should recognize that this is a case of "dense bones." The MR images show that the marrow is diffusely low signal on both T1 and T2, which can be seen with fibrosis. This appearance, together with the history of hepatosplenomegaly, is compatible with either mastocytosis or myelofibrosis. Patients with mastocytosis experience symptoms (flushing, urticaria, syncope, and bronchospasm) related to mast cells' release of vasoactive products (histamine). It would be unusual to have hepatosplenomegaly with osteoblastic metastatic disease and more common to have discrete sclerotic osseous lesions than diffusely dense bones.

Diagnosis

Myelofibrosis

Key Points

- Uncommon myeloproliferative disease characterized by progressive marrow fibrosis and extramedullary hematopoiesis with sclerotic appearing bones.
- Some believe myelofibrosis is a variant of leukemia. It is associated with polycythemia vera, anemias, and chemical exposure (benzene).
- Can be primary (idiopathic) or secondary.
- Found in middle-age to elderly patients, rare in children.
- Weakness, anemia, weight loss, hepatosplenomegaly, and purpura.
- Usually dense bones (patchy or diffuse). Low T1 and T2 signal.
- Spine, pelvis, skull, ribs, and proximal femurs.
- Diagnosis by bone marrow biopsy.
- Degree of marrow fibrosis is indicative of disease severity.
- Poor prognosis (8% disease survival at 6–8 years).
- Differential for diffusely dense bones includes the following: myelofibrosis, osteopetrosis, osteoblastic metastases, mastocytosis, lymphoma, Paget disease, melorheostosis, fluorosis, renal osteodystrophy, and pyknodysostosis.

Suggested Reading

Diamond T, Smith A, Schnier R, Manoharan A. Syndrome of myelofibrosis and osteosclerosis: a series of case reports and review of the literature. Bone. 2002;30:498–501.

Guermazi A, de Kerviler E, Cazals-Hatem D, Zagdanski AM, Frija J. Imaging findings in patients with myelofibrosis. Eur Radiol. 1999;9:1366–75.

Case 22

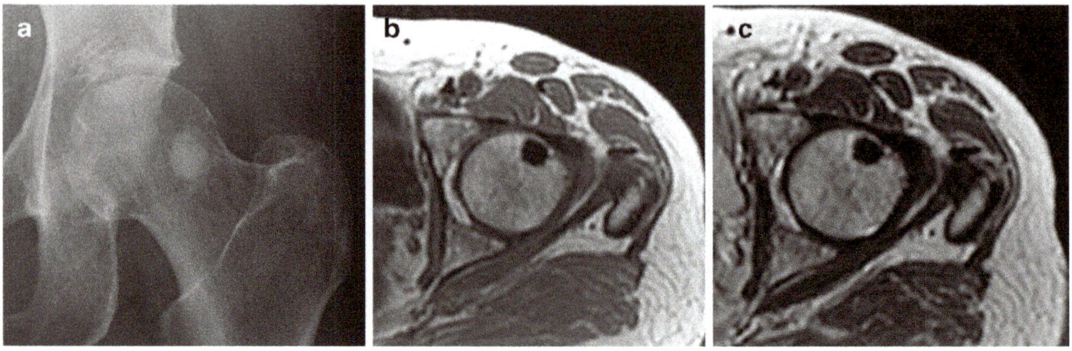

Fig. 10.22

History

A 56-year-old man with left hip pain.

Imaging Findings

Radiograph (a) shows a rounded sclerotic lesion in the femoral neck. The lesion is uniformly low signal on both the T1- (b) and T2-weighted (c) MR images. No perilesional marrow edema is seen.

Differential Diagnosis (Best 3)

Bone island
Sclerotic metastasis (prostate)
Low grade osteosarcoma

Discussion

Bone islands are low signal on T1 and T2 and very common; therefore, they should be highest on the differential list. However, sclerotic metastases can have a similar appearance. In a man with a PSA <10 ng/mL, prostate cancer bone metastasis is highly unlikely. However, following prostatectomy, any detectable serum PSA level implies the presence of metastatic disease. Low grade osteosarcomas are typically larger than this and can be painful, whereas bone islands are asymptomatic.

Diagnosis

Bone island

Key Points

- A bone island occurs when compact (cortical) bone develops in the medullary cavity, thus they are hamartomas and not true tumors.
- They typically occur next to joints, are oval, have a slightly spiculated border, parallel the long axis of the host bone, and should not have perilesional edema.
- They should be painless and need to be distinguished from osteoblastic metastases.

Suggested Reading

Greenspan A, Steiner G, Knutzon R. Bone island (enostosis): clinical significance and radiologic and pathologic correlations. Skeletal Radiol. 1991;20:85–90.
Greenspan A. Benign bone-forming lesions: osteoma, osteoid osteoma, and osteoblastoma. Clinical, imaging, pathologic, and differential considerations. Skeletal Radiol. 1993;22:485–500.

Case 23

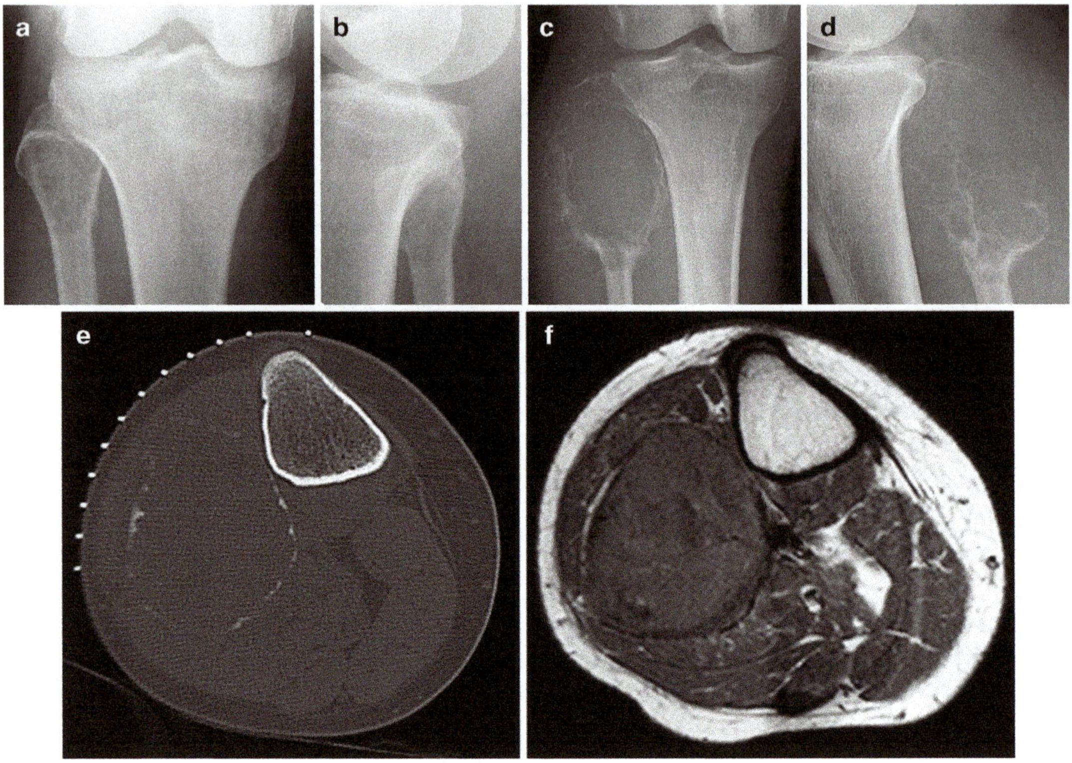

Fig. 10.23 (**a**, **b**) Initial presentation and (**c**, **d**, **e**, **f**) 5 years later

History

A 43-year-old man with slowing progressive knee pain and swelling over 5 years.

Imaging Findings

On the radiographs of the knee (a and b) at initial presentation, there is a lucent lesion without internal matrix in the proximal fibular head. There is subtle periosteal reaction along the medial cortex, best seen on the AP view, probably related to a healing pathologic fracture. Radiographs performed 5 years later (c and d) when the patient experienced more pain, show marked interval increase in the size of the lesion. The lesion is extremely expansile and has a "blown out" appearance, with marked cortical thinning, irregularity, and fenestration. There is a pathologic fracture at the base of the lesion, with associated periosteal new bone formation. CT image (e) demonstrates marked expansion and thinning of the cortex and the T1-weighted MRI image (f) shows low signal soft tissue extending beyond the cortex, anteriorly and posterolaterally.

Differential Diagnosis

Lytic metastases (renal cell or thyroid)
Giant cell tumor (GCT)
Aneurysmal bone cyst (ABC)

Discussion

On the later images, the lesion is clearly aggressive and will require biopsy. A bubbly lytic metastasis, such as renal cell or thyroid carcinoma, could have this appearance. However, it is unlikely that a metastasis could progress over 5 years, without presenting with overwhelming, widespread, metastatic disease. Moreover, expansion, rather than frank destruction, of the fibular head implies that the bone has had time to accommodate the growth of the lesion, which is also less likely in a metastasis. Giant cell tumor can be locally aggressive and can be very expansile when it occurs in a small caliber bone, such as the fibula. As expected with GCT, the lesion is arising in the metaphysis and extending to the epiphysis. ABC can cause significant expansion of a bone and can have cortical penetration, but it generally creates a smoother shell of expanded bone. Cortical penetration is rare in ABC and, when it occurs, is usually more localized. Moreover, ABC often shows fluid–fluid levels on cross-sectional imaging and none are seen here.

Diagnosis

Giant cell tumor

Key Points

- Relatively common lesion: 4–5% of all primary bone tumors.
- GCTs are slightly more common in women, but aggressive GCTs are three times more common in men.
- Campanacci described three types of GCTs: while most are Type II lesions that are well-defined but lack a sclerotic rim, Type III lesions appear aggressive and often have cortical destruction and soft tissue extension.
- The radiographic appearance is not thought to be predictive of histology or clinical behavior.
- "Malignant GCTs" are a heterogeneous group of giant-cell containing lesions that are capable of malignant behaviors; 5–10% of GCTs are malignant.
- CT is good for showing cortical detail, periosteal new bone, fluid levels, and to confirm absence of matrix.
- MRI is good for showing extension into the joint or surrounding soft tissues.

Suggested Reading

Turcotte RE. Giant cell tumor of bone. Orthop Clin N Am. 2006;37:35–51.

Case 24

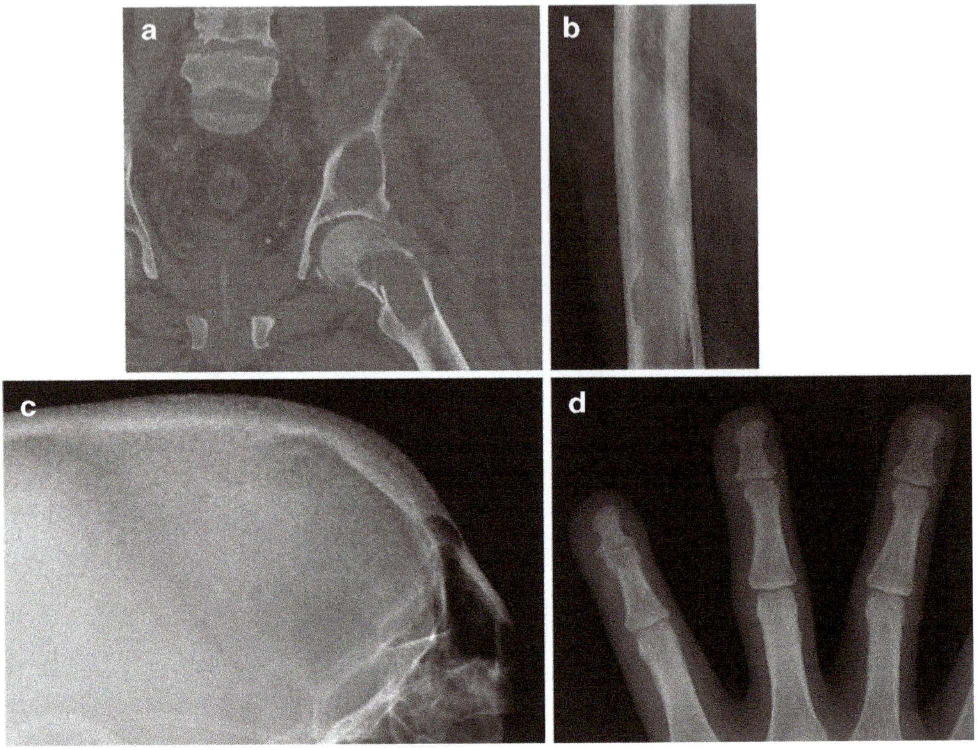

Fig. 10.24

History

A 64-year-old man with acute left hip pain.

Imaging Findings

The coronal CT image (a) of the pelvis shows well-circumscribed lytic lesions without internal matrix in the left acetabulum and the left proximal femur, which has a displaced femoral neck fracture. The radiograph (b) of the right femoral shaft shows several lytic lesions with cortical scalloping. The lateral skull (c) shows numerous small punctate lucent lesions, mostly in the frontal bone, producing a "salt and pepper" appearance. Finally, the AP view of the hand (d) shows osteopenia and subperiosteal cortical resorption along the radial aspects of the middle phalanges of the second to fourth fingers.

Differential Diagnosis (Best 3)

Lytic metastases
Multiple myeloma
Hyperparathyroidism (brown tumor)

Discussion

It is difficult to arrive at an exact diagnosis for this case without additional clinical history and laboratory results. The main teaching point is to recognize that when there are multiple lesions, one needs to consider other diseases besides metastases. Multiple myeloma, infection, fibrous dysplasia, Langerhans cell histiocytosis (in a young patient), and brown tumors from hyperparathyroidism could be considered. Performing a 24 h urine collection and urine and serum protein electrophoresis (UPEP/SPEP) can help to diagnosis multiple myeloma. Elevated levels of parathyroid hormone (PTH), elevated total and ionized calcium, and identifying a parathyroid adenoma on ultrasound or sestamibi scan help make the diagnosis of hyperparathyroidism. In this case, the thyroid ultrasound revealed a parathyroid adenoma and the sestamibi scan was also positive.

Diagnosis

Hyperparathyroidism (brown tumor)

Key Points

- Three types of hyperparathyroidism: (1) primary—increased PTH due to hyperfunctioning gland from parathyroid hyperplasia, adenomas, or carcinoma; (2) secondary—increased PTH due to hyperfunctioning of the parathyroid glands from hypocalcemic stimuli, often due to renal failure or malabsorption; and (3) tertiary (rare)—autonomous parathyroid glands from longstanding renal failure or malabsorption.
- Secondary hyperparathyroidism will have low or normal levels of calcium, whereas primary and tertiary hyperparathyroidism will have elevated levels.
- Brown tumors (osteoclastomas) can occur with all subtypes of hyperparathyroidism and represent accumulation of fibrous tissue and giant cells related to microfracture and hemorrhage from bone resorption.
- The brownish blood products in the lesions give rise to the name.
- With treatment, the lytic lesions should become sclerotic, and lack of a change with treatment should raise suspicion for an alternative diagnosis.
- Pseudohyperparathyroidism refers to a syndrome of hypercalcemia without signs of primary hyperparthryoidism or skeletal findings.

Suggested Reading

Meydan N, Barutca S, Guney E, et al. Brown tumors mimicking bone metastases. J Nat Med Assoc. 2006;98(6):950–3.
Davies AM, Evans N, Mangham DC, Grimer RJ. MR imaging of brown tumour with fluid-fluid levels: a report of three cases. Eur Radiol. 2001;11:1445–9.

Case 25

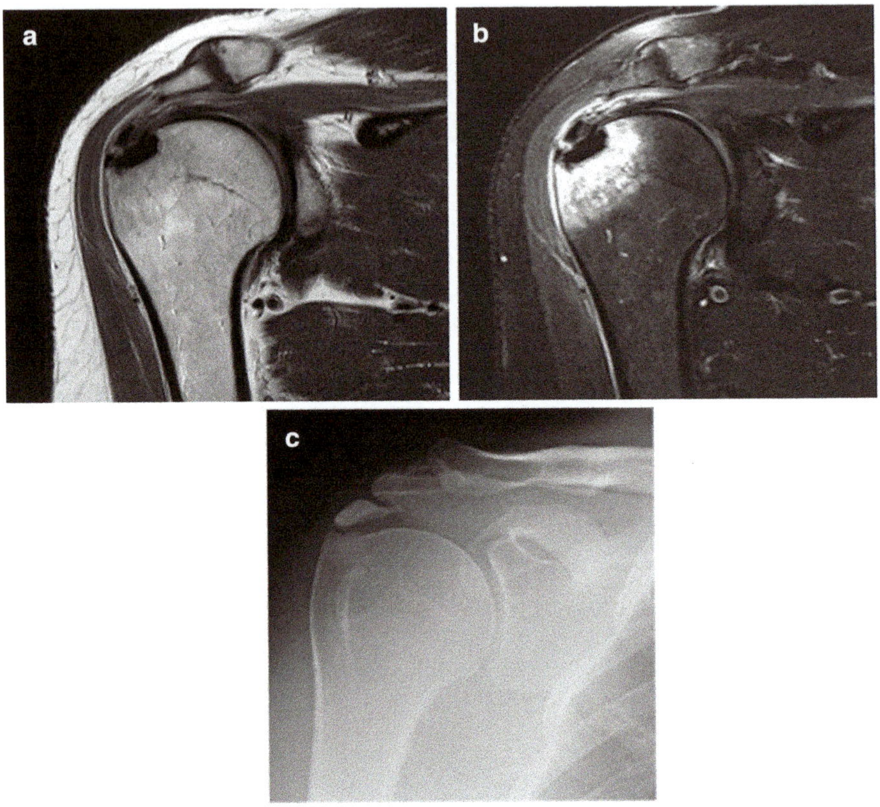

Fig. 10.25 (c) Six months earlier

History

A 47-year-old woman with severe acute on chronic shoulder pain.

Imaging Findings

The T1- (a) and fat-saturated T2-weighted (b) MR images show areas of marked low signal in the greater tuberosity and distal supraspinatus tendon. On the fat-saturated T2 image, prominent edema in the humeral head and distal supraspinatus tendon is seen surrounding the foci of low signal. The shoulder radiograph (c) performed 6 months earlier show an ossific density in the distal supraspinatus tendon near the greater tuberosity.

Differential Diagnosis (Best 3)

Calcific tendinitis (resorptive phase)
Trauma
Surface osteosarcoma

Discussion

The location of the findings is the key to this case. The most common location for calcific tendinitis is the shoulder, with the supraspinatus being the most common tendon affected. Calcific tendinitis has a varied appearance, depending on its stage. In this case, the acute resorptive phase shows marrow edema and irregularity of the calcifications in the osseous insertion of the tendon. The differential diagnosis includes direct trauma to the greater tuberosity with resultant marrow edema and ossific densities related to myositis ossificans. A surface osteosarcoma would be much less likely, because the marrow signal remains normal on the T1 MR image and the calcifications are separate from the bone, centered within the supraspinatus tendon.

Diagnosis

Calcific tendinitis (resorptive phase)

Key Points

- Due to deposition of hydroxyapatite crystals in the tendons.
- Acute clinical symptoms can be severe and can mimic infection or trauma.
- On imaging, calcific tendinitis can mimic aggressive processes such as infection or neoplasm.
- Self-limited, with analgesics for pain relief.
- Fluoroscopic or US guided percutaneous needle aspiration and/or injection of anesthetics can be performed.

Suggested Reading

Siegal DS, Wu JS, Newman JS, del Cura JL, Hochman MG. Calcific tendinitis: a pictorial review. Can Assoc Radiol J. 2009;60:263–72.
Flemming DJ, Murphey MD, Shekitka KM, et al. Osseous involvement in calcific tendinitis: a retrospective review of 50 cases. AJR. 2003;181:965–72. Case 25.

Case 26

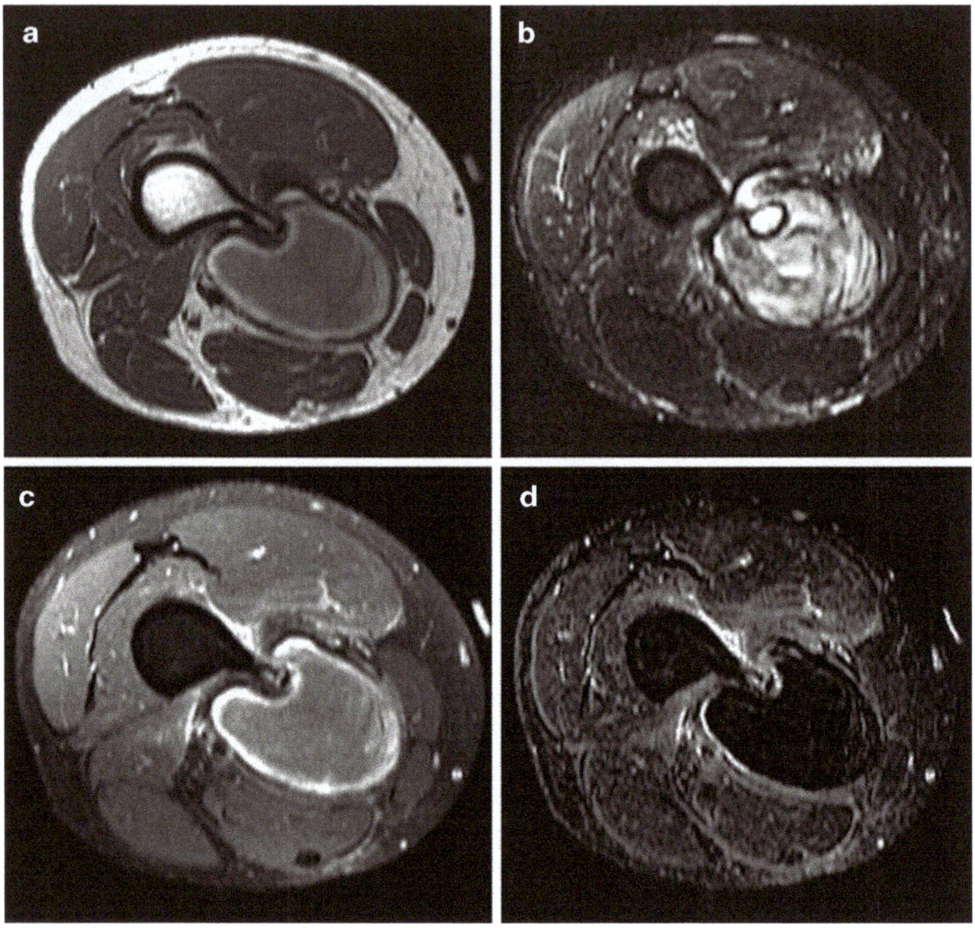

Fig. 10.26 (**a**) T1; (**b**) STIR; (**c**) postcontrast T1 fat-saturated; and (**d**) subtraction

History

A 47-year-old man with palpable medial thigh mass and pain.

Imaging Findings

MR of the right thigh shows a bony excrescence arising from the posteromedial femoral cortex at the level of the mid thigh. The medullary cavity and cortex of the lesion are continuous with the host femur, best seen on the T1 MR image (a). There is a lesion in the soft tissues adjacent to the exostosis which has a peripheral rim of hyperintensity on T1 and central heterogeneous hyperintensity on the STIR image (b). Although the soft tissue component has peripheral hyperintensity on the postcontrast fat-saturated T1-weighted image (c), the subtraction image (d) shows that there is no enhancement with contrast administration.

Differential Diagnosis (Best 3)

Osteochondroma with malignant transformation of the cartilaginous cap
Osteochondroma with reactive bursitis/hematoma
Surface osteosarcoma

Discussion

The first step to this case is to recognize that the bony lesion is an osteochondroma. The medullary cavities of the bone lesion and of the femur are continuous. The next step is to determine the significance of the C-shaped soft tissue mass. Given that there is a lack of enhancement, reactive bursitis should be considered. The presence of a high signal rim on the T1 and fat-saturated T1-weighted images supports a diagnosis of hemorrhagic bursitis or hematoma. The MRI appearance of this lesion is not good for an osteochondroma with malignant transformation of the cartilage cap, because there is no enhancement of the "cartilage cap." The cartilage cap in this osteochondroma has involuted, which typically occurs with age.

Diagnosis

Osteochondroma with reactive bursitis/hematoma

Key Points

- Osteochondromas are the most common benign tumor of bone.
- Complications are related to local mass effect (bursitis and aneurysms), fractures, and malignant transformation of the cartilaginous cap into chondrosarcoma (1% of lesions).
- Pedunculated osteochondromas have a higher association with fracture from direct trauma than sessile osteochondromas.
- Reactive bursal collections can become complicated by infection or hemorrhage.

Suggested Reading

Woertler K, Lindner N, Gosheger G, Brinkschmidt C, Heindel W. Osteochondroma: MR imaging of tumor-related complications. Eur Radiol. 2000;10:832–40.
Lee KC, Davies AM, Cassar-Pullicino VN. Imaging the complications of osteochondromas. Clin Radiol. 2002;57:18–28.
Murphey MD, Choi JJ, Kransdorf MJ, Flemming DJ, Gannon FH. Imaging of osteochondroma: variants and complications with radiologic–pathologic correlation. Radiographics. 2000;20:1407–34.

Case 27

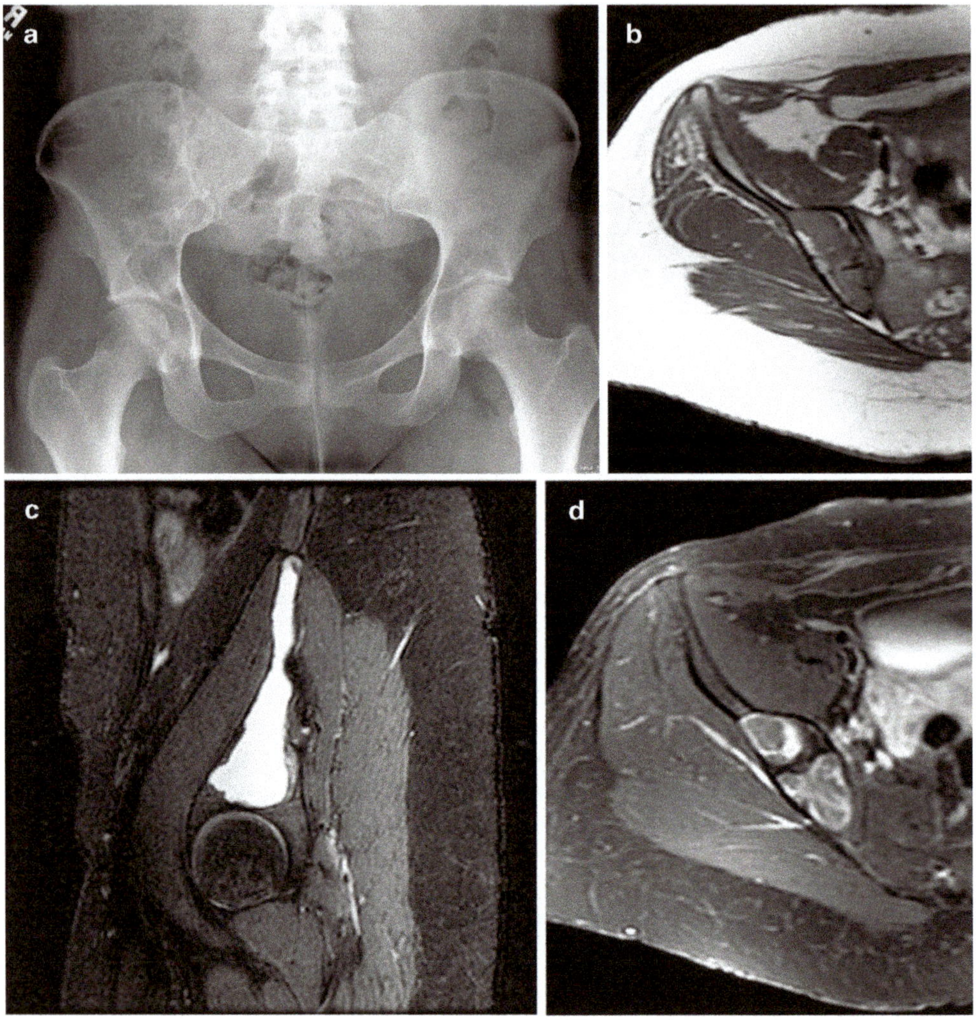

Fig. 10.27 Images courtesy of Dr. Jennifer Son, Boston, MA

History

A 25-year-old woman with groin pain and incidental finding on pelvis radiograph.

Imaging Findings

Radiograph (a) shows a large lytic lesion in the right iliac bone. Margins are not well seen radiographically. MRI shows a slightly expansile geographic lesion with well-defined margins, without reactive edema or soft tissue extension. There is a single, unilocular lesion, best delineated on the sagittal image. (Partial volume artifact on the postcontrast image (d) misleadingly suggests two separate, adjacent foci.) The lesion is homogeneous and isointense to muscle on T1 (b), homogeneously hyperintense on fat-saturated T2-weighted images (c), and has peripheral enhancement postcontrast (d).

Differential Diagnosis (Best 3)

Simple bone cyst (SBC)
Aneurysmal bone cyst (ABC)
Giant cell tumor (GCT)

Discussion

The key is recognizing that this is a unilocular cystic lesion. SBCs have well-defined borders, a thin sclerotic rim, and peripheral (but no internal) enhancement. In patients over 20 years old, SBC can occur in the iliac bone. ABC can occur in the same age group, but is more expansile and is multiloculated, often with multiple fluid levels. GCT rarely occurs in the iliac bone, but is in the differential, because the lesion can extend to the subchondral portion of the acetabulum. On MRI, GCT would appear more complex, either solid or solid and cystic. Metastases and plasmacytoma are the most common tumors in the bony pelvis, but the patient is young and the lesion is cystic, making these both unlikely.

Diagnosis

Simple bone cyst

Key Facts

- Formerly known as unicameral or solitary bone cyst.
- Single chamber, filled with simple fluid (if fractured, can contain serosanguinous fluid).
- Metaphysis or diaphysis of long bones; central; 90% in proximal humerus, femur, or tibia.
- Eighty percent of patients with SBC are <20 years old; asymptomatic or found due to fracture.
- Over 20 years old, may be found incidentally in the iliac bone, calcaneus, or talus.

Suggested Reading

Lee JHE, Reinus QR, Wilson AJ. Quantitative analysis of the plain radiographic appearance of unicameral bone cysts. Invest Radiol. 1999;34(1):28–37.
Margau R, Babyn P, Cole W, et al. MR imaging of simple bone cysts in children: not so simple. Pediatr Radiol. 2000;30:551–7.

Case 28

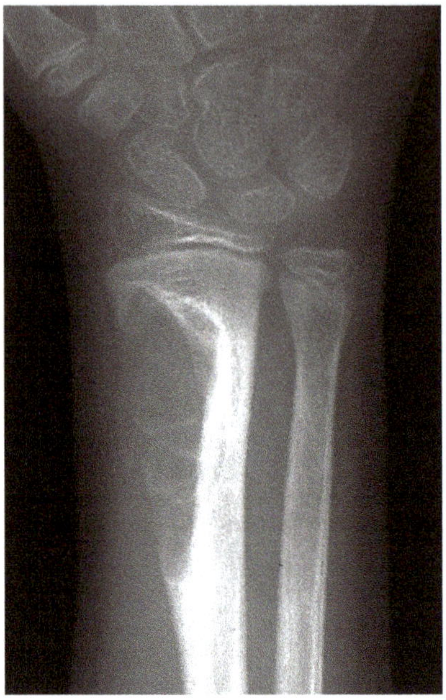

Fig. 10.28

History

A 14-year-old boy with pain and swelling in the distal forearm.

Imaging Findings

AP radiograph shows an elongated, geographic, slightly expansile, eccentric lucent lesion in the distal radial metadiaphysis of a skeletally immature individual. The lesion appears multiloculated, and the overlying cortex is markedly thinned, without periosteal new bone formation. There is dense sclerosis in the medullary cavity of the distal radius.

Differential Diagnosis (Best 3)

Aneurysmal bone cyst (ABC)
Hemophiliac pseudotumor
Non-ossifying fibroma (NOF)

Discussion

Patient history is central to making this diagnosis. Secondary signs, including characteristic findings in joints, can be helpful (radiodense effusions, periarticular osteoporosis, erosions and cysts, epiphyseal overgrowth, and accelerated skeletal maturation). ABC might have a similar appearance, but is not associated with reactive sclerosis. NOF might have a similar appearance on radiographs, but is uncommon in the distal radius and could be distinguished on MRI, since it lacks the hemorrhagic components seen in hemophiliac pseudotumors.

Diagnosis

Hemophiliac pseudotumor

Key Facts

- Hemophiliac pseudotumors are thought to be due to intraosseous or subperiosteal hemorrhage.
- Pseudotumors are relatively uncommon (<2% of patients with severe factor VIII or factor IX deficiency) and are much less common than hemarthrosis, which occurs in 75–90% of hemophiliacs.
- Relatively well-circumscribed radiolucent lesions, ranging from small to very large; can appear aggressive with cortical thinning and interruption, periosteal new bone, and soft tissue extension; trabeculae can extend across the lesions; surrounding bone is often sclerotic.
- Can manifest as bubbly lesions or as multiple osteolytic lesions of varying sizes and can mimic primary and metastatic tumors, osteomyelitis, and other bone lesions.
- Subperiosteal forms can cause periostitis and mimic Ewing sarcoma or osteomyelitis.
- Favor the pelvis and femur; but may be central or eccentric in long bones, as seen here.
- Can arise in soft tissues and cause pressure erosions of bone.
- MRI appearance is variable and can include high T1 hemorrhage, high T2 fluid, and low signal peripherally due to fibrosis and/or hemosiderin.

Suggested Reading

Kerr R. Imaging of musculoskeletal complications of hemophilia. Semin Musculoskelet Radiol. 2003;7(2):127–36.
Jaovisidha S, Ryu KN, Hodler J, Schweitzer ME, Sartoris DJ, Resnick D. Hemophilic pseudotumor: spectrum of MR findings. Skeletal Radiol. 1997;26(8):468–74.

Case 29

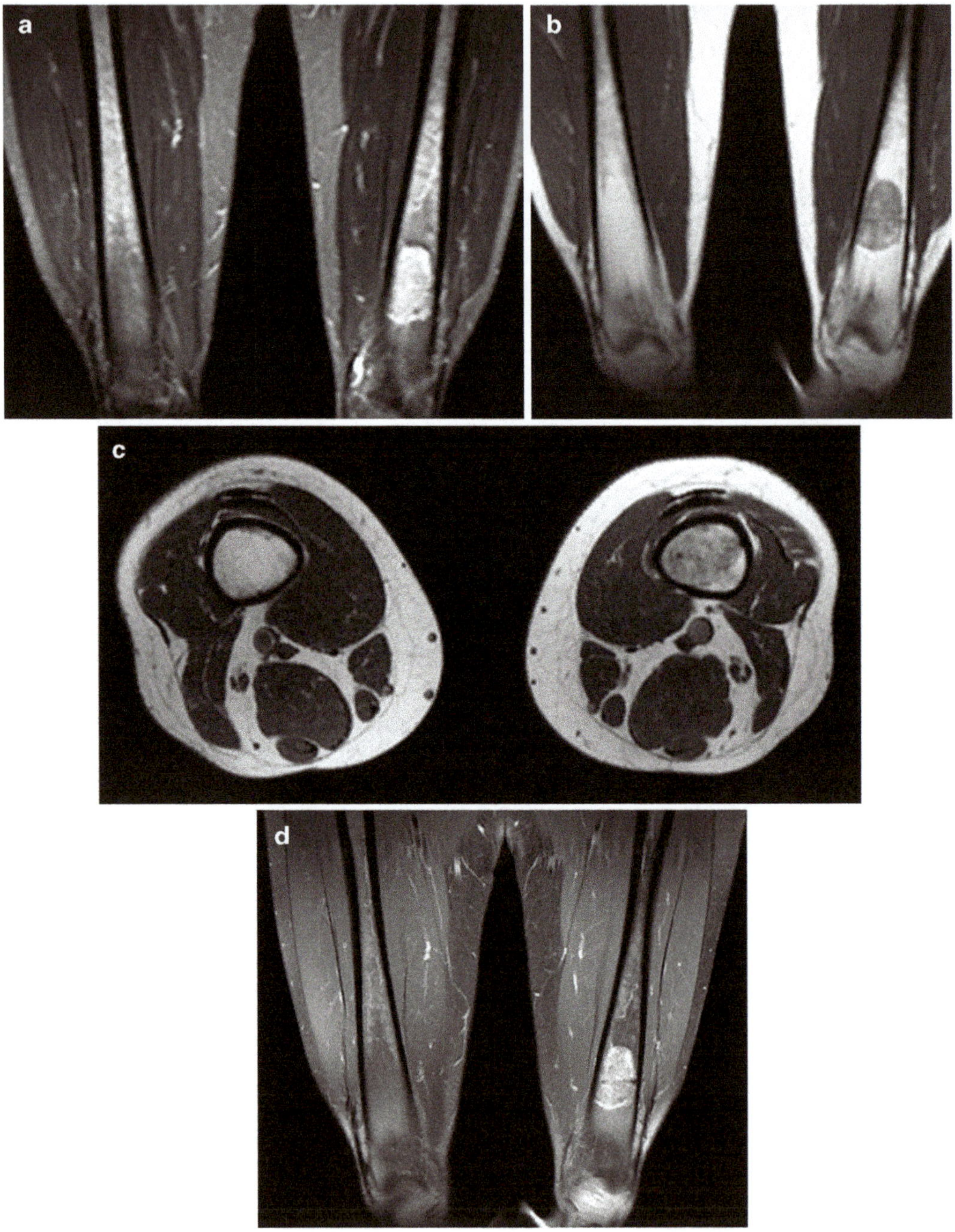

Fig. 10.29

History

A 48-year-old woman with follow-up thigh MRI to assess a lesion in the femur incompletely evaluated on a knee MRI performed for pain following a fall.

Imaging Findings

On the coronal T2-weighted MR image (a), there is a mass-like area of hyperintensity in the distal left femoral metaphysis. The coronal (b) and axial (c) T1-weighted MR images show that the lesion is hypointense to fat, but hyperintense relative to skeletal muscle. The lesion enhances on the postcontrast fat-saturated T1-weighted MR image (d).

Differential Diagnosis (Best 3)

Hematopoietic marrow (red marrow)
Metastasis
Osteonecrosis (early stage)

Discussion

The key to this case is the signal intensity on the T1-weighted images. On the T2-weighted image the lesion is hyperintense and nonspecific. The T1 image shows that the lesion is hyperintense relative to skeletal muscle. Metastases are typically isointense/hypointense to skeletal muscle on T1-weighted images, replacing the underlying fatty marrow. Osteonecrosis early in the disease process can present simply with edema; however, the edema is typically not well-circumscribed and mass-like as seen here. Peripheral areas of low and high signal on T2 weighted images will occur with osteonecrosis disease progression.

Diagnosis

Hematopoietic marrow (red marrow)

Key Points

- Contains the hematopoietic elements (erythrocytes, granulocytes, and thrombocytes).
- Highly vascular.
- Should be hyperintense to skeletal muscle on T1-weighted images.
- Red marrow should demonstrate signal drop out on out-of-phase T1 images due to internal fat content. This will not occur if the lesion does not contain fat, such as with metastases.
- Often occurs in the metaphysis (first area for marrow reconversion) and should not cross the physeal scar into the epiphysis. However, red marrow in a subarticular location in the femoral and humeral heads can be a normal finding.
- Reconversion into red marrow can occur due to anemia (hemolytic and chronic disease), GCSF therapy, obesity, high altitude living, vigorous exercise, smoking, and physiologic stress.
- Reconversion into red marrow begins in the metaphysis, then diaphysis, and finally epiphysis (the reverse of fatty conversion).

Suggested Reading

Kung JW, Yablon CM, Eisenberg RL. Bone marrow signal alterations in the extremities. AJR. 2011;196:W492–510.
Swartz PG, Roberts CC. Radiological reasoning: bone marrow changes on MRI. AJR. 2009;193 Suppl 3:S1–4.

Case 30

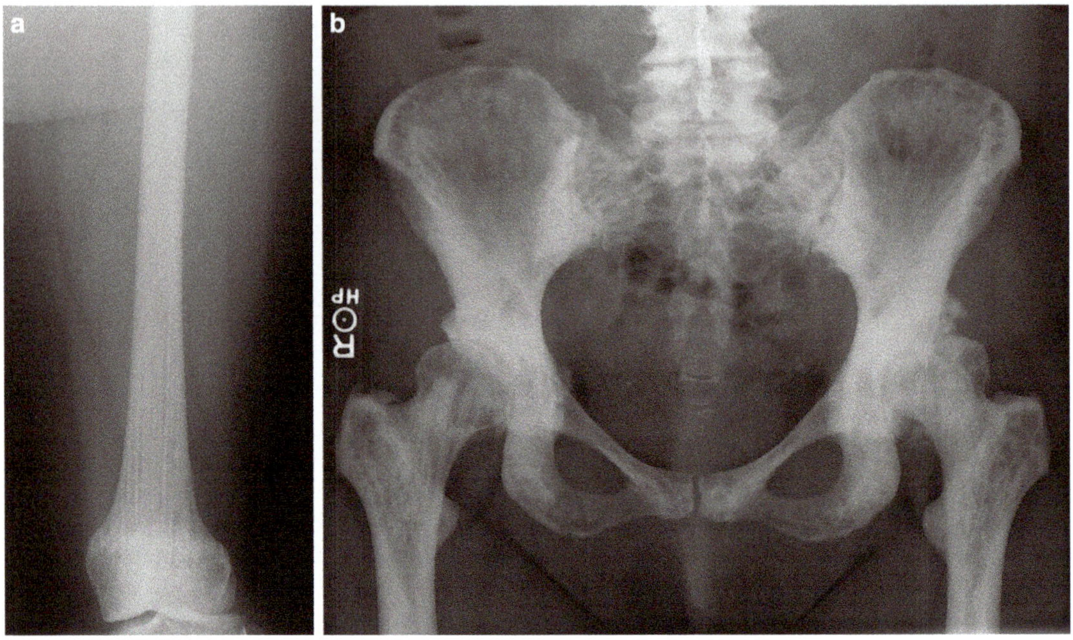

Fig. 10.30

History

A 52-year-old woman with left hip pain.

Imaging Findings

Radiographs show vertically oriented linear bands of increased density in the distal femur (a) and radiating fan-like bands of radiodensity in the ilium and proximal femurs (b). There are osteoarthritic changes in bilateral hips, left worse than right.

Differential Diagnosis (Best 3)

Osteopathia striata
Osteopetrosis
Paget disease

Discussion

The case is essentially an "Aunt Minnie." The vertical striations in the long bones and fan-like linear densities are virtually pathognomonic for osteopathia striata. Osteopetrosis can cause increased density of the bones; however, striations or bands of sclerosis are not present. Paget disease can also cause increased bone density and poor differentiation of the cortex and medullary cavity, but there is no bone expansion or cortical thickening in this case.

Diagnosis

Osteopathia striata (Voorhoeve's disease)

Key Points

- Benign sclerosing dysplasia of bone characterized by vertically oriented linear and band-like radiodense striations.
- Autosomal dominant transmission.
- Patients typically are asymptomatic, but occasionally present with joint pain.
- Osteopathia striata with cranial sclerosis is a variant that is associated with facial deformities, deafness, and mental retardation.
- Femur and ilium are the most commonly affected sites. The disease is typically bilateral.
- Minimal, if any, uptake on bone scan is seen.
- Can occur with other sclerosing bone dysplasias, e.g., osteopoikilosis, osteopetrosis, and melorheostosis.

Suggested Reading

Lee RD. Clinical images of osteopathia striata. Pediatr Radiol. 2004;34(9):753.
Gay BB, Jr, Elsas LJ, Wyly JB, Pasquali M. Osteopathia striata with cranial sclerosis. Pediatr Radiol. 2004;24:56–60.

Case 31

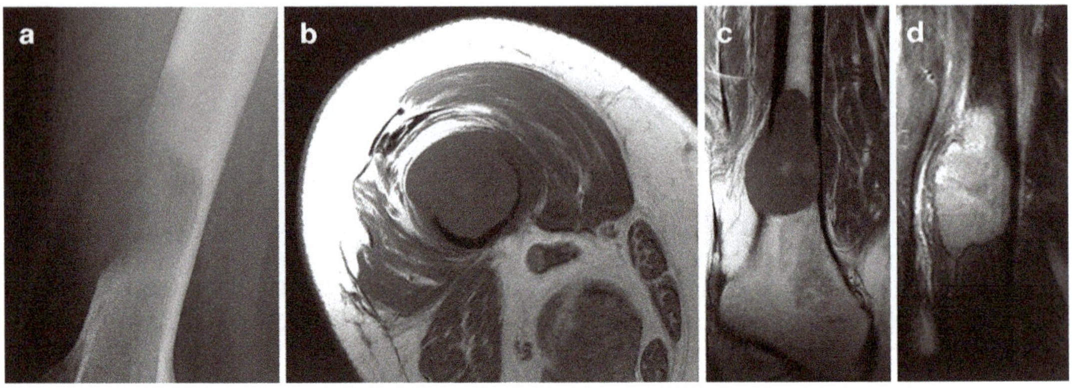

Fig. 10.31

History

A 71-year-old woman with severe debilitating right distal femur pain.

Imaging Findings

The radiograph of the femur (a) shows an aggressive lytic lesion involving the distal femoral diametaphysis. There is a wide zone of transition without discernable osseous or cartilaginous matrix. The MR images (b, c, d) confirm the presence of a low T1, high T2 lesion replacing the marrow cavity and extending outward. There is extensive circumferential cortical destruction, >2/3 of the circumference, best seen on the axial image. On the coronal T1 MR image, there is a sharp distinction between the periphery of the lesion and the normal fatty marrow.

Differential Diagnosis (Best 3)

Osteomyelitis
Plasmacytoma
Lytic metastasis

Discussion

The imaging characteristics are nonspecific but are aggressive and the lesion is at high risk for pathologic fracture. Thus, even if one cannot arrive at a specific diagnosis based on imaging, this lesion will require biopsy and stabilization. This lesion would have a Mirels pathologic fracture score of 11 out of 12 (lower extremity site—2, functional pain—3, lytic lesion—3, >2/3 circumferential involvement—3). Statistically, a lytic metastasis should be highest on the differential as metastases are the most common bone tumor. Moreover, the lesion has a "cookie-bite" appearance with destruction of the cortex and a large soft tissue component which is associated with lung cancer. Osteomyelitis is a possibility; however, given the amount of bone destruction, one would expect more perilesional edema. A plasmacytoma is another good consideration given the large soft tissue component.

Diagnosis

Lytic metastasis (lung cancer)

Key Points

- Metastatic disease should be considered in almost any bone lesion encountered in the elderly.
- The most common lytic metastases include lung, renal, thyroid, and breast.
- Assessment for pathologic fracture is important. Lesions with >50% circumferential involvement (assessed axially) have a 60–70% chance of fracture.
- Lucency in the bone is not evident on radiographs until 50% of the cortical thickness is involved and MRI will better assess the marrow involvement.
- Bony destruction and soft tissue components are indicative of an aggressive process requiring further workup.

Suggested Reading

Mirels H. Metastatic disease in long bones. A proposed scoring system for diagnosing impending pathologic fractures. Clin Orthop Relat Res. 1989;249:256–264.
Rosenthal DI. Radiologic diagnosis of bone metastases. Cancer. 1997;80:1595–607.
Hipp JA, Springfield DS, Hayes WC. Predicting pathologic fracture risk in the management of metastatic bone defects. Clin Orthop Relat Res. 1995;312:120–35.

Case 32

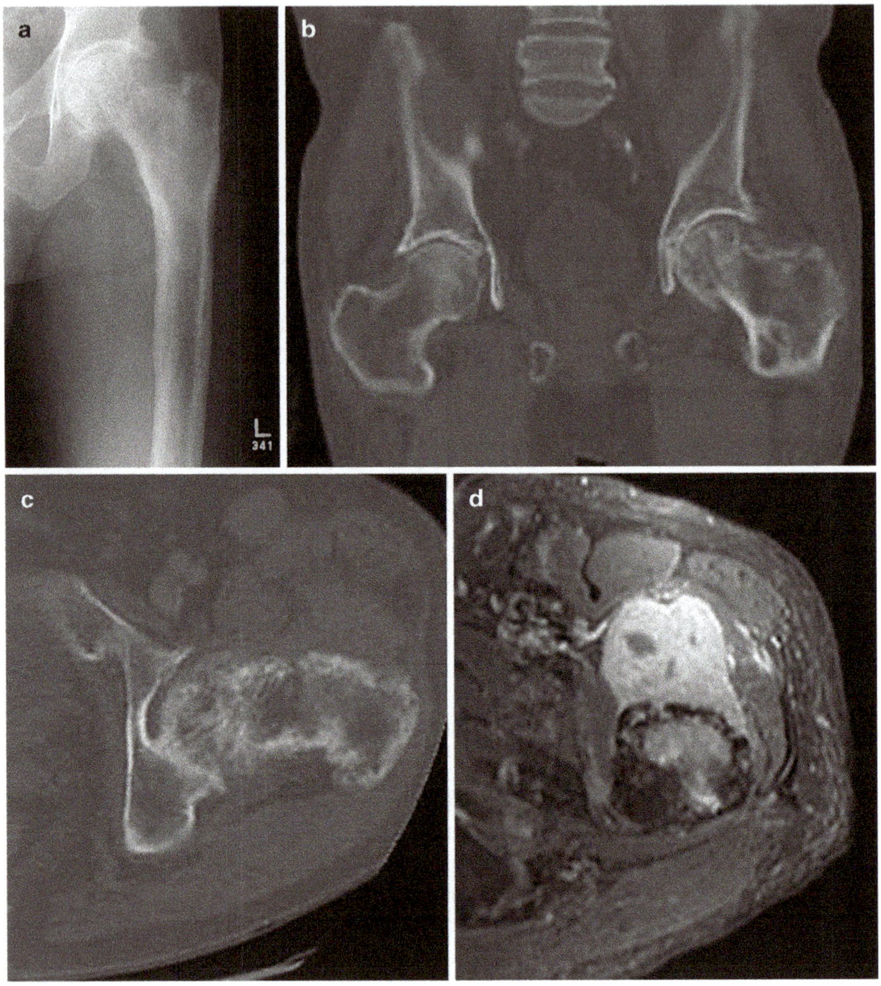

Fig. 10.32

History

A 79-year-old man with new onset acute on chronic left hip pain.

Imaging Findings

The AP radiograph (a) and coronal CT image (b) show cortical and trabecular thickening and enlargement of the left proximal femur as well as mixed lucency and sclerosis in the femoral head and neck. The changes do not involve the acetabulum, although there is joint space narrowing and degenerative spurring consistent with osteoarthritis. The axial CT (c) redemonstrates the thickened cortex, bony expansion, and coarse trabecular pattern. However, there are aggressive areas of cortical breakthrough anteriorly and posteriorly. Contrast enhanced fat-saturated T1 MR image (d) shows an enhancing soft tissue mass emanating from the femur anteriorly, as well as abnormal increased marrow signal and cortical irregularity.

Differential Diagnosis (Best 3)

Paget disease with sarcomatous transformation
Infection
Metastasis

Discussion

The key to this case is recognizing that the femur is involved with Paget disease on the radiograph and CT. The enhancing soft tissue mass on the MRI should then raise suspicion of sarcomatous transformation. Chronic infection may produce this mixed lytic and sclerotic appearance, but typically will not have bony expansion or a large soft tissue mass without surrounding edema. The enhancing mass with cortical breakthrough automatically makes this an aggressive lesion requiring tissue sampling. Metastases also would not be associated with the bone expansion.

Diagnosis

Paget disease with sarcomatous transformation

Key Points

- Paget disease is found in 3% of the population and the incidence increases with age.
- 1% of Paget cases undergo sarcomatous transformation, most commonly to osteosarcoma.
- Malignant transformation is more common in men, polyostotic Paget disease, and longer duration of disease.
- Previous fracture may also predispose to sarcomatous transformation.
- The most common sites for transformation are the femur, pelvis, and humerus.
- Imaging shows areas of cortical destruction and osteolysis within pagetoid bone; often with a soft tissue component.
- Giant cell tumors can also develop in pagetoid bone, usually in the skull and facial bones.
- Myeloma and metastases can also occur in pagetoid bone, hypothesized to be related to increased blood flow in pagetoid bone metastases.
- Sarcomas arising in Paget have very poor prognosis.

Suggested Reading

Deyrup AT, Montag AG, Inwards CY, Xu Z, Swee RG, Krishnan Unni K. Sarcomas arising in Paget disease of bone: a clinicopathologic analysis of 70 cases. Arch Pathol Lab Med. 2007;131:942–6.

Moore TE, King AR, Kathol MH, el-Khoury GY, Palmer R, Downey PR. Sarcoma in Paget disease of bone: clinical, radiologic, and pathologic features in 22 cases. AJR Am J Roentgenol. 1991;156: 1199–203.

Case 33

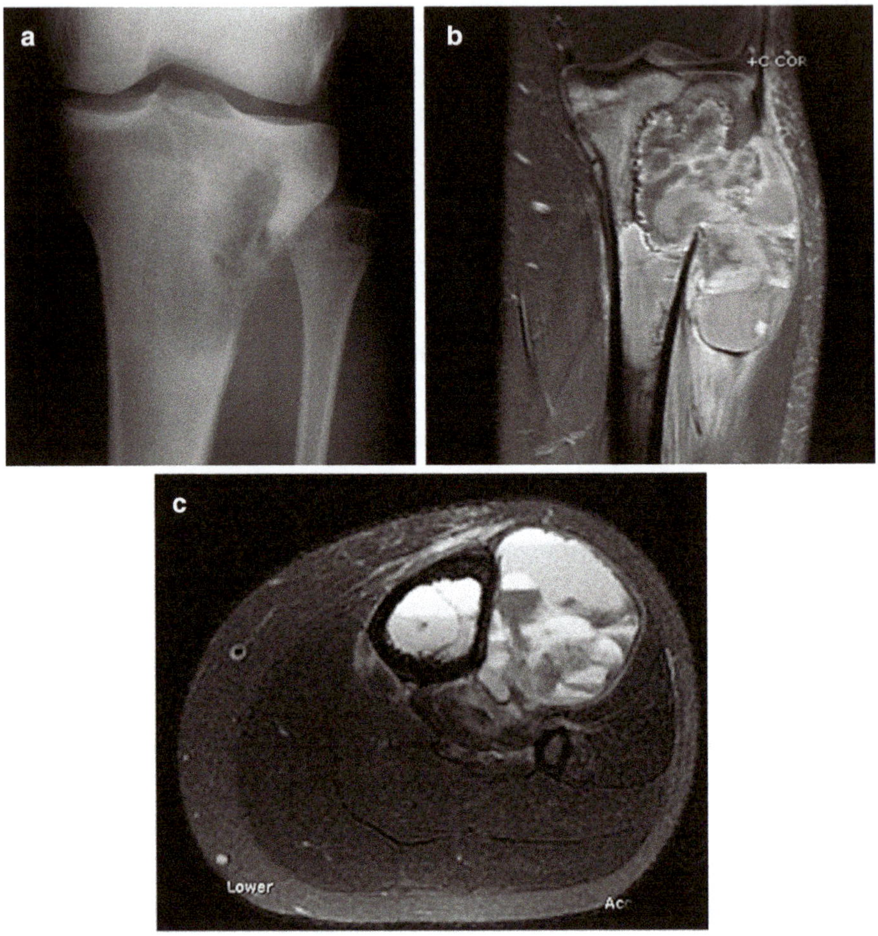

Fig. 10.33 Images courtesy of Dr. Daniel Siegal, Detroit, MI

History

A 17-year-old boy with severe lateral knee pain and swelling.

Imaging Findings

The AP radiograph (a) shows an aggressive lucent lesion in the tibial metaphysis with cortical breakthrough along the lateral aspect. The coronal (b) and axial (c) fat-saturated T2-weighted MR images show a destructive lesion with a large soft tissue component exiting the lateral cortex. Prominent perilesional edema is seen in the bone and soft tissue. There are layering fluid–fluid levels on the axial image.

Differential Diagnosis (Best 3)

Aneurysmal bone cyst (ABC)
Telangiectatic osteosarcoma
Infection

Discussion

The main features of the case are the aggressive nature of the lesion and the layering fluid–fluid levels. Fluid–fluid levels can be seen in many bone lesions but are most commonly associated with aneurysmal bone cysts and telangiectatic osteosarcomas. The large soft tissue component and aggressive cortical breakthrough makes the latter more likely. Osteomyelitis could be considered based on the radiograph, but the discrete soft tissue mass and fluid–fluid levels make it unlikely. Either way, the lesion is aggressive and requires biopsy/treatment.

Diagnosis

Telangiectatic osteosarcoma

Key Points

- Malignant bone forming neoplasm containing cystic cavities with necrosis and hemorrhage.
- Unlike conventional osteosarcoma, there is little osseous mineralization.
- Can differentiate telangiectatic osteosarcoma from an aneurysmal bone cyst (ABC) based on:
  - Thick, solid nodular tissue surrounding the cystic spaces.
  - Matrix mineralization in the periphery, best seen on CT (but can be subtle).
  - Cortical destruction with associated nonencapsulated soft tissue mass.
- Fluid–fluid levels occur when there are layering densities (hemorrhage, tumor necrosis, and fat) in a cavity and can also be seen in simple bone cysts, chondroblastomas, giant cell tumors, and metastases.

Suggested Reading

Murphey MD, wan Jaovisidha S, Temple HT, Gannon FH, Jelinek JS, Malawer MM. Telangiectatic osteosarcoma: radiologic–pathologic comparison. Radiology. 2003;229:545–53.
Keenan S, Bui-Mansfield LT. Musculoskeletal lesions with fluid-fluid level: a pictorial essay. J Comput Assist Tomogr. 2006;30:517–24.
Van Dyck P, Vanhoenacker FM, Vogel J, et al. Prevalence, extension and characteristics of fluid–fluid levels in bone and soft tissue tumors. Eur Radiol. 2006;16:2644–51.

Case 34

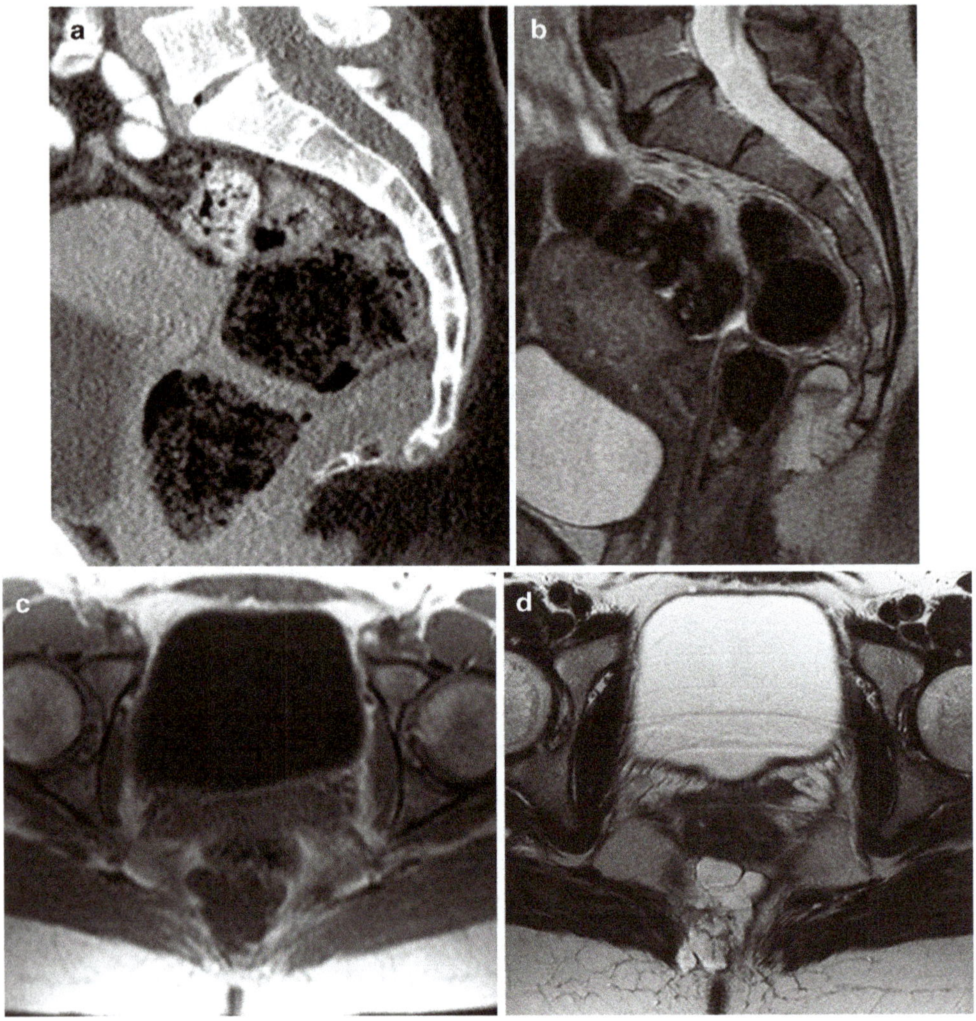

Fig. 10.34

History

A 50-year-old woman with coccygeal pain for 1 year.

Imaging Findings

Sagittal CT image (a) shows a soft tissue mass anterior to the coccyx, centered at a corticated fracture through the C2 level. MRI images demonstrate a lobulated, well-circumscribed mass lying anterior to the coccyx that abuts and displaces the rectum. Sagittal T2-weighted MR image (b) shows that the lesion is either extending out of or eroding into the C2 coccygeal segment. The mass is near-isointense to muscle on the axial T1 (c) and hyperintense with subtle scattered nodular areas of low signal on the axial T2-weighted (d) MR images.

Differential Diagnosis

Chordoma
Developmental cyst
Sacral neurilemoma (schwannoma)

Discussion

The appearance is most compatible with chordoma: a tumor arising in the sacroccoccygeal region, in the midline along the notochordal tract, destroying bone, with a large soft tissue mass. High T2 signal suggests a chordoma with myxoid content. Developmental cysts are well-defined retrorectal uni- or multilocular cysts, with high T2 signal and a thin rim of enhancement. Thickened peripheral enhancement (smooth) should only occur if infected and irregular peripheral enhancement or internal enhancement should not be present unless there is rare malignant degeneration. Associated sacral bone defect and calcifications are rare. Sacral schwannomas arise from peripheral sheaths of sacral nerves and typically occur as rounded, well-defined, heterogeneously enhancing solid lesions that contain some cystic necrotic areas. Evaluation should include a search for association with a nerve or neural foramen, including possible neural foraminal enlargement. When small, schwannomas should be lateral to midline along the course of a nerve, although large tumors may appear to be in the midline.

Diagnosis

Chordoma

Key Facts

- Chordoma originates from notochordal remnants and occurs along the spine in the midline, most often in the sacrococcygeal region or clivus.
- Slow-growing malignancy, often with nonspecific symptoms, that vary with location.
- Expansile, highly destructive lytic lesion, with irregular or scalloped borders, often with large lobulated soft tissue mass and bony debris. Tends to spare the disc and posterior elements.
- Can rarely occur as a mass without bone involvement.
- In the appropriate location, very high T2 MRI signal (due to myxoid composition) and lobulated morphology suggests the diagnosis.
- CT can help assess bone margins and osseous fragmentation; MRI can help assess for soft tissue mass and local invasion.
- Locally aggressive, with frequent microscopic soft tissue infiltration and local recurrence.
- Long term prognosis is poor; distant metastases can occur late in disease.
- Developmental cysts include a spectrum of epidermoid, dermoid, and enteric (tailgut cysts and cystic rectal duplication) lesions. The majority are benign, with rare malignant degeneration.

Suggested Reading

Rosenthal DI, Scott JA, Mankin HJ, et al. Sacrococcygeal chordoma: magnetic resonance imaging and computed tomography. Am J Roentgenol. 1985;145:143–7.
Sze G, Uichanco LS, Brant-Zawadzki MN, et al. Chordomas: MR imaging. Radiology. 1988;166: 187–91.
Dahan H, Arrive L, Wendum D, et al. Retrorectal developmental cysts in adults: clinical and radiologic–histopathologic review, differential diagnosis, and treatment. Radiographics. 2001;21:575–84.

Case 35

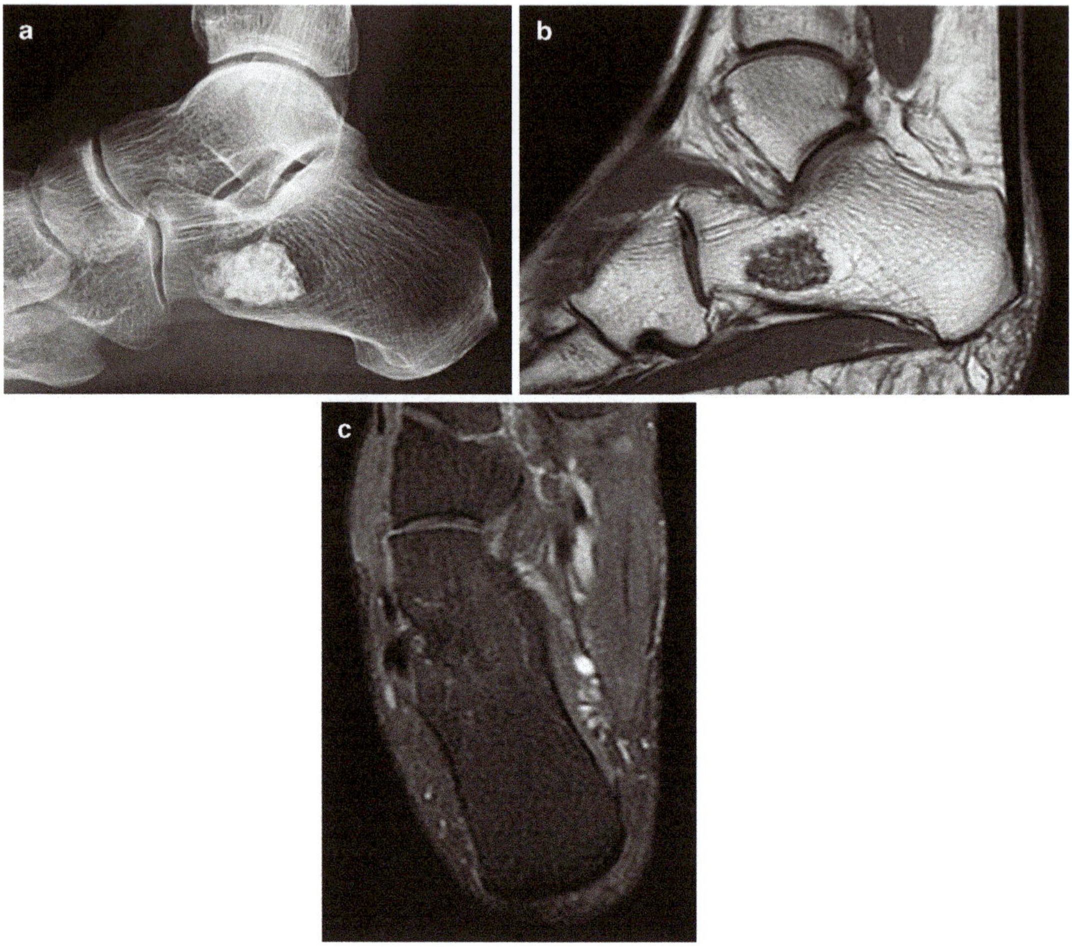

Fig. 10.35

History

A 42-year-old woman with ankle pain following trauma.

Imaging Findings

On the lateral radiograph (a), there is what at first appears to be a simple ovoid sclerotic lesion, in the body of the calcaneus, not typical for either chondroid or osseous matrix mineralization. On closer inspection, there is a thin lucent rim surrounding the density. The lesion is predominantly low signal on the sagittal T1-weighted MR image (b), corresponding to the density on the radiograph, but it also has a surrounding thin rim of high T1 signal, that lacks normal trabeculation. This peripheral high T1 tissue loses signal on the frequency selective fat-saturated T1-weighted postcontrast MR image (c), confirming that it is fat.

Differential Diagnosis (Best 3)

Enchondroma
Intraosseous lipoma
Bone infarct

Discussion

Correct diagnosis depends on recognizing that (1) there is a characteristic differential for lesions that occur in the body of the calcaneus, (2) the lesion is actually a fatty lesion that has calcified, and (3) intraosseous lipomas can be heterogeneous, with internal calcification. Lesions that like to occur in the body of the calcaneus include: normal variant pseudotumor, intraosseous lipoma, and simple bone cyst. This lesion is comprised of fat, but has dense central mineralization. Enchondromas do not typically occur in this location and the central mineralization seen here does not have a typical chondroid pattern. Bone infarcts are also not typical in this location and tend to be more densely mineralized at their periphery. Moreover, infarcts have a more characteristic serpentine, "puzzle piece" MR appearance, with high T2 lines. (Having said that, some authors argue that most of what we call intraosseous lipomas are actually sequela of bone infarcts.) The normal variant pseudotumor of the calcaneus is centered in the body, composed of homogeneous fat on all modalities, and does not contain fluid or calcification. It has a paucity of trabeculae compared to the rest of the calcaneus.

Diagnosis

Intraosseous lipoma

Key Facts

- Intraosseous lipomas are benign and usually an incidental, asymptomatic finding.
- Classically, an intraosseous lipoma appears as a well-circumscribed, geographic, lucent lesion with a narrow zone of transition and a small central or ring-like calcification in the body of calcaneus.
- On MRI, fat within the lipoma may be slightly higher T1 signal than nearby marrow fat.
- Unlike soft tissue lipomas, an intraosseous lipoma need not be pure fat—presence of high T2 fluid and low signal calcification/ossification is common.

Suggested Reading

Propeck T, Bullard MA, Lin J. Radiologic–pathologic correlation of intra-osseous lipomas. AJR Am J Roentgenol. 2000;175:673–8.
Campbell RS, Grainger AJ, Mangham DC, Beggs I, Teh J, Davies AM. Intraosseous lipoma: report of 35 new cases and a review of the literature. Skeletal Radiol. 2003;32(4):209–22.
Milgram JW. Intraosseous lipomas: radiologic and pathologic manifestations. Radiology. 1988; 167(1):155–60.

Case 36

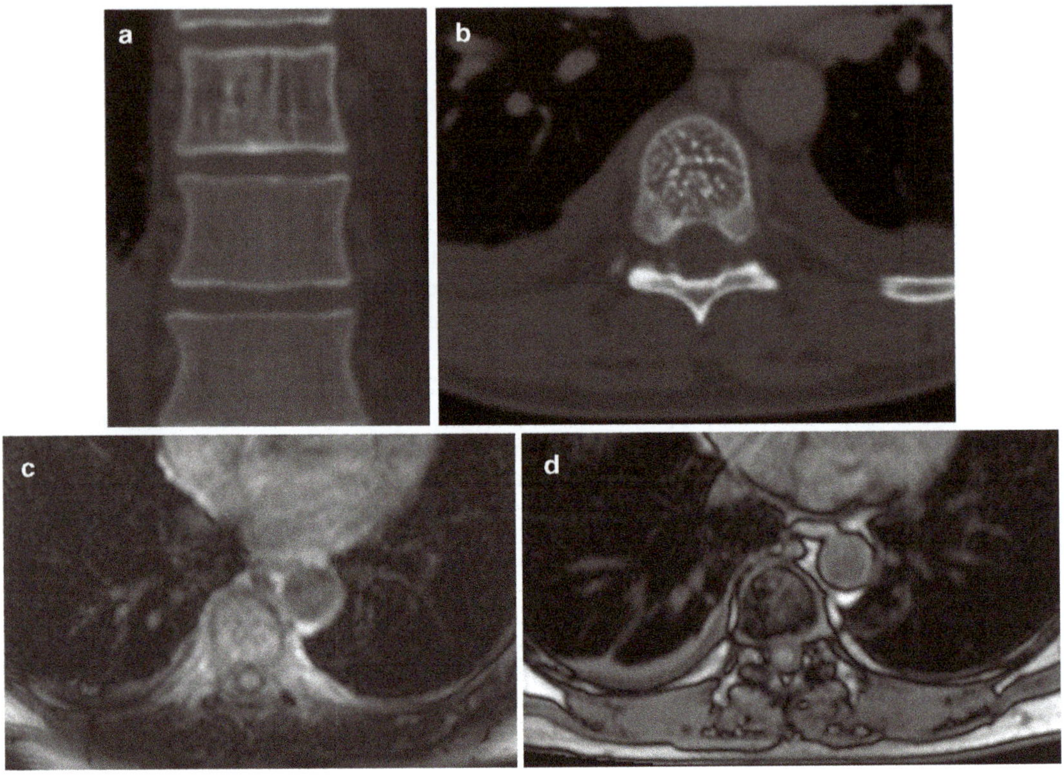

Fig. 10.36

History

Back pain.

Imaging Findings

Coronal (a) and axial (b) CT images show prominent vertical striations in a lower thoracic vertebral body. Axial CT demonstrates a discrete rounded lesion, with thickened vertical trabeculae, surrounded by lucent fatty marrow, giving a "corduroy" (longitudinal) or "polka dot" (axial) appearance. On MRI, the same rounded lesion is bright on the T1 weighted in-phase image (c) and loses signal on the out-of-phase image (d), due to the presence of fat.

Differential Diagnosis (Best 3)

Intraosseous hemangioma
Paget disease
Metastasis

Discussion

The appearance is pathognomonic for a vertebral hemagioma given the accentuation of vertical trabeculae in a "corduroy" (longitudinal) or "polka-dot" (axial) pattern and diffuse intralesional fat content. Trabecular coarsening in Paget disease is less uniform and is accompanied by cortical thickening and vertebral body enlargement, features that are not seen here. Metastasis can cause a lytic vertebral lesion, but does not contain significant fat and destroys, rather than thickens, intralesional trabeculae.

Diagnosis

Intraosseous hemangioma

Key Facts

- Commonly encountered benign hamartoma with characteristic imaging appearance.
- Most often occurs in vertebral bodies and calvarium (frontal and parietal), usually incidental.
- CT appearance can be diagnostic: fat density, "polka dot" appearance of thickened trabeculae in cross section; may have "spoke wheel" appearance in flat bones like the skull.
- Classic MRI appearance is also diagnostic: high T1 due to fat and high T2 due to slow-flowing blood; mild to marked contrast enhancement; and loss of signal on out-of-phase T1-weighted images.
- Some hemangiomas do not demonstrate high T1 signal and cannot be distinguished from other lesions on MRI, including metastases; CT or in-phase/out-of-phase MRI may help.

Suggested Reading

Ross JS, Masaryk TJ, Modic MT, et al. Vertebral hemangiomas: MR imaging. Radiology. 1987;165:165–9.
Disler DG, McCauley TR, Ratner LM, et al. In-phase and out-of-phase MR imaging of bone marrow: prediction of neoplasia based on the detection of coexistent fat and water. AJR Am J Roentgenol. 1997;169:1439–47.
Long SS, Yablon CM, Eisenberg RL. Bone marrow signal alteration in the spine and sacrum. AJR Am J Roentgenol. 2010;195(3):W178–200.

Case 37

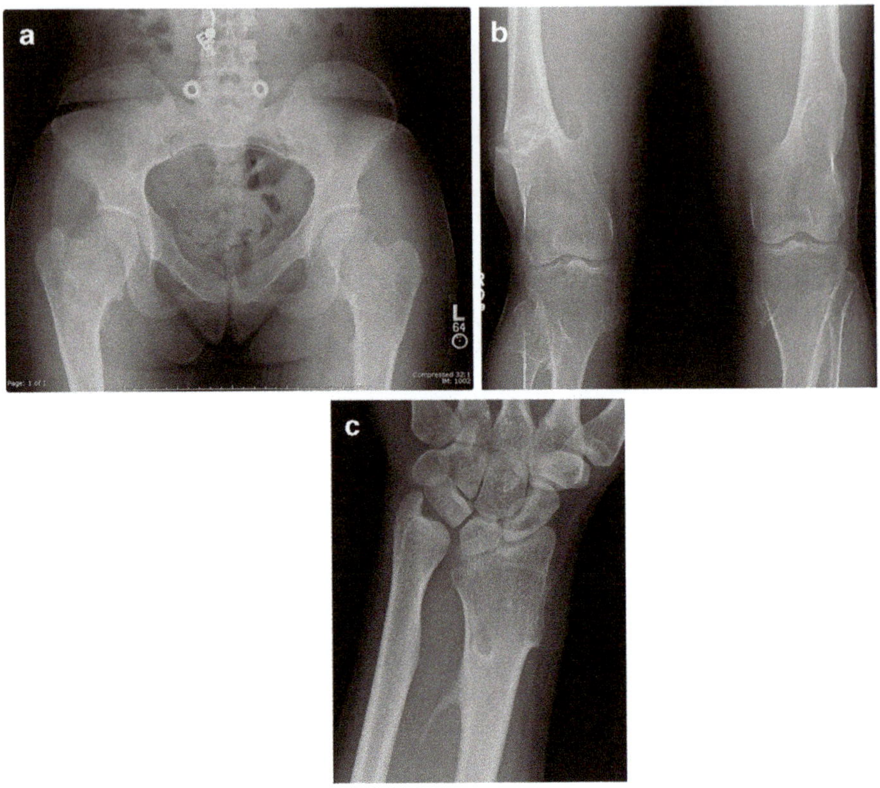

Fig. 10.37

History

A 33-year-old woman with short stature and chronic hip, knee, and wrist pain.

Imaging Findings

AP views of the pelvis (a), knees (b), and wrist (c) demonstrate numerous osseous excrescences arising from the cortical surface. Notice the continuity of the lesions with the host bone, metaphyseal location, and the fact that the lesions point away from the joint. There is deformity (Madelung) of the radiocarpal joint due to growth disturbances. Moreover, several of the lesions seen en face can be mistaken for intramedullary lytic lesions.

Differential Diagnosis (Best 3)

Hereditary multiple exostoses (HME)
Sequela of multiple trauma
Metachondromatosis

Discussion

In this case, it is important not to be distracted by the deformities and to scrutinize each lesion individually. Recognizing that the lesions are all osteochondromas (both sessile and pedunculated) will lead to the diagnosis of HME. Although chronic fractures could result in severe deformities, bony excrescences would be atypical. Metachondromatosis is similar to HME, except that the exostoses point towards the joint space instead of away and is also associated with multiple enchondromas.

Diagnosis

Hereditary multiple exostoses (HME)

Key Points

- Autosomal dominant disease characterized by multiple osteochondromas (exostoses).
- 2/3 of patients have a family history of the disease.
- Most lesions in HME are sessile instead of pedunculated. However, if >90% of lesions are sessile, then higher degree of skeletal deformities.
- Knees and pelvis are the most common sites.
- Numerous clinical manifestations and potential complications: fracture, limited motion, bursitis, joint pain due to mechanical impingement, neurovascular compromise, growth disturbances leading to mild short stature and limb deformities, malignant transformation to chondrosarcoma.
- Sarcomatous transformation (3–5%) is higher than solitary osteochondromas (<1%), but less than previously described (25%).
- Baseline studies (radiographs and bone scan) are useful for comparison if symptoms develop.

Suggested Reading

Pannier S, Legeai-Mallet L. Hereditary multiple exostoses and enchondromatosis. Best Pract Res Clin Rheumatol. 2008;22:45–54.
Bovee JV. Multiple osteochondromas. Orphanet J Rare Dis. 2008;3:3.

Case 38

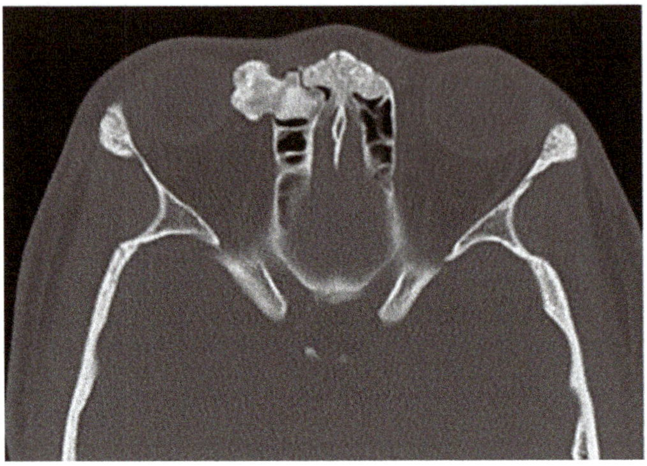

Fig. 10.38 Image courtesy of Dr. Gul Moonis, Boston, MA

History

A 45-year-old woman with vision problems.

Imaging Findings

There is a lobulated sclerotic lesion with smooth borders in the right ethmoid sinus which extends laterally and abuts the right eye.

Differential Diagnosis (Best 3)

Bone island
Osteoma
Surface osteosarcoma

Discussion

The exophytic nature of the lesion can help distinguish it from a bone island which is confined to the intramedullary space. The nonaggressive features (smooth borders, sclerotic rim, and absence of periosteal new bone) and location are more typical of an osteoma than a surface osteosarcoma.

Diagnosis

Osteoma

Key Points

- Normal cortical bone arising from the periosteum (hamartoma).
- Very dense lesion on the surface of the bone, without significant trabecular bone.
- Most commonly found in the skull and sinuses.
- Typically asymptomatic, but can cause cosmetic issues or injure adjacent structures due to mass effect (headaches, vision loss, and sinusitis).
- Usually no or very mild uptake on bone scintigraphy.
- Associated with Gardner's syndrome (desmoid tumors, GI polyps, and osteomas) and tuberous sclerosis (seizures, mental retardation, skin lesions, cortical tubers, subependymal giant cell astrocytomas, and renal angiomyolipomas).

Suggested Reading

Greenspan A. Benign bone-forming lesions: osteoma, osteoid osteoma, and osteoblastoma. Clinical, imaging, pathologic, and differential considerations. Skeletal Radiol. 1993;22:485–500.

Case 39

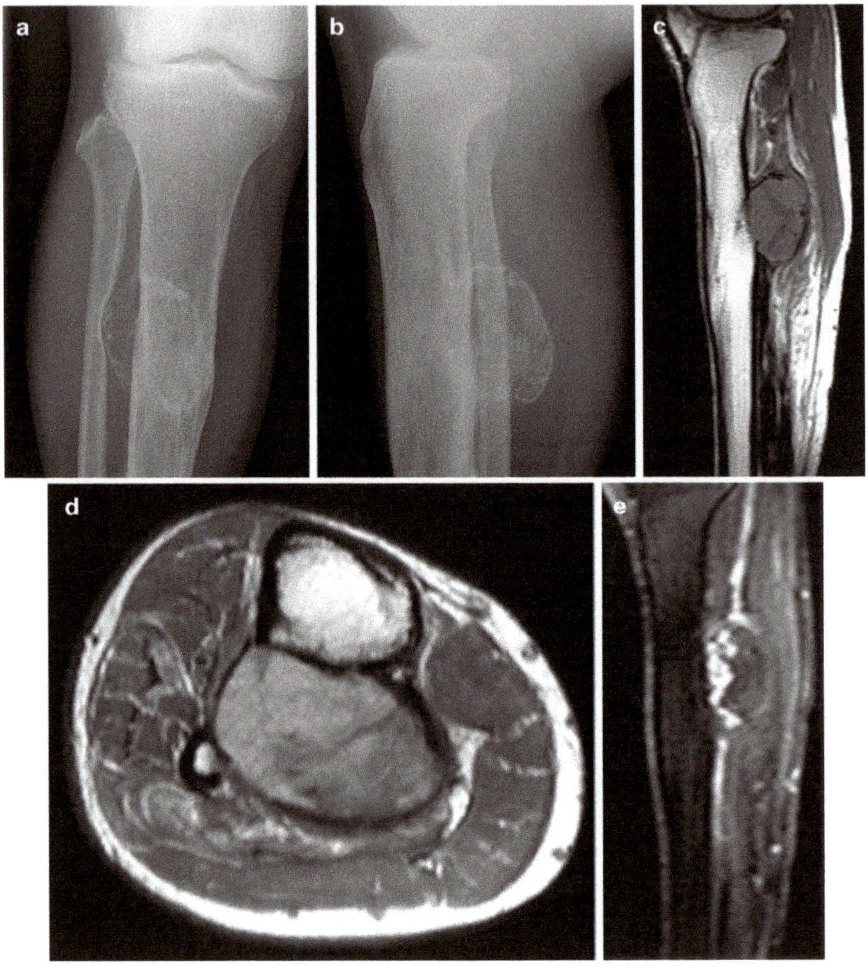

Fig. 10.39

History

A 37-year-old man with painful lump in the posterior calf. In a "car accident"15 years ago in which he sustained multiple injuries.

Imaging Findings

AP (a) and lateral (b) radiographs of the proximal tibia/fibula show an oval calcified lesion adjacent to the posterior tibia. There is smooth remodeling of the fibula on the AP view, suggesting that the fibula has had time to adapt to the growth of the mass. There is also irregularity of the tibial shaft, consistent with a healed fracture. Based on the radiographs it is unclear whether the mass is arising from the tibia or is separate from bone, isolated to the soft tissues. The sagittal (c) and axial (d) T1-weighted MR images show preserved T1 fatty signal in the tibia and that the mass does not extend into the tibia beyond its cortex. The sagittal MR angiogram image (e) shows the popliteal artery entering the mass superiorly with abnormal vessels in the center of the lesion.

Differential Diagnosis (Best 3)

Myositis ossificans
Surface osteosarcoma
Pseudoaneurysm (popliteal artery)

Discussion

In this case, the history of prior trauma and identifying the popliteal artery entering the mass are most helpful. Although the peripheral calcification pattern and traumatic history would be good for myositis ossificans, the vascular findings and adherence to the bone would not be typical. However, some cases of myositis ossificans can be adherent to the cortical surface. Surface osteosarcoma or chondrosarcoma are possibilities, although they typically have more pronounced cortical changes and are not typically associated with a major artery.

Diagnosis

Pseudoaneurysm (popliteal artery)

Key Points

- A pseudoaneursym results when there is a focal defect in the wall of an artery leading to a hematoma that is confined by the adjacent soft tissues. This is different from a "true aneurysm" where all layers of the artery wall bulge outward or from an arterial dissection where there is separation of the artery wall layers.
- Pseudoaneurysms can result from blunt or penetrating trauma after a long time delay, as with this case.
- Pseudoaneurysms in the popliteal fossa can present as a pulsatile mass and can be associated with fixed flexion contractures from fibrosis and shortening of the knee flexors and cruciate ligaments, as well as shrinkage of the joint capsule.
- Reversed saphenous vein grafts or vein patch closure are effective treatment options.
- When pseudoaneursyms calcify, they can be mistaken for surface bone lesions (parosteal osteosarcomas and periosteal chondrosarcomas) and soft tissue lesions (myositis ossificans and synovial sarcoma).
- Identifying an artery entering and exiting the mass and history of prior trauma are helpful distinguishing features.

Suggested Reading

Woolgar JD, Reddy DS, Robbs JV. Delayed presentation of traumatic popliteal artery pseudoaneurysms: a review of seven cases. Eur J Vasc Endovasc Surg. 2002;23:255–9.
Megalopoulos A, Siminas S, Trelopoulos G. Traumatic pseudoaneurysm of the popliteal artery after blunt trauma: case report and a review of the literature. Vasc Endovascular Surg. 2006;40(6): 499–504.

Case 40

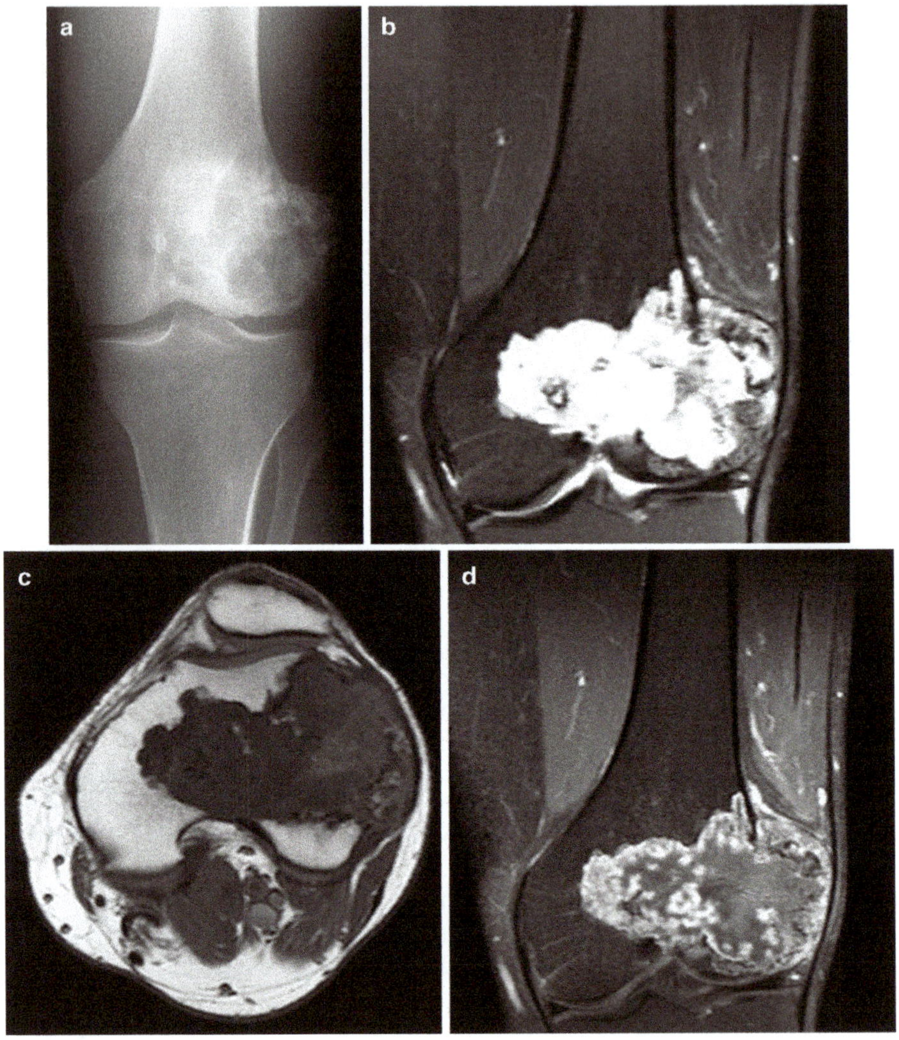

Fig. 10.40

History

A 62-year-old man with knee pain.

Imaging Findings

The AP radiograph (a) shows a mixed lytic and sclerotic lesion in the lateral femoral epiphysis extending to the articular cartilage. There is suggestion of chondroid matrix with punctuate areas of calcification. The MRI shows that the lesion is hyperintense on the T2 weighted image (b), hypointense on the T1 weighted image (c), and has peripheral and central enhancement on the postcontrast fat-saturated T1-weighted MR image (d). Note the lobulated peripheral margin and the area of cortical breakthrough at the superolateral aspect of the distal femur.

Differential Diagnosis (Best 3)

Giant cell tumor (GCT)
Chondroblastoma
Chondrosarcoma (clear cell)

Discussion

An important feature of this case is recognizing that the lesion contains cartilaginous matrix. Although the location is good for a giant cell tumor, GCTs typically have no appreciable matrix. The epiphyseal location is a feature of both clear cell chondrosarcomas and chondroblastomas; however, the patient's older age, large size of the lesion, and the area of cortical breakthrough should suggest a clear cell chondrosarcoma over a chondroblastoma.

Diagnosis

Clear cell chondrosarcoma

Key Points

- Very rare low grade chondrosarcoma subtype.
- Contain large cells with clear and eosinophilic cytoplasm.
- Treated with en bloc resection.
- Important distinguishing features from a chondroblastoma:
  - Large size
  - More likely to extend outside the epiphysis
  - Older population

Suggested Reading

Collins MS, Koyama T, Swee RG, Inwards CY. Clear cell chondrosarcoma: radiographic, computed tomographic, and magnetic resonance findings in 34 patients with pathologic correlation. Skeletal Radiol. 2003;32:687–94.

Kaim AH, Hugli R, Bonel HM, Jundt G. Chondroblastoma and clear cell chondrosarcoma: radiological and MRI characteristics with histopathological correlation. Skeletal Radiol. 2002;31:88–95.

Case 41

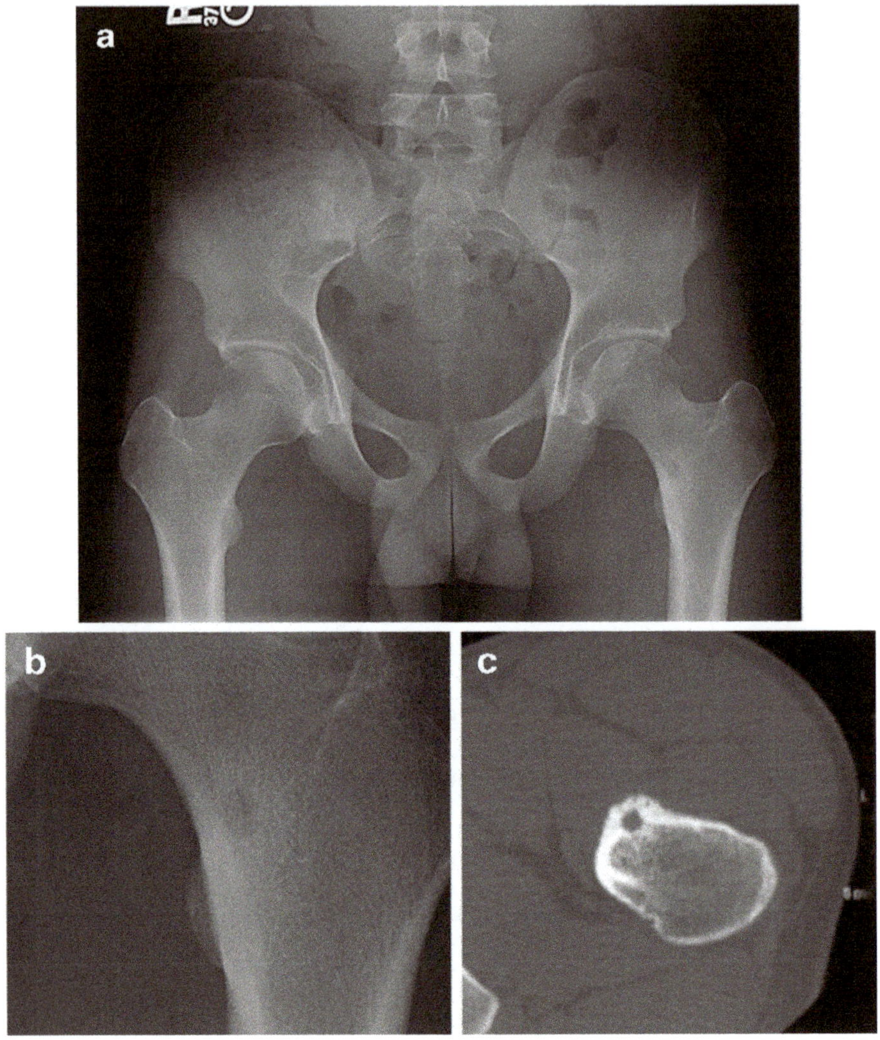

Fig. 10.41

History

A 22-year-old man with left hip pain.

Imaging Findings

AP pelvis (a) and magnified image (b) of the left hip shows a small, 6 mm, lucency in the left femoral neck medially with subtle surrounding sclerosis. CT scan (c) shows a small focal lucency in the anteromedial femoral cortex with surrounding periosteal reaction.

Differential Diagnosis (Best 3)

Osteoid osteoma
Brodie's abscess
Synovial herniation pit (Pitt's pit)

Discussion

This case highlights the fact that intra-articular osteoid osteoma can have minimal reactive bony changes due to the absence of overlying periosteum. Thus, the intra-articular nidus is poorly seen on the radiograph in this case. Radiographically, the lesion is difficult to distinguish from infection. On cross-sectional imaging, osteoid osteomas are typically cortically based whereas Brodie's abscesses are typically intramedullary and may show a cloaca or sinus tract. A synovial herniation pit is typically centered in the femoral neck anteriorly and has a thin sclerotic border without periosteal reaction. If the patient were older, multiple myeloma could be considered, based on the radiograph.

Diagnosis

Osteoid osteoma (intra-articular)

Key Points

- Osteoblastic neoplasm with central core of highly vascularized connective tissue.
- Almost always painful, consider a different diagnosis if pain is not present.
- Pain worse at night and relieved quickly by aspirin (aspirin interferes with prostaglandin release by the tumor).
- Intra-articular lesions can have less sclerosis due to absence of overlying periosteum and can have synovitis with joint effusion, mimicking a septic joint.
- Lesions typically resolve spontaneously in 4–5 years without treatment. Can be treated definitively with resection or radiofrequeny ablation.

Suggested Reading

Chai JW, Hong SH, Choi JY, et al. Radiologic diagnosis of osteoid osteoma: from simple to challenging findings. Radiographics. 2010;30:737–49.

Case 42

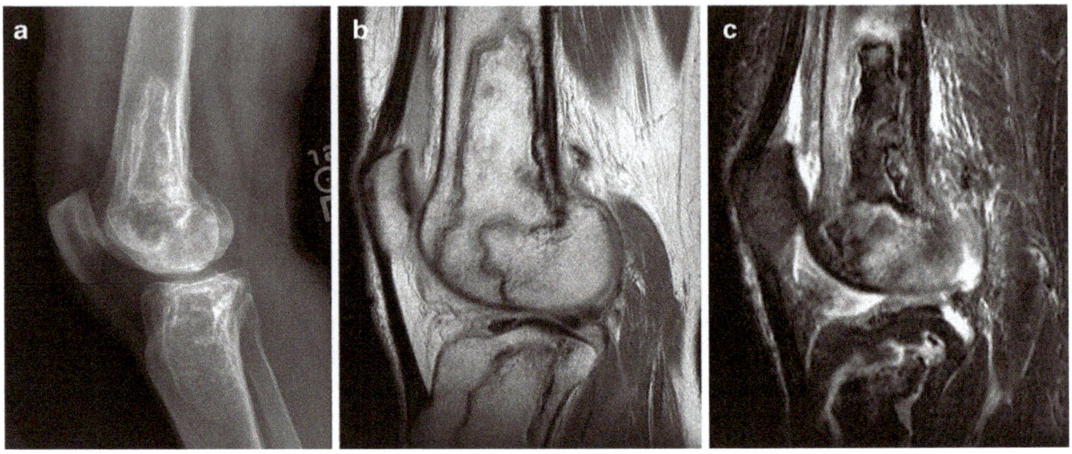

Fig. 10.42

History

A 56-year-old woman with systemic lupus erythematosis (SLE) and knee pain.

Imaging Findings

The lateral knee radiograph (a) shows areas of mixed lucency and peripheral sclerosis in the distal femur and proximal tibia. There is no bony expansion, cortical breakthrough, or joint space narrowing. The MR (b) images show well-demarcated serpentine areas of low and high signal in a "puzzle-piece" configuration. There is fatty signal in the center of the lesion on the T1-weighted MR image (b) and perilesional edema on the STIR image (c).

Differential Diagnosis (Best 3)

Osteonecrosis
Enchondromas (based on radiograph)
Intraosseous lipomas

Discussion

Osteonecrosis classically has peripheral serpentine sclerosis with central lucency, whereas enchondromas have central calcifications with subtle peripheral lucency. The MR appearance is pathognomonic for avascular necrosis with its irregular serpentine borders of low and high signal. Intraosseous lipomas are rarely multiple and have a round/oval appearance. Chronic steroid use and underlying SLE were the presumed causes of osteonecrosis in this patient.

Diagnosis

Osteonecrosis (avascular necrosis)

Key Points

- Osteonecrosis results from ischemic necrosis of the bone from lack of blood supply.
- There is variability in terminology, however, in general "avascular necrosis" refers to osteonecrosis affecting the epiphysis and extending to the articular surface whereas "bone infarct" refers to intramedullary areas of osteonecrosis in the metaphysis or diaphysis.
- Causes include: trauma (#1), steroids (#2), hemoglobinopathies, alcoholism, pancreatitis, Gaucher's disease, irradiation, chemotherapy, and Caisson disease.
- Steroids are believed to increase fat content in the marrow, leading to increased intraosseous pressure or fat emboli.
- Appearance varies with the stage of disease and findings on radiographs lag behind findings on MRI and bone scintigraphy.
- Gadolinium enhanced MRI can aid in detecting early cases and to assess need for revascularization.

Suggested Reading

Jaramillo D. What is the optimal imaging of osteonecrosis, Perthes, and bone infarcts? Pediatr Radiol. 2009;39 Suppl 2:S216–9.
Assouline-Dayan Y, Chang C, Greenspan A, Shoenfeld Y, Gershwin E. Pathogenesis and natural history of osteonecrosis. Semin Arth Rheum. 2002;32(2);94–124.

Case 43

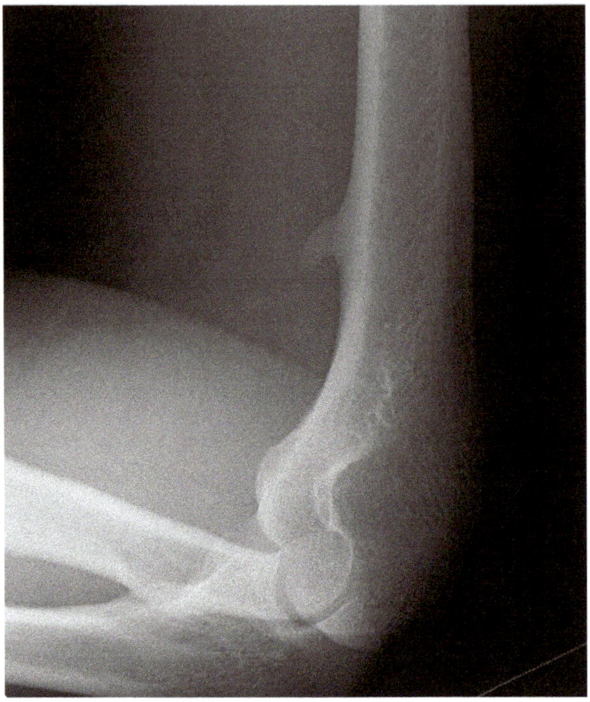

Fig. 10.43

History

A 36-year-old woman with elbow pain following fall.

Imaging Findings

There is a beak-like bony exostosis arising front the anterior cortex of the distal humerus. The apex of the exostosis points towards the elbow joint.

Differential Diagnosis (Best 3)

Supracondylar process
Osteochondroma
Surface osteosarcoma

Discussion

Given its classic location and appearance, this congenital variant supracondylar process should not be mistaken for an aggressive surface lesion such as a surface osteosarcoma. Unlike an osteochondroma, a supracondylar process should point towards the elbow joint, instead of away from it.

Diagnosis

Supracondylar process

Key Points

- First described by Struthers in 1848.
- Bony process that arises from the anteromedial aspect of the humerus in about 1–3% of the population.
- Two subtypes (tubercle and spine).
- Phylogenetic vestige of the supracondyloid foramen seen in some reptiles and mammals.
- A ligament of Struthers can arise from the spur and attach to the medial humeral epicondyle creating a fibroosseous tunnel that can compress the median nerve and, sometimes, the brachial artery, as they pass through it.

Suggested Reading

Natsis K. Supracondylar process of the humerus: study on 375 caucasian subjects in Cologne, Germany. Clin Anat. 2008;21:138–41.

Case 44

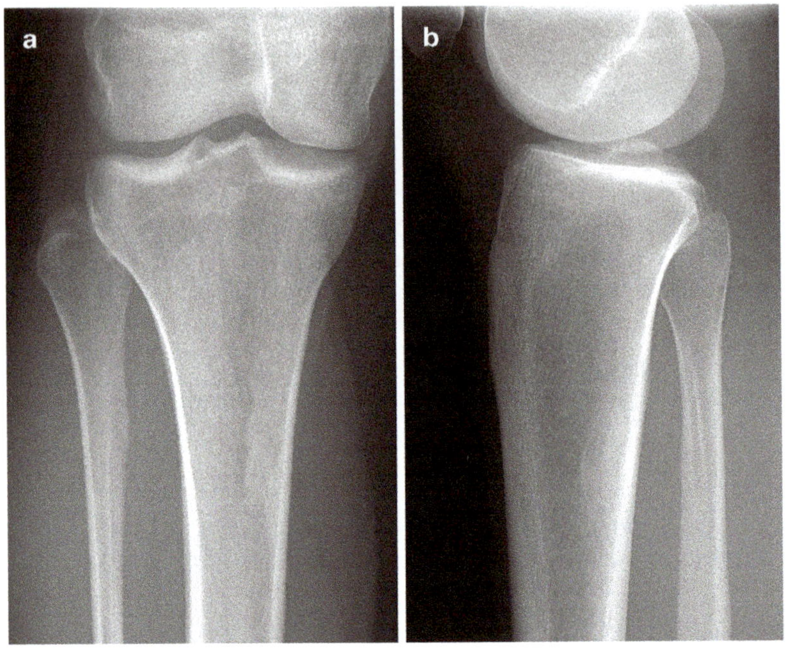

Fig. 10.44

History

A 27-year-old man with knee pain.

Imaging Findings

AP (a) and lateral (b) radiographs show a focal, elongated, predominantly sclerotic area in the proximal tibial diaphysis, abutting the posteromedial cortex. The margins are somewhat indistinct. Overlying cortex is intact.

Differential Diagnosis (Best 3)

Fibrous dysplasia
Osteoid osteoma
Healed non-ossifying fibroma (NOF)

Discussion

This appearance is pathognomonic for a healed NOF that has filled in. The location seen here, eccentric and abutting the posterior cortex, is highly suggestive of an NOF. While fibrous dysplasia might have a similar radiographic appearance and can also occur in the metadiaphysis, it tends to be central, rather than eccentric, when in a long bone. Osteoid osteoma commonly occurs in the tibia and in the diaphysis, where it can generate sufficient sclerosis to obscure the nidus. However, osteoid osteomas almost invariably present with pain, usually worse at night.

Diagnosis

Healed non-ossifying fibroma (NOF)

Key Points

- Classic "don't touch" lesion; benign and possibly posttraumatic.
- Should not have soft tissue mass.
- Migrate from metaphysis to diaphysis with age.
- Most "heal," i.e., spontaneously fill-in with trabecular bone, partially or completely, over 4+ years, beginning at the end of adolescence.
- Lesion should not appear de novo in an adult—if so, it is not a NOF.
- MRI appearance is heterogeneous and variable, with low T2 sclerotic rim.

Suggested Reading

Jee WH, Choe BY, Kang HS, et al. Non-ossifying fibroma: characteristics at MR imaging with pathologic correlation. Radiology. 1998;209:197–202.

Case 45

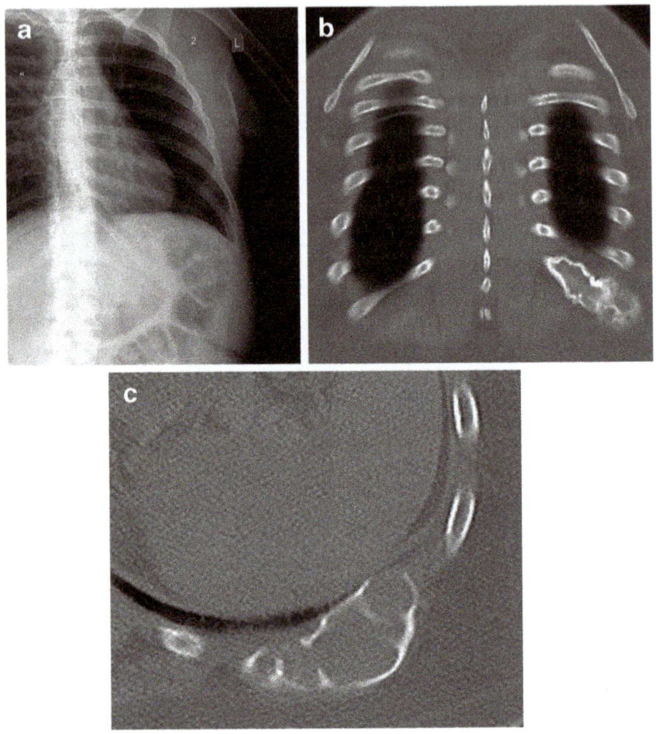

Fig. 10.45

History

A 37-year-old man with pleuritic left back pain after minor trauma.

Imaging Findings

On the radiograph (a), a long segment of the left tenth posterior rib is lucent, expanded, and lobulated, with cortical thinning. Coronal (b) and axial (c) CT images better depict the lesion and demonstrate faint ground glass density within it. There is a nondisplaced fracture, accounting for a small area of cortical interruption. There is no soft tissue mass.

Differential Diagnosis (Best 3)

Fibrous dysplasia
Metastasis
Myeloma

Discussion

Each diagnosis is the most common rib lesion in its category: benign lesions—fibrous dysplasia; malignant—metastasis; and primary bone malignancy—multiple myeloma. Fibrous dysplasia tends to be a long lesion in a long bone, with ground glass density, and can cause expansion and cortical thinning when in a small bone. It should have no cortical interruption, periosteal new bone, or surrounding soft tissue abnormality, unless there is a fracture. Metastases and myeloma tend to involve smaller segments of rib, appear more aggressive, and may have soft tissue extension.

Diagnosis

Fibrous dysplasia (with non-displaced fracture)

Key Points

- Benign lesion; malignant transformation is extremely rare.
- ≤20% of monostotic cases and 55% of polyostotic cases have fibrous dysplasia in the ribs.
- Can occur anywhere along the rib; expansion and mineralization may vary along the lesion.
- Most lesions, including ribs, cease or slow growth at puberty.

Suggested Reading

Fitzpatrick KA, Taljanovic MS, Speer DP, et al. Imaging findings of fibrous dysplasia with histopathologic and intraoperative correlation. AJR Am J Roentgenol. 2004;182:1389–98.

Case 46

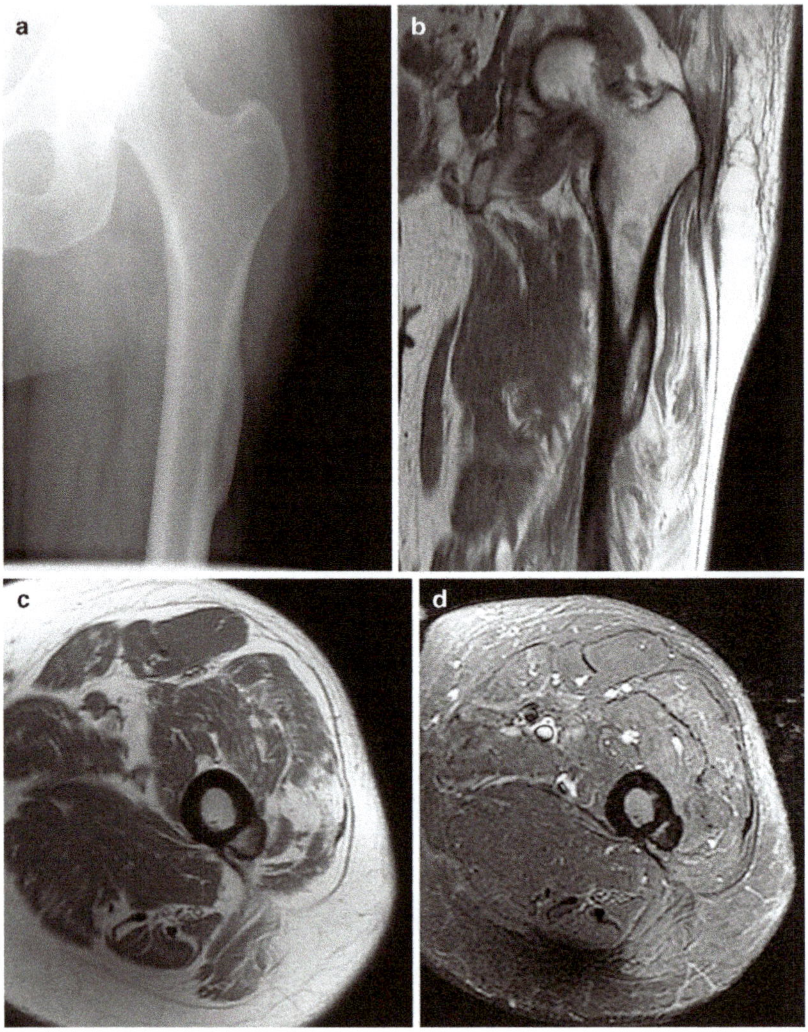

Fig. 10.46

History

A 68-year-old man with hip pain.

Imaging Findings

The AP radiograph (a) shows a lesion arising from the lateral cortex of the proximal femur. The lesion has a smooth nonaggressive appearance and there is an area of lucency between the normal femoral cortex and the lateral surface of the lesion. On the MRI images, there is high T1 signal (b and c) within the lesion, which follows fat signal on all MR sequences. There is also a lack of marrow edema on the fat-saturated T2 image (d). The lateral thigh muscles show focal atrophy and fatty replacement.

Differential Diagnosis (Best 3)

Osteochondroma
Surface osteosarcoma
Chronic periosteal hematoma

Discussion

The lesion has a nonaggressive appearance and could be mistaken for a sessile osteochondroma. However, there is no connection between the medullary cavities of the femur and the lesion, making an osteochondroma unlikely. The nonaggressive nature and lack of hyperintense signal on the fat-saturated T2 image makes a surface osteosarcoma unlikely. Moreover, the center of the lesion follows fat on all sequences, compatible with the fatty marrow that can be seen with a chronic periosteal hematoma that has gone on to ossify.

Diagnosis

Chronic periosteal hematoma

Key Points

- The periosteum is a fibrous membrane which is closely adherent to the nonarticular surface of the bone and only visible when injured.
- Infection, trauma, and tumor can all elevate the periosteum, which can then form new bone.
- Since the periosteum is highly vascular, subperiosteal hematomas can form, dissecting the periosteal membrane away from the bone, forming a focal mass.
- Often, these lesions will resolve with no sequela; however, subperiosteal hematomas that persist can ossify.
- The lesions can be recognized by their nonaggressive appearance, subperiosteal location, and the fact that they often contain fatty marrow.

Suggested Reading

Choi HJ, Lee CC, Lim TH, Singer AJ. Traumatic subperiosteal pseudoaneurysm: a rare case of subperiosteal hematoma. Am J Emerg Med. 2009;27(9):1172.

Case 47

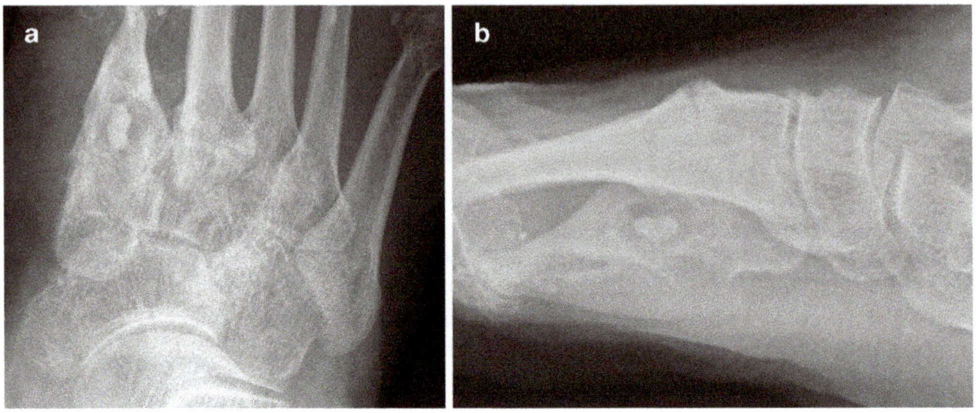

Fig. 10.47 Images courtesy of Dr. Manjiri Didolkar, Boston, MA

History

A 50-year-old man with intermittent pain, swelling, and drainage in the medial right foot.

Imaging Findings

Radiographs (a and b) show a lobulated, homogeneously dense, calcific density lying within a well-defined lucent lesion in the proximal first metatarsal. There is an incomplete sclerotic rim, an area of cortical interruption inferiorly, and soft tissue stranding. The proximal first metatarsal is irregular (expanded proximally and tapered distally from prior surgery).

Differential Diagnosis (Best 3)

Chronic osteomyelitis
Osteoid osteoma
Lymphoma

Discussion

The key is recognizing that the density represents a bony sequestrum. It lies within a well-circumscribed cavity, with a cloaca (tract through the bone), consistent with chronic osteomyelitis. An osteoid osteoma in the metaphysis should have more surrounding sclerosis (though lesions in the joint space may have minimal periostitis). Sequestra can be seen in lymphoma and Langerhans cell histiocytosis, but lymphoma is a more aggressive, moth-eaten or permeative lytic lesion, and LCH sequestra are usually seen in the skull. Neither osteoid osteoma or LCH should have a cloaca interrupting the bone, although, recently, a "vascular groove" has been described in osteoid osteomas.

Diagnosis

Chronic osteomyelitis with bony sequestrum

Key Points

- Chronic osteomyelitis can have quiescent periods, punctuated by recurrent episodes of swelling and purulent drainage. Features are well demonstrated by CT.
- Sequestrum in chronic osteomyelitis—necrotic, devascularized bone fragment, surrounded by granulation tissue and normal bone. Can harbor live infectious organisms. Not treatable with antibiotics and requires surgery.
- Involucrum—reactive bone that surrounds the sequestrum.
- Cloaca—focal channel through the involucrum.
- On MRI, the sequestrum is low signal. Surrounding granulation tissue can enhance.
- "Sequestrum" can also refer to an island of bone within an osteolytic lesion, regardless of vascular status, and can be seen in Langerhans cell histiocytosis, lymphoma, fibrosarcoma, MFH, and metastatic carcinoma. Differential diagnosis includes lesions with matrix calcification that simulates sequestra: osteoid osteoma, osteoblastoma, chondroma, chondroblastoma, lipoma, and some benign fibrous tumors.

Suggested Reading

Jennin F, Bousson V, Parlier et al. Bony sequestrum: a radiologic review. Skeletal Radiol. 2011:40:963–75.
Wells PO. The button sequestrum of eosinophilic granuloma of the skull. Radiology. 1956;67:746–7.

Case 48

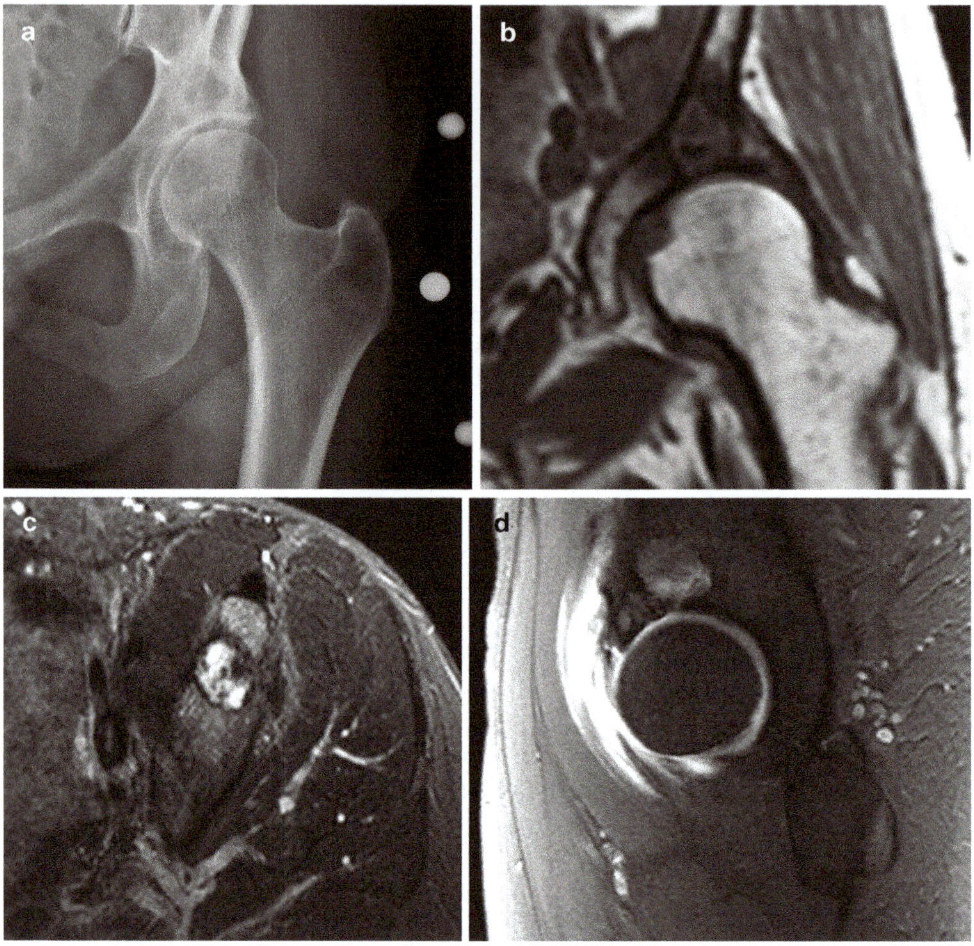

Fig. 10.48

History

A 65-year-old with left hip pain.

Imaging Findings

Radiograph (a) shows a large lobulated subchondral lucency with sclerotic rim in the supraacetabular left iliac bone, isointense to muscle on the T1-weighted MR image (b) and hyperintense with surrounding edema on the axial fat-saturated T2-weighted MR image (c). Sagittal image from an MR arthrogram (d) shows high signal gadolinium contrast extending from the joint space into the lesion, with cartilage thinning, additional subchondral changes, and labral tear anteriorly.

Differential Diagnosis (Best 3)

Langerhans cell histiocytosis (LCH)
Eggers cyst (osteoarthritis)
Metastasis

Discussion

In most cases, when large subchondral cysts occur, there will be additional radiographic evidence of osteoarthritis. If those features are not present, then the differential might include lucent lesions that involve the epiphysis, such as Langerhans cell histiocytosis or even metastasis. A sclerotic rim is uncommon in LCH, but might be seen in the early phases of healing. Because subchondral cysts occur with degenerative changes, the patients are usually older and metastatic disease is often a consideration. Typically metastatic lesions lack a sclerotic rim and can occur in the absence of osteoarthritis changes. In this case, MRI reveals cartilage thinning and additional subchondral changes that were not apparent on the radiograph and also demonstrates that the lesion communicates with the joint, confirming a subchondral cyst.

Diagnosis

Eggers cyst (osteoarthritis)

Key Points

- Eggers cysts are acetabular cysts associated with osteoarthritis of the hip.
- Subchondral cysts (geodes) can show some internal enhancement after IV contrast. The etiology is controversial, possibly due to seepage of joint fluid through cortical fissures, enhancement of synovium extending into the cyst, or diffusion from subchondral bone.
- Lesions that arise in or extend into the epiphysis include: osteoarthritic cysts (geodes), erosions due to PVNS or rheumatoid arthritis, osteomyelitis secondary to septic arthritis, LCH, chondroblastoma, clear cell chondrosarcoma, and giant cell tumor (extending into epiphysis).

Suggested Reading

Eggers GWB, Evans EB, Blumel JJ, et al. Cystic changes in the iliac acetabulum. J Bone Joint Surg Am. 1963;45:669–86.
Stark DD, Genant HK, Spring DB. Primary cystic arthrosis of the hip. Skeletal Radiol. 1984;11:124–7.
Crema MD, Roemer FW, Marra J, et al. Contrast-enhanced MRI of subchondral cysts in patients with or at risk for knee osteoarthritis: the MOST study. Eur J Radiol. 2010;75(1):e92–6.

Case 49

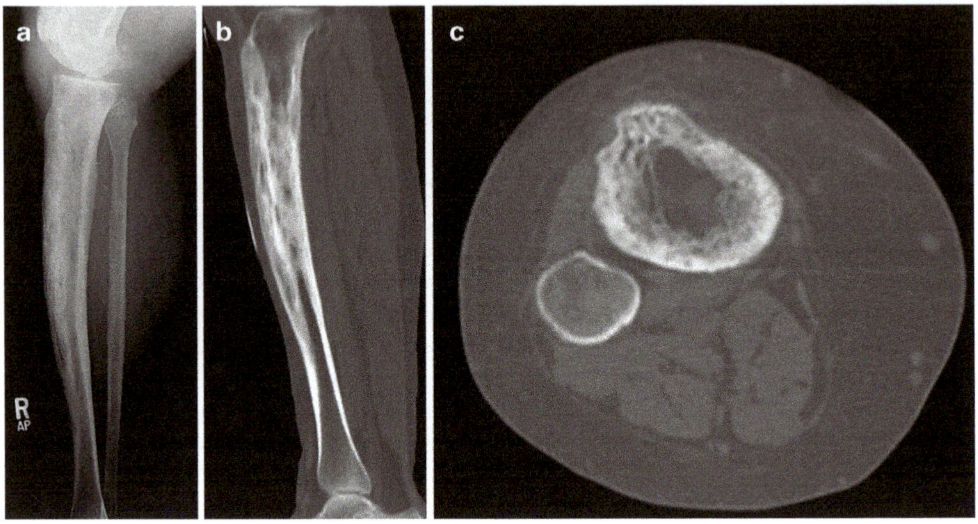

Fig. 10.49

History

A 63-year-old man with leg pain.

Imaging Findings

Lateral radiograph (a) of the tibia shows mixed lucent and sclerotic changes in the tibial shaft with mild anterior bowing of the bone. There is sparing of the proximal and distal ends of the tibia. Although the changes are mostly in the anterior cortex on the radiograph, the sagittal CT image (b) shows that the changes extend to the posterior aspect as well. The axial CT image (c) shows that the findings are circumferential and there is cortical and medullary expansion. No cortical breakthrough is seen.

Differential Diagnosis (Best 3)

Adamantinoma
Osteomyelitis
Paget disease

Discussion

Several disease processes can occur in the tibia, particularly the anterior tibia. Adamantinomas occur almost exclusively in the anterior cortex of the tibia and occur from invagination of epitheliod cells into the tibial cortex during development. Here, circumferential involvement makes adamantinoma unlikely. Osteomyelitis is possible, although the uniform cortical enlargement would be unusual. While Paget disease characteristically begins at the end of a long bone and progresses contiguously from the epiphysis into the diaphysis, Paget disease in the tibia is unique in that it can arise in the middle of the bone, without involving the epiphysis.

Diagnosis

Paget disease

Key Points

- Unknown cause, possibly viral (paramyxovirus).
- Disease of the elderly and more common in men.
- Characterized by excessive bony remodeling with active and latent phases.
- Causes thickening of the medullary trabeculae and bone cortex with overall bony enlargement.
- Three phases: (1) lytic—excessive bone resorption, (2) mixed—increased bone formation due to osteoblastic activity, and (3) blastic—osteoblastic activity declines and disease becomes less active.
- Symptoms: fractures, pain, hearing loss, and sarcomatous transformation (osteosarcoma) in <1%.
- Hydroxyproline can be elevated during the lytic phase due to bone resorption; alkaline phosphatase increased in mixed and blastic phases due to osteoblastic activity.
- Pelvis, skull, and long bones are most commonly affected sites.
- Paget disease in the tibia can be localized to the mid-shaft (as in this case) instead of beginning at one end of the bone.
- Bisphosphonates (alendronate) and calcitonin can be effective treatment medications.

Suggested Reading

Levine SM, Lambiase RE, Petchprapa CN. Cortical lesions of the tibia: characteristic appearances at conventional radiography. Radiographics. 2003;23:157–77.
Ocguder A, Tecimel O, Firat A, Bozkurt M. Silent swelling of the tibia in a 43-year-old man. Clin Orthop Relat Res. 2008;466:2565–9.

Case 50

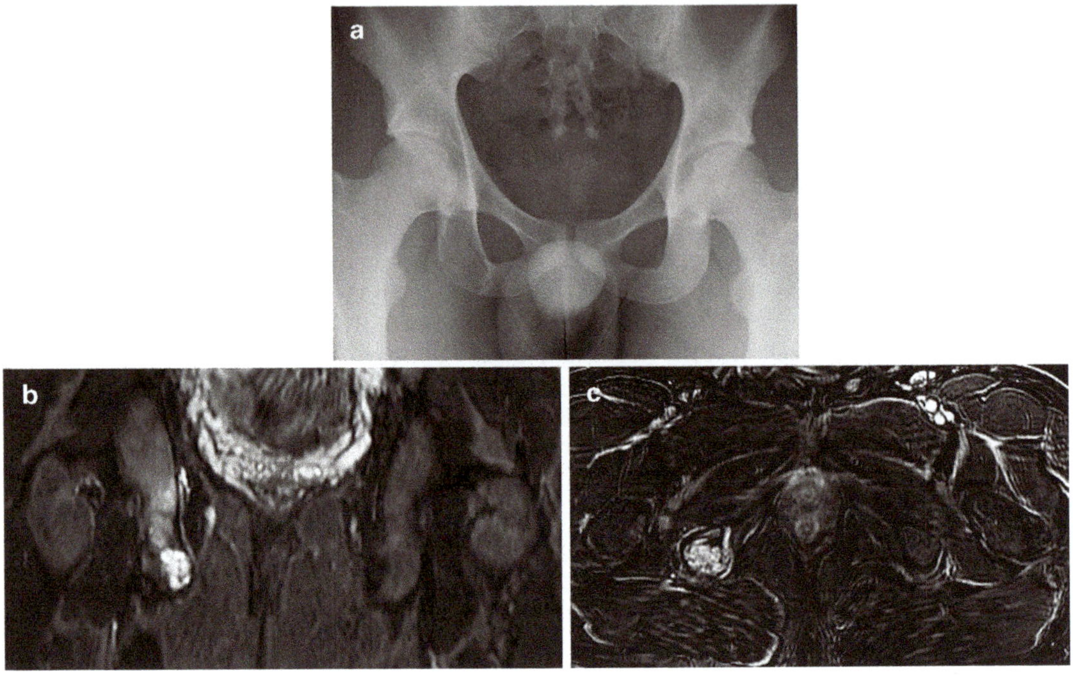

Fig. 10.50

History

A 21-year-old man with posterior right hip pain.

Imaging Findings

AP radiograph (a) shows a well-circumscribed, geographic, lucent lesion in the right ischial tuberosity. The lesion is slightly expansile, with cortical thinning, but no matrix mineralization or periosteal new bone. On MRI, the lesion is hyperintense on the coronal STIR image (b) with surrounding edema, and has diffuse homogeneous enhancement on the postcontrast subtraction MR image (c).

Differential Diagnosis (Best 3)

Aneurysmal bone cyst (ABC)
Simple bone cyst (SBC)
Giant cell tumor (GCT)

Discussion

The radiographic appearance and young age could include all three diagnoses, although ABC is more expansile. Most ABCs, SBCs, and GCTs occur in long bones; however, ABC and SBC can be seen about the pelvis in older individuals. Recognizing that the ischial tuberosity is an apophysis helps support a diagnosis of GCT, since GCT can occur in apophyses and other epiphyseal equivalents. MRI helps drive the diagnosis: the lesion is solid, not cystic, excluding SBC, and there are no fluid levels to suggest ABC. Campanacci Type III GCTs can be locally aggressive. Absence of chondroid calcification makes clear cell chondrosarcoma unlikely. In an older person, the differential could include a metastasis or multiple myeloma.

Diagnosis

Giant cell tumor at ischial apophysis

Key Facts

- GCT can be a primary or secondary lesion.
- Also known as "osteoclastoma," similar histologically to brown tumors.
- Though majority are in long bones about knee, can also occur in apophyses, e.g., ischial tuberosity, and in epiphyseal equivalents.
- T2 signal on MRI is variable: low/intermediate due to hemosiderin or fibrosis; high due to cystic areas; fluid levels due to secondary ABC component.
- Can see high T2 signal and contrast enhancement in the marrow surrounding the lesion, due to inflammatory changes in lesions with high prostaglandin levels.

Suggested Reading

Herman SD, Mesgarzadeh N, Bonakdarpour A, Dalinka MK. The role of magnetic imaging in giant cell tumor of bone. Skeletal Radiol. 1987;16:635–43.
Yamamura S, Sato K, Sugiura H, et al. Prostaglandin levels of primary bone tumor tissues correlate with peritumoral edema demonstrated by magnetic resonance imaging. Cancer. 1997; 79(2)255–61.

Case 51

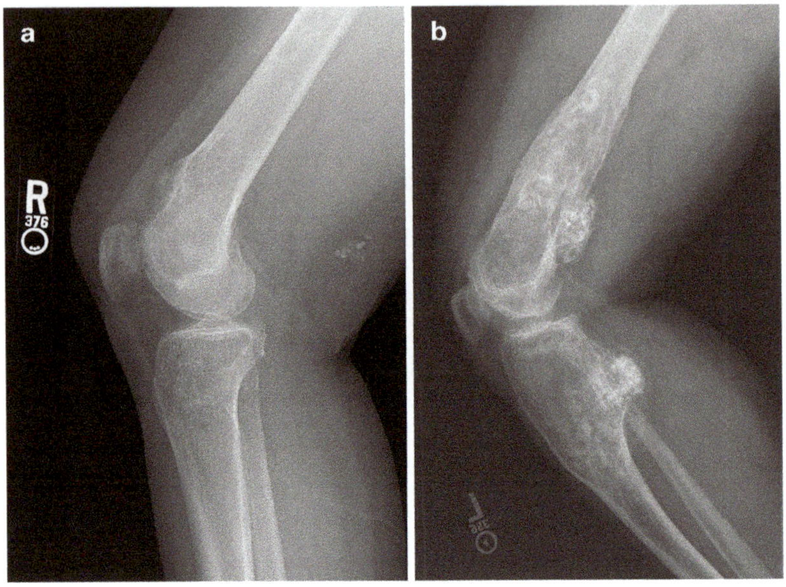

Fig. 10.51

History

A 46-year-old woman with bilateral chronic knee pain and short stature.

Imaging Findings

Lateral radiographs of both knees (a and b) show multiple lesions arising from both femurs and tibias. These lesions cause expansion and osseous deformity, left worse than right, and although several lesions are exophytic, they involve the medullary cavity. The lesions have punctuate and lobulated areas of calcification consistent with chondroid matrix. In the right knee, rounded calcifications with lucent centers (phleboliths) are seen in the posterior soft tissues.

Differential Diagnosis (Best 3)

Hereditary multiple exostoses (HME)
Ollier disease
Maffucci syndrome

Discussion

Given that there are multiple bilateral lesions, a systemic process should be considered. The pattern of involvement is similar to a patient with HME; however, the lesions are centered in the medullary cavity, not arising from the cortical surface as would be expected of an osteochondroma (exostosis). The posterior calcifications in the right knee are phleboliths from a cavernous hemangioma, which helps distinguish Maffucci syndrome from Ollier disease.

Diagnosis

Maffucci syndrome

Key Points

- Congenital, nonhereditary disorder characterized by multiple enchondromas and cavernous hemangiomas (or less commonly with lymphangiomas).
- Risk of transformation into chondrosarcoma is 10–25%.
- Associated with pain, limited range of motion and growth disturbances.
- Patients often require multiple surgeries to correct growth deformities and painful lesions.
- Multiple enchondromatosis includes several rare disorders associated with enchondromas: metachondromatosis (has both enchondromas and osteochondromas), genochondromatosis, and spondyloenchondrodysplasia.

Suggested Reading

Pannier S, Legeai-Mallet L. Hereditary multiple exostoses and enchondromatosis. Best Pract Res Clin Rheumatol. 2008;22:45–54.

Pansuriya TC, Kroon HM, Bovée JV. Enchondromatosis: insights on the different subtypes. Int J Clin Exp Pathol. 2010;3(6):557–69.

Case 52

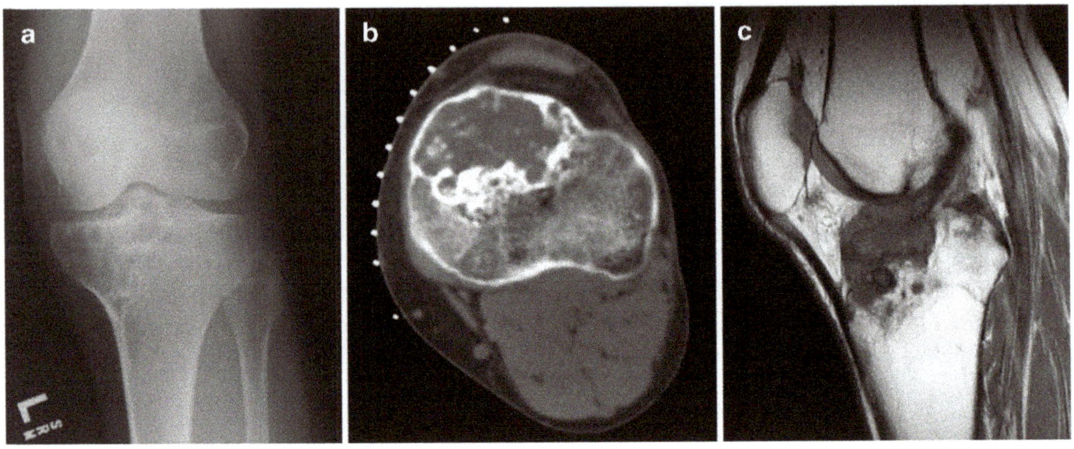

Fig. 10.52

History

A 27-year-old man with severe non-traumatic knee pain.

Imaging Findings

The radiograph (a) shows a mixed lytic and sclerotic lesion in the medial tibial plateau extending to the articular surface. On the CT image (b), the chondroid matrix in the lesion is better visualized than on the radiograph. The T1-weighted MR image (c) shows the aggressive nature of the lesion. There is cortical breakthrough superiorly into the joint space, with involvement of the anterior cruciate ligament, compatible with extracompartmental disease.

Differential Diagnosis (Best 3)

Subchondral cyst (based on the radiograph)
Chondrosarcoma (clear cell)
Chondroblastoma

Discussion

Although a large subchondral cyst is possible, the lack of significant osteoarthritis and corresponding changes in the femur make it unlikely. The CT is helpful in demonstrating the chondroid matrix. Since the lesion is in an epiphyseal location, a clear cell chondrosarcoma or chondroblastoma should be considered. The MR shows the aggressive nature of the lesion with intra-articular spread, suggesting a chondrosarcoma. At resection, most of the specimen showed high grade chondrosarcoma; however, a small percentage of the tumor was composed of high grade malignant osteoid producing cells. Thus, the final diagnosis was a osteosarcoma, chondroblastic type.

Diagnosis

Osteosarcoma, chondroblastic type

Key Points

- Although the majority of the tumor in this case was chondrosarcoma, any mesenchymal sarcoma that produces osteoid matrix is termed an "osteosarcoma," even if only 1% of the lesion produces bone.
- The tumor is comprised of lobules of malignant cartilage cells and peripheral spindle cells intermixed with lace-like osteoid.
- Most common locations are the femur and tibia.
- The presence of both cartilaginous and osteoid components can lead to sampling error.
- Contrast enhanced MR can help to identify enhancing nodular tissue to target for biopsy.
- Staging is best performed with MR, which can help show extracompartmental spread, such as extension into the joint space.

Suggested Reading

Murphey MD, Robbin MR, McRae GA, Flemming DJ, Temple HT, Kransdorf MJ. The many faces of osteosarcoma. Radiographics. 1997;17:1205–31.
Logan PM, Mitchell MJ, Munk PL. Imaging of variant osteosarcomas with an emphasis on CT and MR imaging. AJR Am J Roentgenol. 1998;171:1531–7.

Case 53

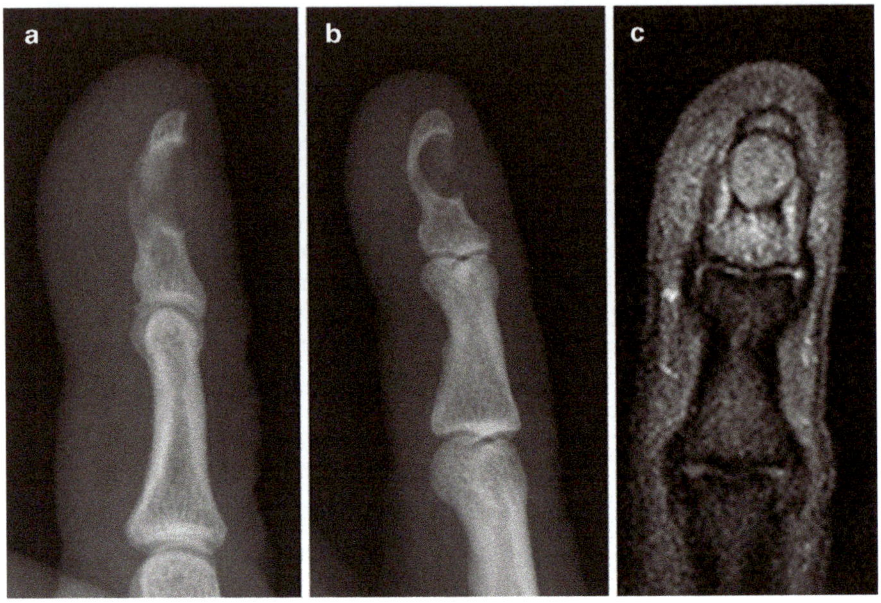

Fig. 10.53 Images courtesy of Dr. Colm McMahon, Dublin, Ireland

History

A 45-year-old man with finger pain.

Imaging Findings

Lateral (a) and oblique (b) radiographs of the small finger show a round lucent lesion with thin sclerotic margin in the distal phalanx. There is cortical breakthrough dorsally, with an apparent soft tissue component. The coronal fat-saturated T2 MR image (c) shows mild bone expansion and perilesional edema in the adjacent marrow and soft tissues.

Differential Diagnosis (Best 3)

Enchondroma
Epidermoid inclusion cyst of bone (EIC)
Glomus tumor

Discussion

Lytic lesions of the hand are common. Enchondromas in the hands and feet often do not have internal cartilaginous calcifications, unlike enchondromas elsewhere in the body. The history of prior trauma would favor an EIC, but often the patient does not recall any trauma. Glomus tumors are benign tumors of the glomus body, a structure which helps with body temperature regulation. They are often found around the nailbed and can cause scalloping of the adjacent bone. Infection and metastases are also considerations, but are less likely to have a sclerotic margin. Moreover, isolated metastases to the digits are rare.

Diagnosis

Epidermoid inclusion cyst of bone (EIC)

Key Points

- EIC in bone results from direct implantation of epidermis into bone, often from direct trauma.
- The distal phalanges of the hand and scalp are the most common locations.
- EIC appears as a lucent lesion with a thin sclerotic border on radiographs.
- At histology, the cyst has a lining of stratified squamous epithelium and contains keratin.
- It is important to remove the entire cyst capsule in order to prevent recurrence.
- Bone grafting is occasionally needed, depending on the amount of bone destruction.
- Metastases distal to the elbow or knees are rare; but when present, the most common cause is lung cancer (squamous cell), followed by renal and breast.

Suggested Reading

Hamad AT, Kumar A, Kumar CA. Intraosseous epidermoid cyst of the finger phalanx. J Ortho Surg. 2006;14(3):340–2.
Momeni A, Iblher N, Herget G. Bley T, Stark GB, Bannasch H. Distal phalangeal bone cysts: differentiation of enchondromata and epidermal cysts. J Hand Surg (Eur). 2010;35E(2):144–5.

Case 54

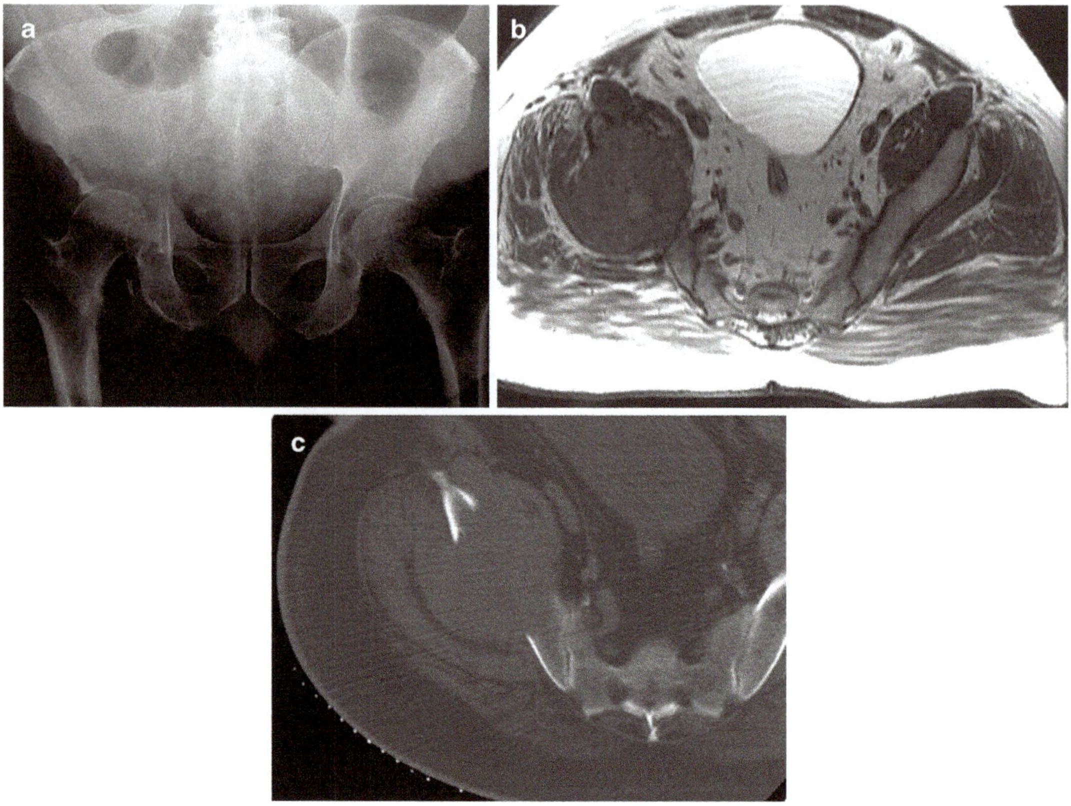

Fig. 10.54

History

A 54-year-old with right hip pain.

Imaging Findings

On close scrutiny, the AP radiograph (a) of the pelvis shows a well-circumscribed, large lucency overlying the supraacetabular portion of the right iliac bone. On first glance, this bone lesion might be mistaken for bowel gas. In retrospect, the radiograph supports the presence of a bone lesion: the normal sclerotic line along the acetabular roof (the acetabular "sourcil") and the ilioischial line are effaced and there is asymmetric narrowing of the right hip joint space. Axial T2-weighted MRI (b) and axial CT (c) images demonstrate a large, nearly isointense-to-muscle soft tissue mass centered in the iliac bone, expanding outward, and destroying cortex, without internal matrix, reactive sclerosis, or periosteal new bone.

Differential Diagnosis (Best 3)

Plasmacytoma
Lytic metastasis
Brown tumor

Discussion

The main point of this case is to show that lesions in certain areas of the body (pelvis, scapula, sternum, and rib) may be difficult to detect on radiographs even if large in size. In these instances, it is important to obtain cross-sectional imaging with CT or MRI. In patients over 40 years old with a lytic lesion, metastasis and plasmacytoma (a form of multiple myeloma) should be considered in the differential. Renal cell carcinoma and thyroid carcinoma are two common lesions that present with large "bubbly" expansile lytic lesions of bone. Renal cell carcinoma not uncommonly presents as a solitary metastasis. Absence of reactive sclerosis is a common feature in metastases. Plasmacytoma can be indistinguishable from metastasis at imaging. While brown tumors might have a similar appearance, they are typically multiple and occur in conjunction with other laboratory and imaging findings of hyperparathyroidism (e.g., resorptive changes about the radial aspects of the middle phalanx of the index and middle fingers, pubic symphysis, SI joints, and chondrocalcinosis).

Diagnosis

Renal cell metastasis

Key Points

- 50% of bone mineralization must be lost before changes are visible at conventional radiography.
- The pelvis, ribs, sternum, and scapula are areas that can be difficult to fully assess with radiographs alone. Cross-sectional imaging with CT or MRI can often help in evaluating occult lesions on radiographs.
- Osseous metastases from renal cell are common; solitary metastases are not infrequent.
- Most renal cell metastases are lytic (90%).
- Limited sensitivity for renal metastasis on bone scan, due to limited reactive bone formation.

Suggested Reading

Chua S, Gnanasegaran G, Cook GJR. Miscellaneous cancers (lung, thyroid, renal, cancer, myeloma, and neuroendocrine tumors): role of SPECT and PET in imaging bone metastases. Semin Nucl Med. 2009;39:416–30.

Cronin CG, Cashell T, NiMhuircheartaigh J, et al. Bone biopsy of new suspicious bone lesions in patients with primary carcinoma: prevalance and probability of an alternative diagnosis. Am J Roentgenol. 2009;193:W407–10.

Case 55

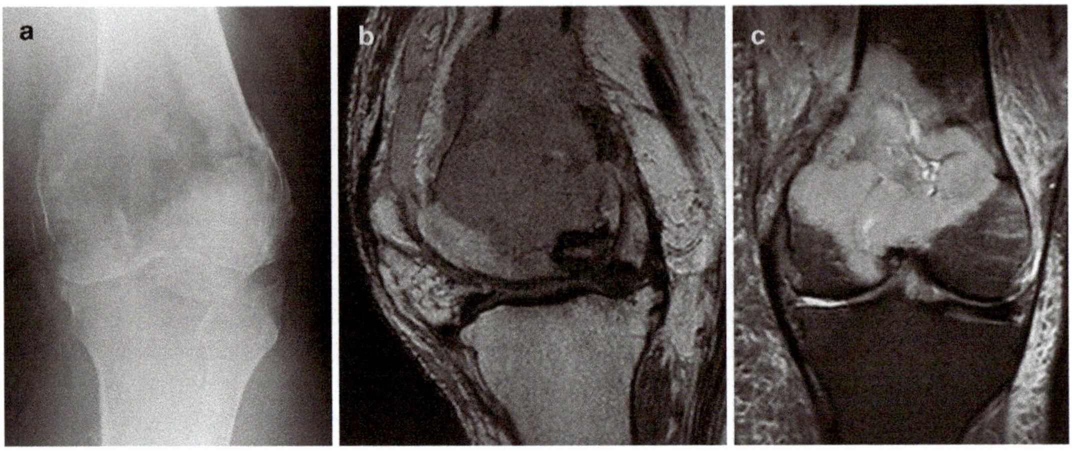

Fig. 10.55

History

A 60-year-old woman with increasing knee pain, worsening over 6 months.

Imaging Findings

The AP radiograph (a) shows an aggressive lytic lesion centered in the distal femoral metaphysis with a pathologic fracture and periosteal new bone formation. On MRI, the normal fatty marrow is replaced by a mass that is near-isointense to muscle on T1 (b), heterogeneously hyperintense on fat-saturated T2W (c) images, extends into the epiphysis, and also extends through the cortex into the surrounding soft tissues. The mass can be seen eroding out of the bone, deep to the proximal MCL.

Differential Diagnosis (Best 3)

Lymphoma
Plasmacytoma
Metastasis

Discussion

All three lesions could account for a large, aggressive, lytic lesion in someone of this age. Metastases and myeloma/plasmacytoma are less likely to demonstrate a permeative or moth-eaten pattern than lymphoma and less likely to have periosteal reaction. Although secondary lymphoma of bone is much more common than primary lymphoma of bone, secondary non-Hodgkin lymphoma (NHL) often occurs in the axial skeleton, while primary NHL occurs most commonly near the ends of long bones, such as the femur and tibia. Primary Hodgkin lymphoma of bone is extremely rare, though secondary involvement can occur in widespread disease. A torso CT would help in identifying a potential primary lesion or other findings suggestive of myeloma. Serum and urine protein electrophoresis could help in diagnosis of a plasmacytoma. In any event, given the aggressive nature, biopsy is warranted.

Diagnosis

Primary lymphoma of bone (large B cell)

Key Points

- Primary non-Hodgkin lymphoma of bone is rare and most cases are diffuse large B cell.
- Considered Stage I non-Hodgkin lymphoma. Should have no distant soft tissue or lymph node involvement and (some say) no extraosseous or nodal involvement for 6 months after diagnosis.
- Older patients, M>F.
- Most commonly presents as a lytic lesion near end of long bone, often large, poorly defined.
- Pathologic fracture, soft tissue extension, periostitis; can spread across joints.
- MRI best for extent of marrow and soft tissue disease, though reactive edema can occur.
- Isointense or slightly hyperintense to muscle on T1; enhancement and T2 signal variable.
- Tumor permeating or "oozing" through cortex into soft tissues, with only limited cortical disruption, is highly suggestive of lymphoma or other round cell tumors.
- Bone scintigraphy usually positive, even if radiographs negative.
- FDG PET/CT is used for staging workup.

Suggested Reading

Kwee TC, Kwee RM, Nievelstein RA. Imaging in staging of malignant lymphoma: a systematic review. Blood. 2008;111(2):504.
Jhanwar YS, Straus DJ. The role of PET in lymphoma. J Nucl Med. 2006;47(8):1326–34.

Case 56

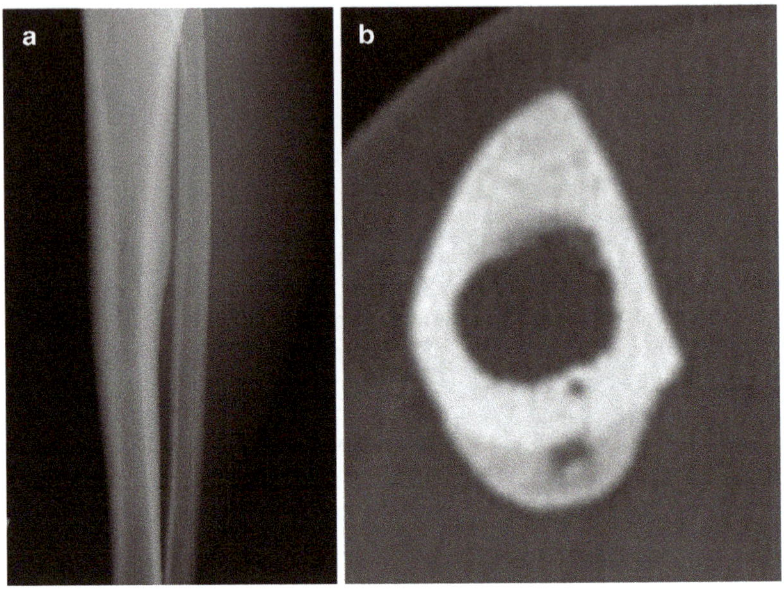

Fig. 10.56

History

A 22-year-old woman with intense posterior leg pain.

Imaging Findings

The radiograph (a) shows an area of nonaggressive mild cortical thickening along the posterior cortex of the tibia. On the CT image (b), there is a smooth periosteal thickening arising from the posterior tibia cortex. A focal lucency is centered within the thickened periosteum, not in the cortex. Incidental note is made of a tiny lucency anterior to the lesion in the tibial cortex from a vascular channel.

Differential Diagnosis (Best 3)

Osteoid osteoma (subperiosteal)
Soleal line
Osteomyelitis

Discussion

The radiographic findings are relatively nonspecific as there are many things that can cause periosteal thickening: tumor, infection, and trauma. The CT is extremely helpful in showing the nidus of the osteoid osteoma; however, the nidus is subperiosteal in location and not cortically based as in the majority of osteoid osteomas. A soleal line is a “tug” lesion due to traction from the attachment of the soleus on the tibia. The soleal line extends lateral to medial down the upper 1/3 of the posterior tibia, should not have a central nidus, and is painless. Osteomyelitis usually has changes based in the medullary cavity. Stress fractures may have a linear lucency representing the fracture line, surrounded by the periosteal reaction.

Diagnosis

Osteoid Osteoma (subperiosteal)

Key Points

- Osteoid osteomas are classified based on location: (1) cortical, (2) medullary (cancellous), and (3) subperiosteal.
- Almost always associated with pain (worse at night and alleviated by salicylates); an alternate diagnosis should be suspected if the lesion is painless.
- CT is very helpful in demonstrating the lucent nidus and its location in the bone.
- Increased use of CT and MRI suggest that the subperiosteal subtype is more common than previously thought.
- Subperiosteal osteoid osteomas typically have less periosteal reaction than cortical osteoid osteomas, making them more subtle and harder to diagnose on radiographs.
- Subperiosteal osteomas are most frequently found in the medial aspect of the femoral neck and in the hands and feet (especially the talus), but can occur in nearly any bone.

Suggested Reading

Chai JW, Hong SH, Choi JY, et al. Radiologic diagnosis of osteoid osteoma: from simple to challenging findings. Radiographics. 2010;30:737–49.
Kransdorf MJ, Stull MA, Gilkey FW, Moser RP. Osteoid osteoma. Radiographics. 1991;11:671–96.

Case 57

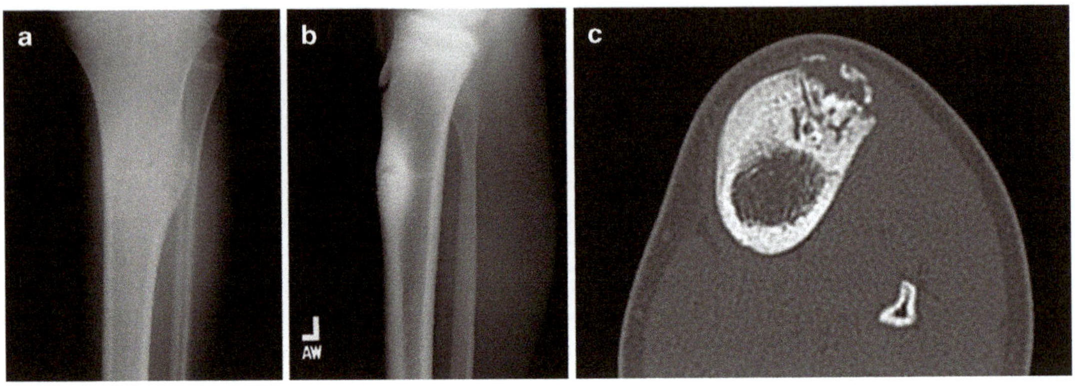

Fig. 10.57 Images courtesy of Dr. Daniel Siegal, Detroit, MI

History

A 15-year-old girl with leg pain and swelling.

Imaging Findings

AP (a) and lateral (b) radiographs of the tibia show an aggressive lesion arising from the anterolateral surface of the tibial cortex. The lesion has multiple lucencies and causes marked cortical thickening of the anterior tibial shaft. There is aggressive breakthrough of the lesion anteriorly but no involvement of the medullary cavity on the CT (c).

Differential Diagnosis (Best 3)

Periosteal chondroma
Periosteal osteosarcoma/chondrosarcoma
Osteomyelitis

Discussion

The surface irregularity and extensive cortical thickening caused by the lesion raises is consistent with an aggressive process, and additional workup is needed. This lesion can be any of the three processes listed in the above differential. Periosteal chondromas typically cause pressure erosions known as "saucerization" and can be very hard to distinguish from periosteal osteosarcomas, periosteal chondrosarcomas, or osteomyelitis. Periosteal chondromas are less likely to the have the hair-on-end periosteal reaction seen in periosteal osteosarcomas and are typically smaller (<3 cm) than periosteal chondrosarcomas. This lesion should not be confused with an osteochondroma, which will have continuity between the medullary cavities of the lesion and the host bone. Moreover, an osteoid osteoma typically has a single discrete lucent nidus.

Diagnosis

Periosteal chondroma

Key Points

- Rare benign cartilage lesion originating at the periosteal surface.
- Identical histology to enchondromas.
- Most common locations are the hands, feet, and long bones.
- Presents as a radiolucent cortically based mass (2–3 cm) with faint calcifications (50%).
- May have a "cuff" or "shelf" of bone at the edges of the lesion—"periosteal buttress sign".
- CT can be helpful to show chondroid matrix.
- Can be difficult to distinguish from periosteal chondrosarcomas; size is most reliable indicator with lesions >3 cm suggestive of chondrosarcomas.

Suggested Reading

Robinson P, White LM, Sundaram M, et al. Periosteal chondroid tumors: radiologic evaluation with pathologic correlation. AJR Am J Roentgenol. 2001;177:1183–8.

Case 58

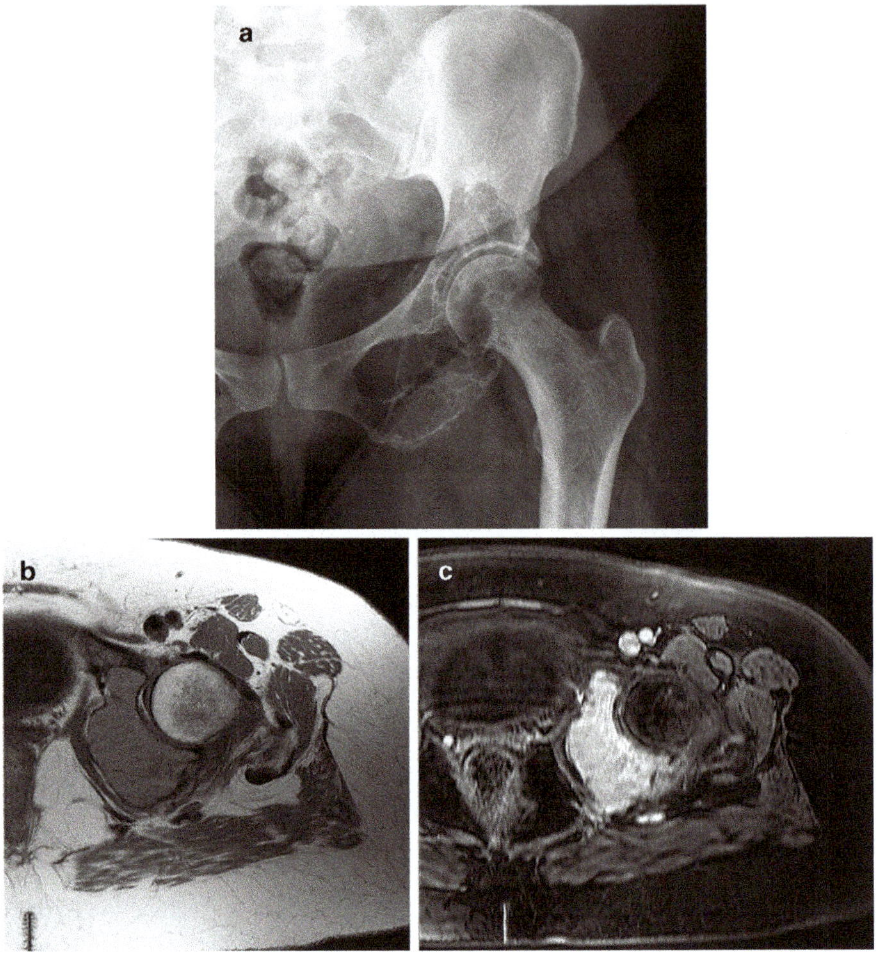

Fig. 10.58

History

A 55-year-old woman with left hip pain.

Imaging Findings

Radiograph (a) shows a large, expansile, geographic lytic lesion centered in the left acetabulum, extending into the iliac and ischial bones. There is pseudotrabeculation and marked cortical thinning, but no internal matrix. The joint space is preserved. On MRI, the lesion expanding the marrow space is relatively homogeneous, near isointense to muscle on the T1W image (b) and has diffuse intense enhancement, with evidence of soft tissue extension beyond the bone, on the post contrast image (c).

Differential Diagnosis

Chondrosarcoma
Lytic metastasis
Plasmacytoma

Discussion

The radiographic differential could include a number of geographic, lytic, and expansile lesions. In any event, the presence of soft tissue extension indicates an aggressive lesion and supports a decision to biopsy. This patient is skeletally mature, with subtle changes of osteoarthritis (suggesting someone older), making plasmacytoma and lytic metastasis most likely. History of malignancy, lab tests for myeloma, and torso CT to evaluate for primary (e.g., renal and thyroid) might help to discriminate among the various diagnoses. Chondrosarcoma occurs commonly in the pelvis and often has chondroid calcifications. In a young person, the differential would include ABC, and MRI would show multiple fluid levels.

Diagnosis

Plasmacytoma

Key Facts

- Solitary plasmacytoma of bone (SPB) represents about 5% of all plasma cell neoplasms.
- SPB is a focal bone lesion caused by neoplastic proliferation of a single clone of plasma cells, in the absence of other features of myeloma (anemia, hypercalcemia, renal insufficiency, or multiple lytic bone lesions).
- Unclear why some patients develop plasmacytoma and others develop myeloma.
- Diagnosis of plasmacytoma requires: biopsy of index lesion showing clonal plasma cells, negative bone survey (radiographic skeletal survey and either PET/CT or MRI of spine and pelvis); bone marrow aspirate and biopsy that is negative for clonal plasma cells; and absence of anemia, hypercalcemia, or renal insufficiency attributable to a clonal plasma cell disorder.
- Mean age 10–15 years younger than for multiple myeloma; twice as common in men.
- Most common in vertebrae (especially thoracic), pelvis, and ribs.
- Bone lesion can have soft tissue extension, but not required for diagnosis.
- Most common in bone, but can also arise in soft tissue (extramedullary plasmacytoma).
- Present with skeletal pain, fracture of affected bone, or, if in spine, neurologic symptoms.
- Treated with radiation therapy; median survival is 10 years.
- 50–60% with plasmacytoma develop multiple myeloma after initial radiation therapy, most within 4 years.

Suggested Reading

Terpos E, Moulopoulos LA, Dimopoulos MA. Advances in imaging and the management of myeloma bone disease. J Clin Oncol. 2011;29(14):1907–15.

Soutar R, Lucraft H, Jackson G, et al. Guidelines on the diagnosis and management of solitary plasmacytoma of bone and solitary extramedullary plasmacytoma. Br J Haematol. 2004;124(6): 717–26.

Delorme S, Baur-Melnyk A. Imaging in multiple myeloma. Eur J Radiol. 2009;70(3):401–8.

Case 59

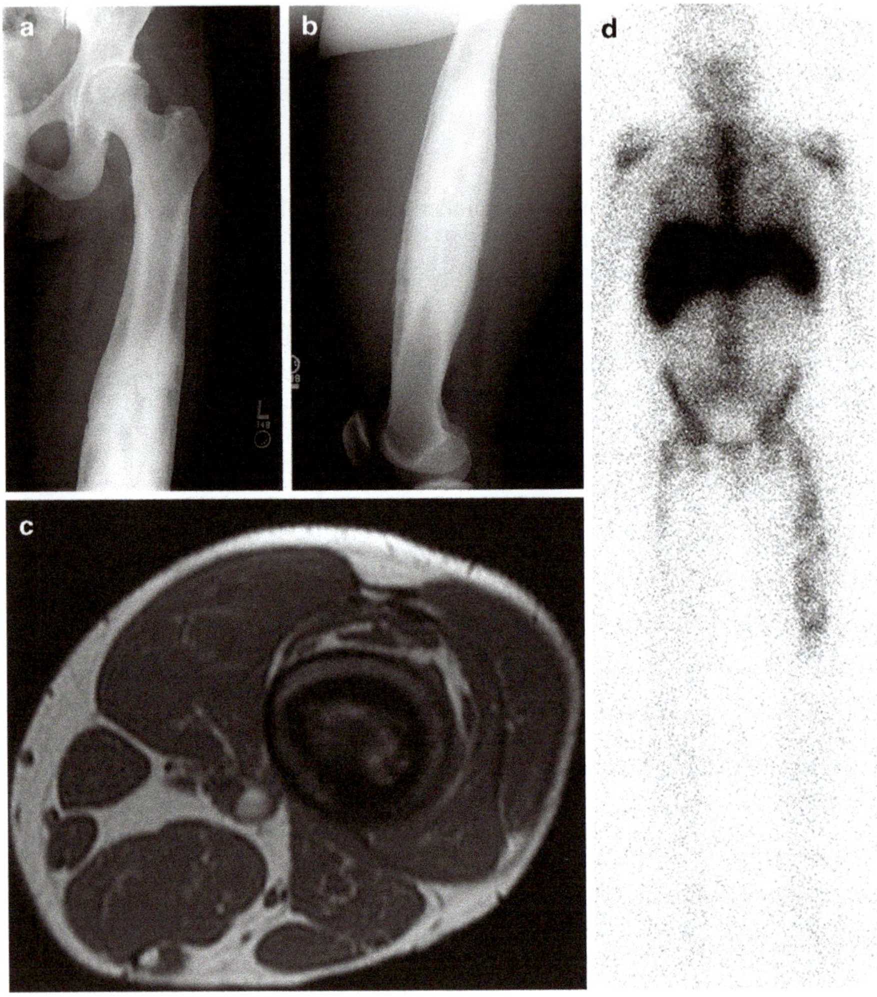

Fig. 10.59

History

A 28-year-old Brazilian man with chronic pain in the left thigh.

Imaging Findings

AP (a) and lateral (b) radiographs of the left femur showed dense bone formation in the mid shaft of the femur. There is laminated periosteal reaction best seen at the proximal aspect. The axial T1 weighted (c) MR image shows the circumferential periosteal reaction surrounding the femoral shaft. There is loss of the normal fatty marrow in the femur. The labeled white blood cell study (d) shows uptake in the femur consistent with osteomyelitis.

Differential Diagnosis (Best 3)

Trauma
Osteosarcoma
Osteomyelitis (chronic)

Discussion

Any insult to bone, including trauma, infection, and tumor can lead to new bone formation. A history of trauma should be easy to determine as the markedly abnormal appearance of the femur would have to be the result of some major trauma. Both infection and tumor can be more indolent. The type of periosteal reaction in this case is helpful. Osteosarcoma typically elicits a more aggressive subtype of periosteal reaction (sunburst, hair-on-end). The smooth and laminated periosteal reaction of the lesion is nonaggressive. However, there is often overlap in the appearance of periosteal reaction caused by benign and malignant lesions and biopsy is often warranted if malignancy can not be excluded.

Diagnosis

Osteomyelitis (chronic)

Key Points

- Osteomyelitis can have a varied imaging appearance depending on its clinical stage.
- In the acute stage, radiographs can reveal areas of aggressive periostitis, cortical destruction, endosteal scalloping, and intracortical tunneling.
- In the laminated subtype of periosteal reaction, multiple layers of new bone are formed concentrically around the cortex, producing a laminated or "onion skin" pattern.
- Originally, it was believed that alternating cycles of rapid and slow injury to bone led to the formation of concentric layers. However, more recent studies suggest that multiple layers form due to modulation of sheets of fibroblasts in the adjacent soft tissue, which develop osteoblastic potential and give rise to sheets of new bone.
- Another suggested mechanism is that, as the new layer of bone is lifted off the cortex, the inner cambium layer is stimulated to form a new bone layer below.
- The laminated appearance is seen in both benign and malignant lesions, including osteosarcomas, osteomyelitis, and chondroblastomas.

Suggested Reading

Rana RS, Wu JS, Eisenberg RL. Periosteal reaction. AJR. 2009;193:W259–72.

Case 60

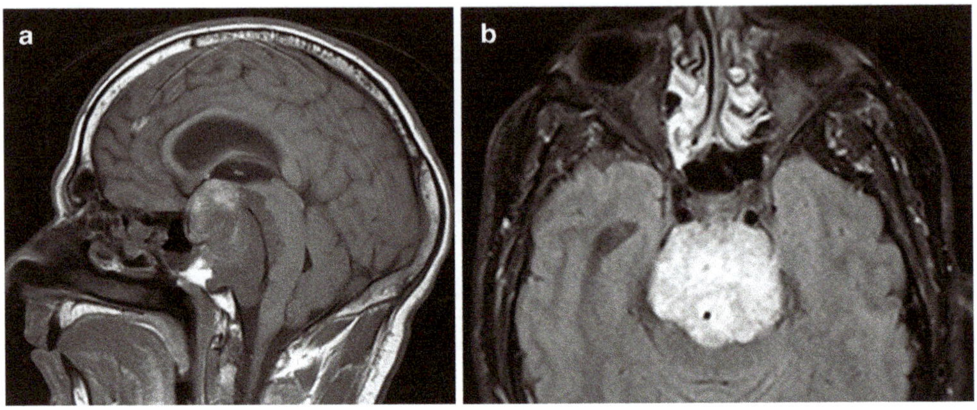

Fig. 10.60 Images courtesy of Dr. Gul Moonis, Boston, MA

History

A 43-year-old male with severe headache for 1 week.

Imaging Findings

Sagittal T1-weighted MR image (a) shows a large heterogeneous mass arising from the clivus and extending posteriorly. The lesion compresses the brainstem and cerebellum. On axial flair MR image (b), the heterogeneously high signal mass erodes the dorsal wall of the clivus, displaces both internal carotid arteries, and encases the basilar artery, with evidence of hydrocephalus.

Differential Diagnosis

Chordoma
Chondrosarcoma
Metastasis/plasmacytoma

Discussion

A midline lesion involving the clivus, with high T2 signal, heterogeneous enhancement, and bone erosion is highly suggestive of chordoma. However, chordoma cannot be conclusively distinguished from chondrosarcoma based on imaging. Chondrosarcoma tends to present at a younger age (mean 21 years). Chondrosarcomas are classically off-midline, involving the petro-occipital synchondrosis, while chordomas are classically midline, but there is significant overlap. MRI characteristics and incidence of calcifications are similar. Distinction among these and metastasis or plasmacytoma ultimately requires tissue sampling.

Diagnosis

Chordoma

Key Points

- Slow-growing, locally aggressive bone neoplasm arising from notochordal remnants.
- Typically in axial skeleton—60% in sacrum and 25% at skull base (mostly clivus).
- Median age is 46 years old, though can occur in children/adolescents.
- Patients often present with chronic headache and diplopia (cranial nerves VI and III).
- CT for bone erosion and tumor mineralization, MRI for relationship to surrounding structures.
- CT can detect erosion of occipital condyle, which requires fusion.
- CT - isodense to slightly hypodense; bone destruction common, though sometimes only a small portion of the clivus; mineralization and bony debris common; and sclerosis unusual.
- MRI - lobulated margins; low to intermediate T1, may have high T1 hemorrhage; heterogeneous high T2, perilesional brain edema very uncommon; enhancement usually heterogeneous, but some tumors show minimal enhancement.
- Extension into surrounding structures common; displacement and encasement of blood vessels common, but luminal narrowing is rare.
- Local recurrence is common. Goal of treatment is 100% surgical resection, but hard to achieve; adjuvant radiotherapy often used.
- Differentiation from chondrosarcoma is difficult on both imaging and histology, but is important, because prognosis is significantly better for chondrosarcomas.

Suggested Reading

Meyers SP, Hirsch WL, Curtin HL, et al. Chordomas of the skull base: MR features. AJNR. 1992;12:1627–36.
Pamir NM, Ozduman K. Analysis of radiological features relative to histopathology in 42 skull-base chordomas and chondrosarcomas. Eur J Radiol. 2006;58:461–70.

Case 61

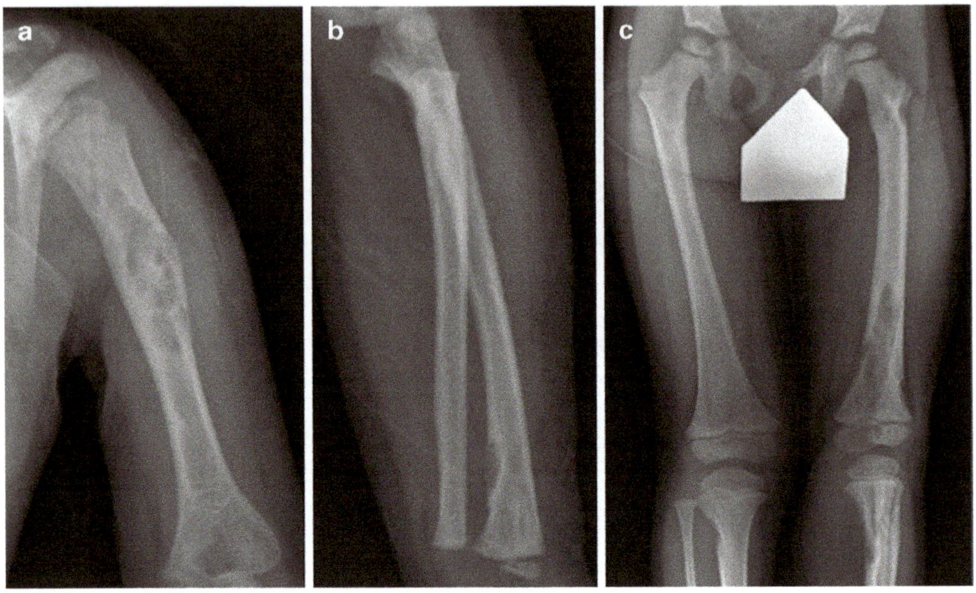

Fig. 10.61 Images courtesy of Dr. Daniel Siegal, Detroit, MI

History

An 11-year-old boy with café au lait spots and mental retardation.

Imaging Findings

The patient is skeletally immature, with multiple elongated, geographic, lucent lesions in both extremities. Lesions in the distal radius, left proximal femur, and both proximal tibiae are small, eccentric, and abut and thin the cortex. Lesions in the left proximal humerus and left distal femur are larger and extend into the central diaphysis. No periosteal new bone formation or soft tissue masses are associated with the lesions.

Differential Diagnosis (Best 3)

Polyostotic fibrous dysplasia
Neurofibromatosis Type 1 (NF1)
Jaffe-Campanacci Syndrome (JC)

Discussion

Findings are compatible with multiple non-ossifying fibromas (NOFs). JC consists of multiple NOFs with "coast of California" café au lait spots (smooth borders) and, in some cases, mental retardation. NOFs and "coast of California" spots can also occur in NF1, though bone lesions in NF1 are most often pressure erosions from neurofibromas. Additional features present in NF1 help distinguish it from JC: neurofibromas, Lisch nodules, axillary freckling, optic gliomas, and family history. Polyostotic fibrous dysplasia can be distinguished based on "coast of Maine" café au lait spots (irregular borders) and the fact that the bone lesions are typically central, diaphyseal, are long lesions, and contain ground glass density.

Diagnosis

Jaffe-Campanacci Syndrome (JC)

Key Points

- Multiple NOFs are unusual-seen in only 8% of cases.
- Jaffe-Campanacci is characterized by multiple NOFs with café au lait spots, without neurofibromas. Some patients have mental retardation.
- Rare, peak 10–15 years old; M = F.
- Majority of cases of JC are sporadic and lack positive family history.
- May present with pathologic fracture, but the lesion's natural history is like other NOFs, remaining benign and resolving over time.
- Controversy: some believe that JC is a subset of neurofibromatosis Type 1.

Suggested Reading

Hau MA, Fox EJ, Cates JM, et al. Jaffe-Campanacci syndrome. A case report and review of the literature. J Bone Joint Surg Am. 2002;84-A(4):634–8.
Colby RS, Saul RA. Is Jaffe-Campanacci syndrome just a manifestation of neurofibromatosis type 1? Am J Med Genet A. 2003;123A(1):60–3.
Moser RP, Jr, Sweet DE, Haseman DB, Madewell JE. Multiple skeletal fibroxanthomas: radiologic–pathologic correlation of 72 cases. Skeletal Radiol. 1987;16(5):353–9.

Case 62

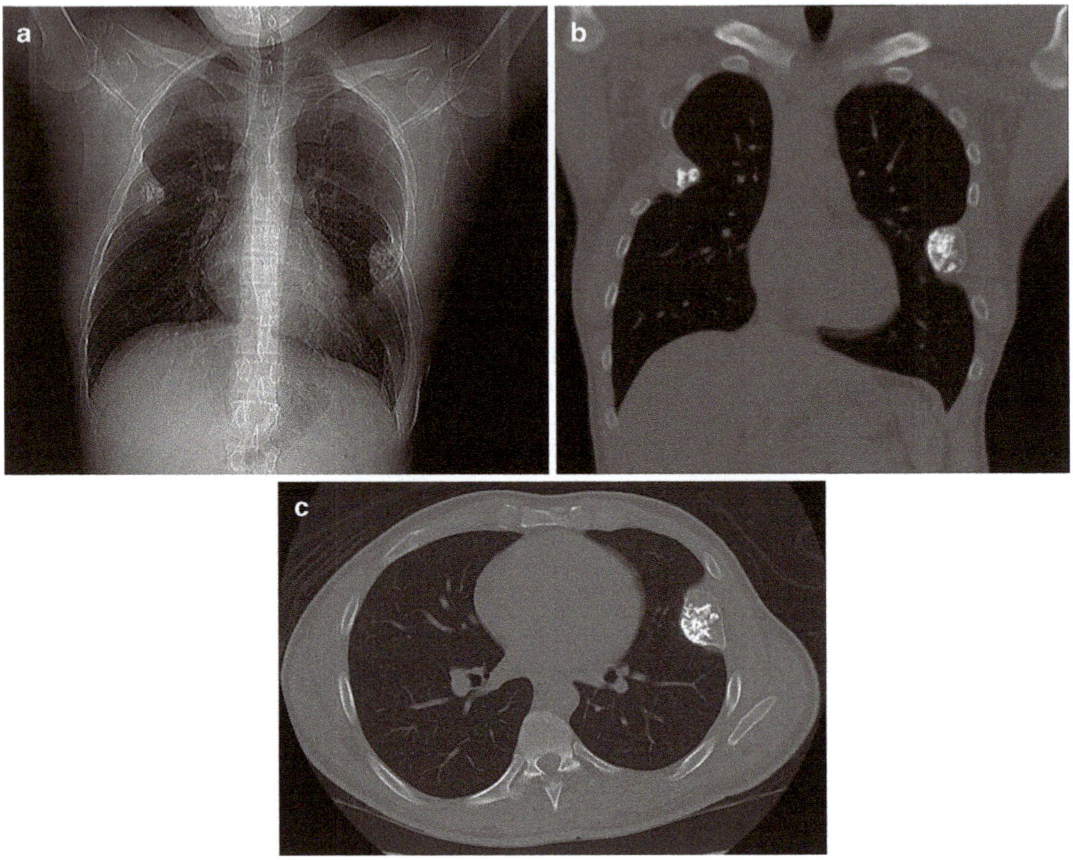

Fig. 10.62

History

A 21-year-old man with painless chest wall deformities.

Imaging Findings

CT scout image (a) shows expansile lesions with calcifications in the anteromedial aspects of the right fourth and left sixth ribs. The coronal (b) and axial (c) CT images demonstrate shortened and medially positioned ribs, likely due to growth disturbance from the underlying lesions. The lesions contain stippled calcifications and lack aggressive features such as cortical breakthrough.

Differential Diagnosis (Best 3)

Healed rib fractures
Hereditary multiple exostoses (HME)
Chondrosarcoma

Discussion

Mild bony expansion and deformity can be seen with traumatic rib fractures; however, the calcifications seen in these lesions would be unusual. The important distinguishing features of this case are the cartilaginous matrix within the lesions and the presence of multiple lesions, both of which support the diagnosis of multiple osteochondromas in a patient with HME. Chondrosarcomas are rarely multifocal and usually occur in older patients.

Diagnosis

Hereditary multiple exostoses (HME)

Key Points

- Autosomal dominant disorder characterized by multiple osteochondromas (exostoses).
- 62% of affected patients have a positive family history.
- Patients can have pain, short stature, limb deformities, joint immobility, and sarcomatous transformation; however, most are asymptomatic.
- Sarcomatous transformation (3–5%) is higher than in patients with solitary osteochondromas (<1%), but less than the previously described 25%.
- Although there are no standard guidelines, lesions are typically followed by radiographs and/or bone scintigraphy every 2–3 years. Symptomatic lesions can be imaged on a more frequent basis.
- Dysplasia epiphysealis hemimelica (Trevor's disease) can have multiple cartilaginous overgrowths involving the epiphyses, most commonly in the lower extremities, is unilateral, and does not undergo malignant transformation.
- Metachondromatosis can have both osteochondromas and enchondromas, typically in the hands and feet, and the osteochondromas point towards the growth plate instead of away.

Suggested Reading

Pannier S, Legeai-Mallet L. Hereditary multiple exostoses and enchondromatosis. Best Pract Res Clin Rheumatol. 2008;22:45–54.
Bovee JV. Multiple osteochondromas. Orphanet J Rare Dis. 2008;3:3.

Case 63

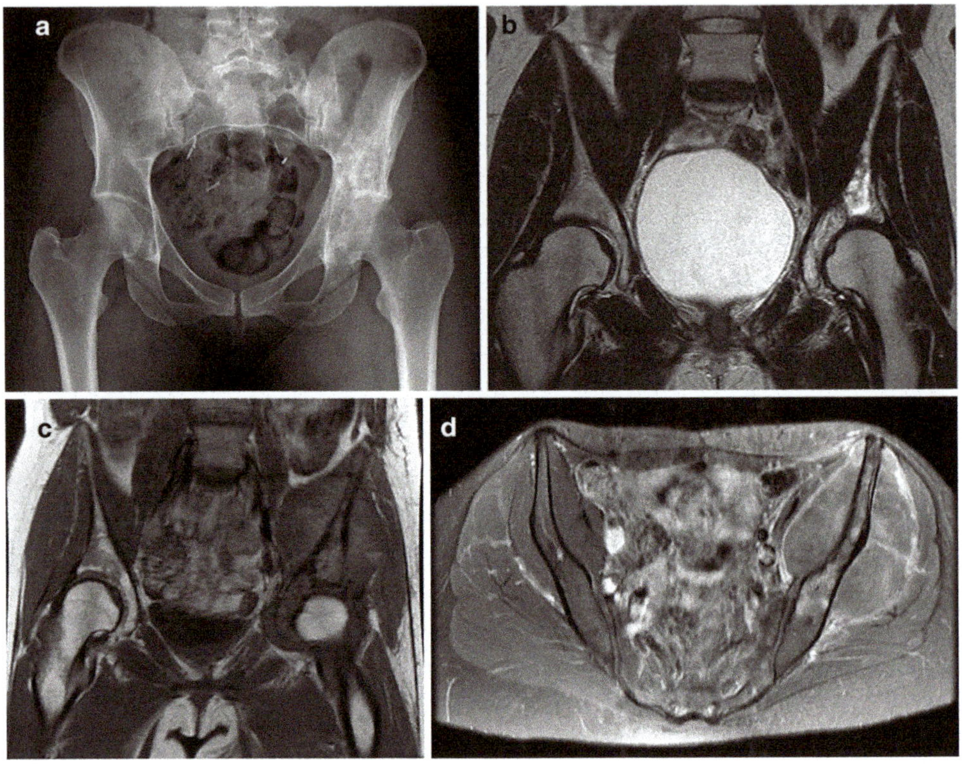

Fig. 10.63 (**a**, **b**) Seven years after treatment and (**c**, **d**) 12 years after treatment

History

A 37-year-old woman with history of Ewing sarcoma at age 25 treated with radiotherapy and chemotherapy. Now with progressive pain in the left hip and pelvis.

Imaging Findings

Seven years after treatment: The AP radiograph (a) of the pelvis shows an area of sclerosis in the left hemipelvis without periostitis or focal soft tissue mass. The coronal T2-weighted MR image (b) shows increased T2 signal in the left ilium. The adjacent muscles are normal in signal intensity and bulk.

Twelve years after treatment: The coronal T1-weighted (c) and axial postcontrast fat-saturated T1-weighted (d) MR images show interval development of a large soft tissue mass emanating from the left iliac bone with a relatively intact cortex. There is replacement of the marrow in the ilium and acetabulum by low T1 signal and heterogeneous enhancement in the bone and surrounding soft tissue mass on the postcontrast MR image.

Differential Diagnosis (Best 3)

Recurrent Ewing sarcoma
Radiation-induced sarcoma
Lymphoma

Diagnosis

Radiation-induced sarcoma

Discussion

The key to this case is the history of prior radiation therapy. The films 7 years following treatment show changes attributable to radiation changes (sclerosis and increased T2 signal); however, the films 12 years after treatment are markedly abnormal with development of a large soft tissue mass. Although recurrence of the Ewing sarcoma is possible, and would have similar imaging characteristics, given the latent period of 12 years, radiation-induced sarcoma should be highly suspected. The large soft tissue component and relatively intact cortex can be seen in small round cell tumors such as lymphoma; however, the prior radiotherapy makes sarcoma more likely. Regardless, the lesion is markedly aggressive and biopsy is needed.

Key Points

- Radiation-induced sarcoma is a rare complication of radiation treatment and can occur as a bone or soft tissue mass.
- Radiation-induced sarcomas most commonly occur in patients following treatment for breast cancer and lymphoma.
- The pelvis is the most commonly affected site.
- Osteosarcoma and malignant fibrous histiocytoma are the most common radiation-induced sarcoma subtypes and usually high grade.
- In a large study, the mean latent interval between radiotherapy and diagnosis of a sarcoma was 17 years (range 4–50 years), after an average dose of 50 Gy. There was no correlation between radiation dose and the time to development of a sarcoma.
- Radiation-induced sarcomas can develop in as short a time as 3–4 years following radiotherapy.
- Sarcoma may also develop following chemotherapy treatment.

Suggested Reading

Patel SR. Radiation-induced sarcoma. Curr Treat Op Oncol. 2000;1:258–61.

Case 64

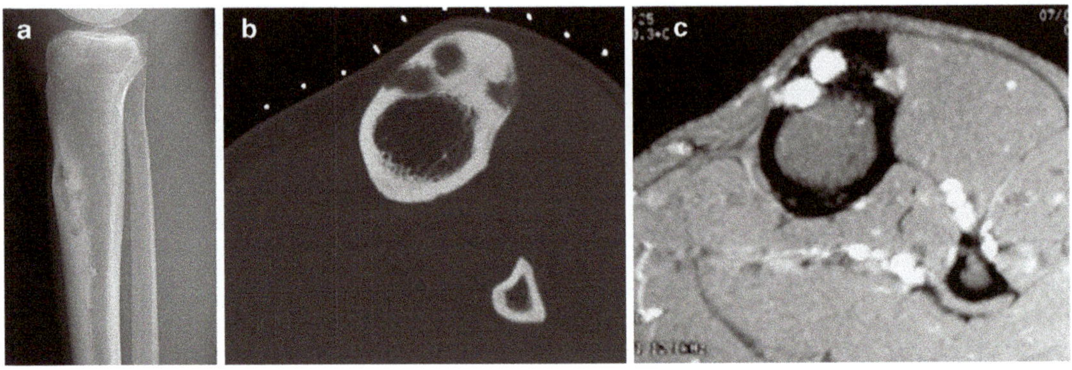

Fig. 10.64

History

A 31-year-old man with intermittent leg pain and swelling since age 8.

Imaging Findings

Radiograph (a) shows multiple rounded, somewhat discrete lucencies, centered in and along an area of dense sclerosis in the anterior cortex of the proximal tibia. CT (b) shows a markedly thickened anterior cortex, but no periostitis or medullary extension. Several lucent foci are present, with thinning of the overlying cortex, but no frank soft tissue extension. On the postcontrast fat-saturated T1-weighted MR image (c), the rounded foci within the area of cortical thickening enhance. The marrow cavity of the tibia is normal.

Differential Diagnosis (Best 3)

Osteomyelitis
Adamantinoma
Osteofibrous dysplasia (OFD)

Discussion

The appearance is consistent with osteofibrous dysplasia, which most often occurs as a multiloculated lesion centered in the anterior cortex of the tibia, often with cortical thickening, though OFD usually occurs in children and typically demonstrates tibial bowing. Chronic osteomyelitis with intracortical abscesses could have a similar appearance, but might be expected to have more reactive edema and enhancement in the surrounding medullary bone and soft tissues. With osteomyelitis, one would also look for sequestra, cloacae, sinus tracts, and periosteal new bone formation. Adamantinoma occurs in older patients (median 25–35 years old) than OFD, tends to be longer and more aggressive, is more likely to have medullary cavity extension, can have soft tissue extension, and is less likely to have tibial bowing. In this case, it is difficult to confidently exclude adamantinoma and biopsy should therefore be considered. Fibrous dysplasia is typically centered in the medullary canal, has cortical thinning rather than thickening, and does not have small bubbly components.

Diagnosis

Osteofibrous dysplasia

Key Points

- Controversial entity—thought to be benign and self-limited, but some believe it is a benign precursor of adamantinoma, which is a malignant lesion. There is also an OFD-subtype of adamantinoma that is distinct, but very difficult to distinguish histologically, from OFD itself.
- Rare, usually boys <15 years old, with swelling or painless bowing deformity.
- 80% in proximal or middle tibia, centered in anterior cortex; 20–25% occur in other bones.
- Anterior bowing in >80% and can be complicated by fracture and pseudarthrosis. Bowing is more common in OFD than adamantinoma.

Suggested Reading

Most MJ, Sim FH, Inwards CY. Osteofibrous dysplasia and adamantinoma. J Am Acad Orthop Surg. 2010;18(6):358–66.

Case 65

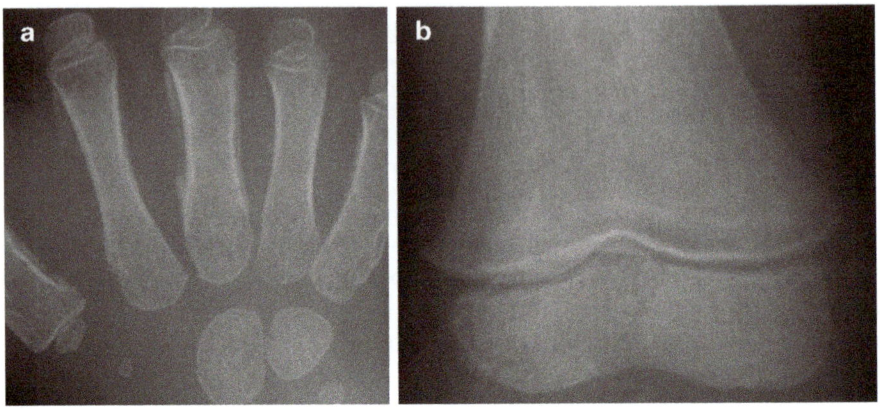

Fig. 10.65

History

A 6-year-old child with fever and hand and knee pain.

Imaging Findings

The hand radiograph (a) shows aggressive periostitis along multiple metacarpal shafts (particularly the third). Knee radiograph (b) shows submetaphyseal linear lucency in the distal femoral metaphysis (radiolucent metaphyseal band), with faint metaphyseal sclerosis parallel and proximal to the lucent band, and subtle subchondral lucency in the medial and lateral distal femoral epiphysis.

Differential Diagnosis (Best 3)

Leukemia
Metastatic neuroblastoma
Rickets

Discussion

Submetaphyseal lucent bands are a nonspecific finding seen in several chronic childhood illnesses. In children older than 2 years, the bands are more suggestive of leukemia. The combination of a radiolucent metaphyseal band in the knee and periosteal new bone in the hand suggests a systemic marrow infiltrating disease such as leukemia, metastatic neuroblastoma, or (unusual) multifocal osteomyelitis. CBC with differential and bone marrow biopsy can help to confirm leukemia. Rickets should include additional findings, such as widened physes and pseudofractures due to unmineralized osteoid, cupping and fraying of metaphyses, cortical spurs, and bowing deformity due to soft bones.

Diagnosis

Acute lymphocytic leukemia with leukemic lines and periostitis

Key Points

- Most common pediatric malignancy—ALL (80%, peak 2–5 years) and AML (15–20%).
- Findings and complications include marrow infiltration, diffuse osteopenia, permeative osteolysis, periostitis, fractures, osteonecrosis, spontaneous hemorrhage, granulocytic sarcoma (chloroma), ostemyelitis, leukemic or infectious arthritis.
- "Leukemic lines"—metaphyseal lucent bands with variable growth arrest sclerosis, paralleling physis, due to decreased enchondral ossification or leukemic infiltration.
- Periostitis secondary to subperiosteal leukemic cells, complicating fracture, or osteomyelitis.

Suggested Reading

Parker, BR. Leukemia and lymphoma in childhood. Radiol Clin N Am. 1997;35:1495–516.
Moulopoulos LA, Dimopoulos MA. Magnetic resonance imaging of the bone marrow in hematologic malignancies. Blood. 1997;90:2127–47.

Case 66

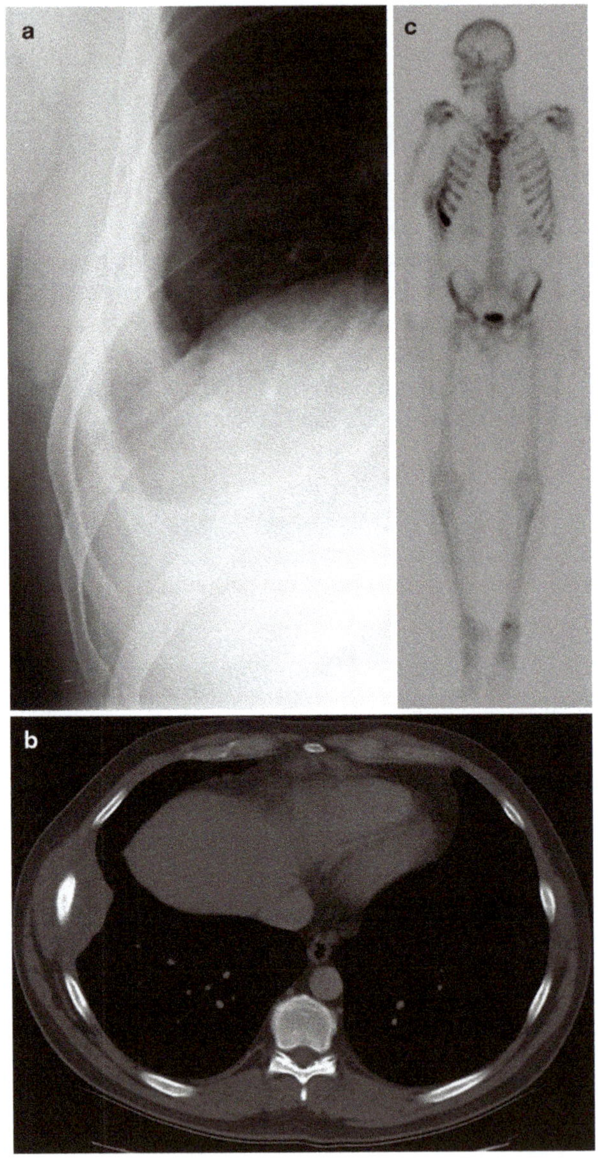

Fig. 10.66

History

A 32-year-old man with right chest pain for several months.

Imaging Findings

Magnified AP chest radiograph (a) shows cortical ill-definition and periosteal new bone formation along a lower right lateral rib. On the CT image (b), the right rib is sclerotic and has a surrounding soft tissue mass. Bone scan (c) shows increased activity along a long segment of the rib, as well as faint uptake in the soft tissue mass component.

Differential Diagnosis (Best 3)

Fibrous dysplasia
Lymphoma
Primitive neuroectodermal tumor (PNET)

Discussion

Fibrous dysplasia is the most common benign rib lesion and typically involves a long segment of the rib, but should not have periosteal new bone (unless fractured) and should not be associated with a soft tissue mass. Lymphoma tends to occur in older patients but is hard to distinguish based on imaging. Primitive neuroectodermal tumor can involve the ribs and is associated with periosteal new bone formation and a soft tissue mass. Metastasis would be less likely, because the patient is young.

Diagnosis

Primitive neuroectodermal tumor (PNET)

Key Points

- Ewing sarcoma family of tumors includes Ewing sarcoma (ES), atypical ES, PNET, and Askin tumor (also known as malignant small cell tumor of the thoracopulmonary region). All share the same chromosomal translocation.
- On imaging, PNET and Ewing are indistinguishable.
- Highly malignant bone tumor, usually age 10–25, M>F.
- Involves almost any bone, approximately half in long bones and half in flat bones.
- Long lesion with disproportionately large soft tissue mass; usually aggressive osteolysis, but can be mixed lucent-and-sclerotic or sclerotic.
- Workup: MRI best for local bone and soft tissue extent; bone scan and chest CT for metastases; potential role for FDG PET; 25% present have metastases at presentation.

Suggested Reading

Grier HE. The Ewing family of tumors: Ewing sarcoma and primitive neuroectodermal tumors. Pediatr Clin N Am. 1997;44:992–1004.
Kaste SC. Imaging pediatric bone sarcomas. Radiol Clin N Am. 2011;49(4):749–65.
Heare T, Hensley MA, Dell'Orfano S. Bone tumors: osteosarcoma and Ewing sarcoma. Curr Opin Pediatr. 2009;21(3):365–72.

Case 67

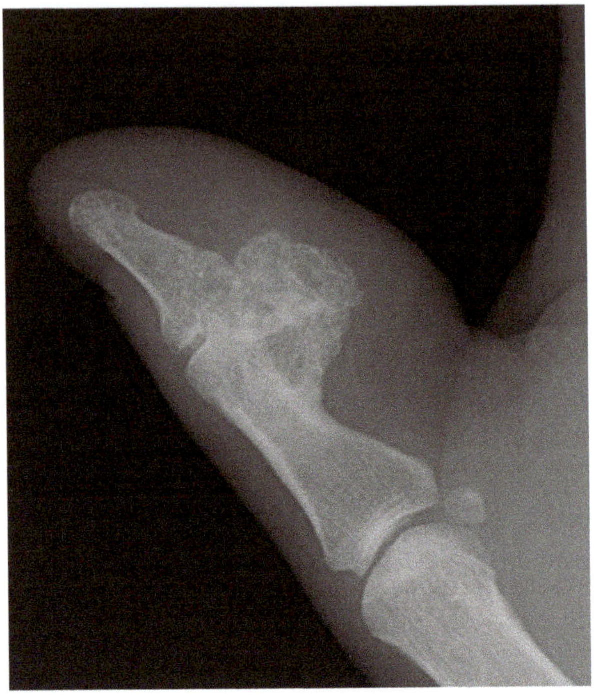

Fig. 10.67

History

A 45-year-old woman with tender, nonmobile, hard "lump" on the thumb.

Imaging Findings

There is a lesion arising from the cortical surface of the proximal phalanx of the thumb. The lesion has well-defined margins, osseous matrix, and distorts the adjacent soft tissues.

Differential Diagnosis (Best 3)

Osteochondroma
Parosteal osteosarcoma
Bizarre parosteal osteochondromatous proliferation (BPOP)

Discussion

Although osteochondromas are very common benign lesions, the medullary cavity of the host bone is not continuous with the lesion, making osteochondroma unlikely. Parosteal osteosarcomas and BPOP can have similar appearances; however, BPOP often occurs in the hands and surface osteosarcomas are not common in this location.

Diagnosis

Bizarre parosteal osteochondromatous proliferation (BPOP) or Nora's lesion

Key Points

- First described by Nora, Dahlin, and Beabout in 1983.
- Benign process characterized by fibroosseous proliferation with a cartilaginous cap, arising from the cortical surface.
- Most common in the hands and feet.
- Unknown cause; however, may be associated with trauma.
- Similar to osteochondromas, but does not have continuation of the cortex and medullary cavity with the host bone.
- Surgical resection is the main treatment; however, recurrence is high.

Suggested Reading

Oviedo A, Simmons T, Benya E, Gonzalez-Crussi F. Bizarre parosteal osteochondromatous proliferation: case report and review of the literature. Pediatr Dev Pathol. 2001;4:496–500.
Dhondt E, Oudenhoven L, Khan S. Nora's lesion, a distinct radiological entity? Skeletal Radiol. 2006;35:497–502.

Case 68

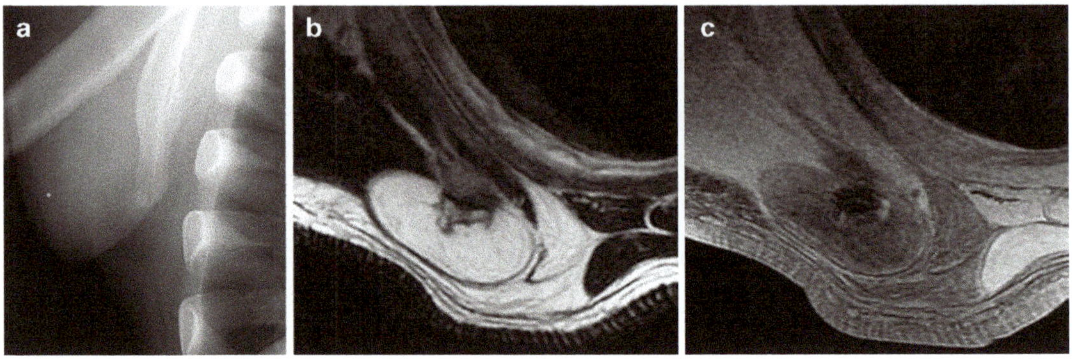

Fig. 10.68

History

A 45-year-old woman with progressively enlarging mass over back.

Imaging Findings

Radiograph (a) shows a small bony excrescence arising from the inferior edge of the scapula, with suggestion of surrounding soft tissue lucency projecting over the axilla. MRI shows the scapular exostosis surrounded by a well-circumscribed, homogeneously high T1 signal (b) ovoid mass, that loses signal on the fat-saturated T1-weighted image (c), and that lacks thickened septae or nodular soft tissue components.

Differential Diagnosis (Best 3)

Parosteal lipoma
Osteochondroma
Enthesis at muscle insertion site

Discussion

The MRI appearance is diagnostic for parosteal lipoma. The remainder of the differential given above should be eliminated, once one recognizes that the lesion consists of both a bony excrescence and an overlying lipoma. Presence of a bony excrescence supports a diagnosis of parosteal lipoma, rather than soft tissue lipoma abutting bone. Unlike osteochondroma, the medullary cavity of the associated bone excrescence is *not* continuous with the host bone.

Diagnosis

Parosteal lipoma

Key Points

- Benign neoplasm, extremely rare (0.3% of all lipomas); formerly called periosteal lipoma.
- Usually arises along long bone diaphyses, especially femur, humerus, tibia, and proximal radius.
- Often asymptomatic; can present due to mass effect or nerve compression.
- May be visible on radiographs as a fatty mass centered on a small bony excrescence.
- Bony findings vary: cartilage, osteoid metaplasia, cortical thickening, cortical excrescence or exostosis, or periosteal reaction.
- Bone erosion and bowing can occur.
- The associated soft tissue lipoma can have thin fibrovascular septae.
- MRI used for pre-surgical planning, shows relationship to muscles and neurovascular bundle.
- Treated with complete surgical resection. If evidence of nerve entrapment, resection should not be delayed, due to potential for irreversible damage. Recurrence is unusual.

Suggested Reading

Murphey MD, Carroll JF, Flemming DJ, et al. From the archives of the AFIP: benign musculoskeletal lipomatous lesions. Radiographics. 2004;24:1433–66.
Bui-Mansfield LT, Myers CP, Chew FS. Parosteal lipoma of the fibula. AJR Am J Roentgenol. 2000;174(6):1698.

Case 69

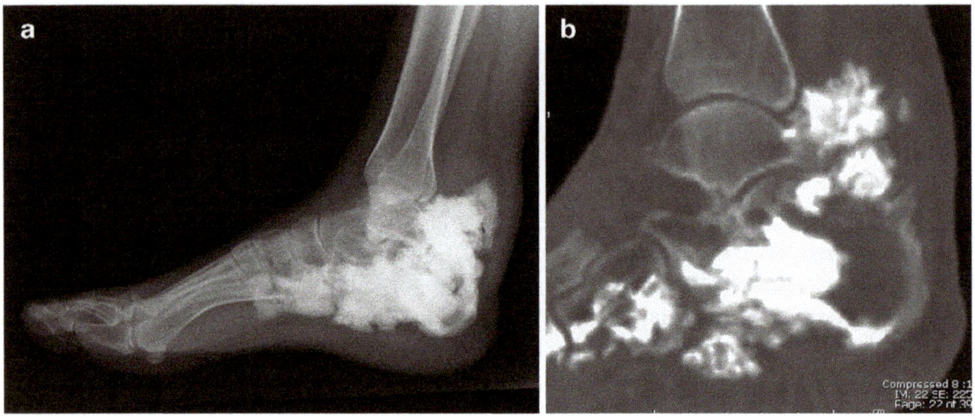

Fig. 10.69

History

A 47-year-old woman with long history of right ankle pain and swelling.

Imaging Findings

Lateral (a) radiograph shows dense sclerotic lesion(s) obscuring the calcaneus and tarsal bones. The CT image (b) shows that there are multiple osseous excrescences arising from several contiguous tarsal bones.

Differential Diagnosis (Best 3)

Parosteal osteosarcoma
Myositis ossificans
Melorheostosis

Discussion

From the radiograph, it is difficult to determine whether the dense sclerotic lesion(s) are in the soft tissues or arising from the bone. This distinction is critical, as the differential diagnosis will vary. If in the soft tissue, possible diagnoses would include myositis ossificans or tumoral calcinosis. If arising from bone, parosteal osteosarcoma and melorheostosis should be considered. The CT shows that there are multiple lesions arising from multiple contiguous bones (along a sclerotome). Since multiple surface osteosarcomas in contiguous bones would be extremely unlikely, melorheostosis is most likely.

Diagnosis

Melorheostosis

Key Points

- Rare sclerosing bone dysplasia, first described in 1922 by Léri and Joanny.
- 40–50% present with symptoms by age 20.
- Typically occurs in a single limb, often in a sclerotomal distribution.
- Appears as wavy areas of cortical thickening, mimicking hot candle wax dripping along the sides of a lit candle; however, at times it can be intramedullary (as in this case).
- Increased uptake (on surface of bone) is typically seen on bone scintigraphy, helping to differentiate from osteopathia striata or osteopoikilosis.
- Histopathologic diagnosis is difficult, as findings are nonspecific.
- Cause is unknown, but postulated to be related to vascular disturbances. However, as the disease often affects a single sclerotome, abnormality of the segmental sensory nerve may be the cause.
- Associated with numerous diseases, including osteopoikilosis, vascular and lymphatic malformations.
- Patients can present with joint pain and swelling. As the disease progresses, there are muscle contractures, tendon and ligament shortening leading to growth disturbances, and soft tissue and skin changes (hyperpigmentation, fibrosis, and shiny skin) leading to severe debilitation.
- Surgical treatment of the soft tissue contractures and bony excrescences can provide some relief.

Suggested Reading

Freyschmidt J. Melorheostosis: a review of 23 cases. Eur Radiol. 2001;11:474–9.
Gagliardi GG, Mahan KT. Melorheostosis: a literature review and case report with surgical considerations. J Foot Ankle Surg. 2010;49(1):80–5.

Case 70

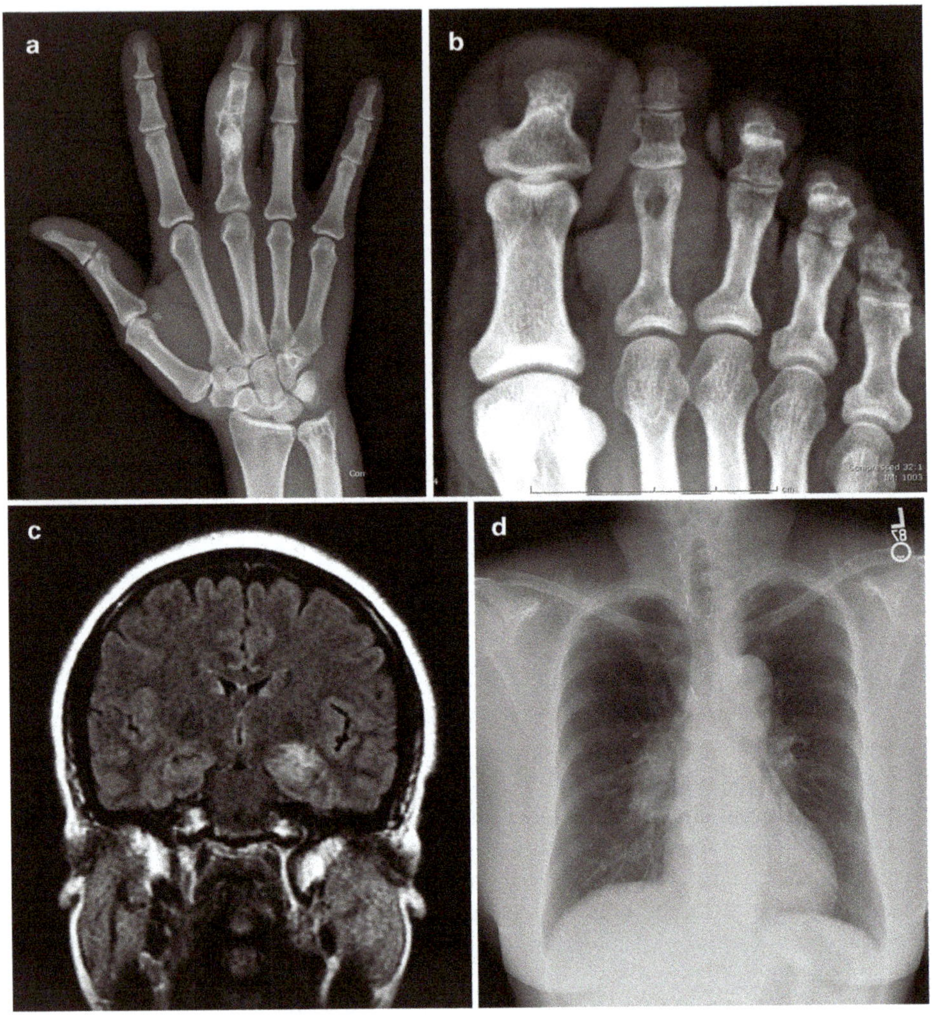

Fig. 10.70

History

A 39-year-old black woman with hand/foot pain and respiratory disease.

Imaging Findings

Radiograph of the hand (a) shows mixed lytic and sclerotic changes to the proximal and middle phalanges of the long finger in a lace-like pattern and with associated soft tissue swelling. Similar findings are seen of the distal ulna. The radiograph of the foot (b) shows a small nonaggressive lucent lesion with a narrow zone of transition and no cortical breakthrough in the second proximal phalanx with surrounding soft tissue swelling. MR FLAIR image of the brain (c) shows edema in the left temporal lobe. Frontal CXR (d) shows hilar prominence consistent with lymphadenopathy.

Differential Diagnosis (Best 3)

Infection (multifocal)
Gout
Sarcoidosis

Discussion

Bony lesions related to infection typically do not have sclerotic margins as seen here in the hand. Sclerotic margins are indicative of a slowly progressive process to which the bone has had time to react. Although the soft tissue swelling and increased density could be due to gouty tophi, there are no periarticular erosions and gout typically has preserved joint space early in the disease process. Given the additional findings in the brain and lungs, sarcoid is the best diagnosis.

Diagnosis

Sarcoidosis

Key Points

- Granulomatous disorder of unknown cause that involves many organ (lungs, lymph nodes, skin, and musculoskeletal) systems and is characterized by noncaseating granulomas.
- Although sarcoidosis is more common in blacks, bony involvement is more common in whites.
- Lesions are classically lytic with a fine reticular "lace-like" pattern, and are often multiple.
- Less commonly, sarcoidosis can present with "punched out" cystic lesions, osteoporosis, or, very rarely, with osteosclerosis.
- Bones of the feet and hands are most commonly involved.
- Lesions are can be painful, restrict motion, and lead to pathologic fracture.
- 1–13% of patients with sarcoidosis have osseous abnormalities and they typically occur late in the disease process.
- Osseous findings rarely occur without corresponding pulmonary findings and skin changes (lupus pernio).
- Affected sites typically have uptake on bone scintigraphy.

Suggested Reading

Anakwenze OA, Kancherla V, Hatch M, Brooks JS, Ogilvie CM. Primary musculoskeletal sarcoidosis. Orthopedics. 2010;33(5):308.
Moore SL, Teirstein A, Golimbu C. MRI of sarcoidosis patients with musculoskeletal symptoms. AJR. 2005;185:154–9.

Case 71

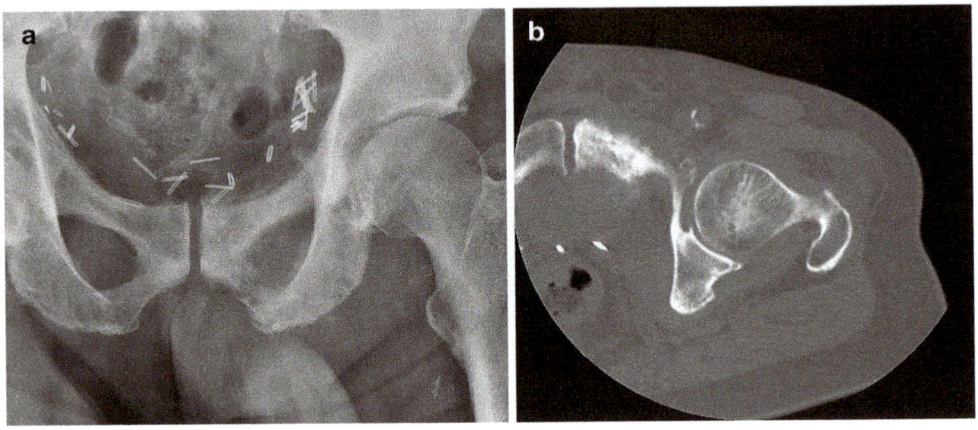

Fig. 10.71

History

A 66-year-old man with left hip pain.

Imaging Findings

AP radiograph (a) of the pelvis shows increased density of the left superior and inferior pubic rami when compared to the right side. There is abnormal aggressive periosteal reaction elevating the periosteum and a fracture of the inferior pubic ramus. Surgical clips in the pelvis are consistent with prostatectomy. Axial CT image (b) of the left hip shows abnormal sclerosis of the left superior pubic ramus with sunburst periosteal reaction.

Differential Diagnosis (Best 3)

Infection
Metastasis (prostate cancer)
Osteosarcoma

Discussion

The sunburst periosteal reaction is indicative of an aggressive process and can be seen with infection, osteosarcoma, and Ewing sarcoma. However, certain metastases can also have this pattern of new bone formation, most commonly prostate cancer. Give the man's age and surgical clips in the pelvis, metastasis from prostate cancer would be the most likely diagnosis.

Diagnosis

Metastasis (prostate cancer)

Key Points

- Prostate metastases are rarely seen with a PSA <10 ng/mL.
- Other entities that can produce multifocal or diffusely dense bones include: mastocytosis, myelofibrosis, treated metastatic disease, fluorosis, and renal osteodystrophy.
- Periosteal reaction is rare with metastatic disease, but can occur in a subset of primary malignancies: prostate, bronchus, colon, carcinoid, neuroblastoma, and retinoblastoma.
- The sunburst pattern of periosteal new bone is believed to be related to invasion of the periosteum, with formation of bone along small vessels perpendicular to the cortex.
- Although metastases rarely occur distal to the elbow or knee, 20% of metastases with sunburst periosteal reaction occur in these distal locations.
- Metastases with sunburst periosteal new bone are extremely rare in the spine (one case report).

Suggested Reading

Bloom RA, Libson E, Husband JE, Stoker DJ. The periosteal sunburst reaction in bone metastases. Skeletal Radiol. 1987;16:629–34.
Nguyen BD. Bilateral iliac metastases with sunburst pattern from prostate cancer. Clin Nucl Med. 2003;28:931–2.

Case 72

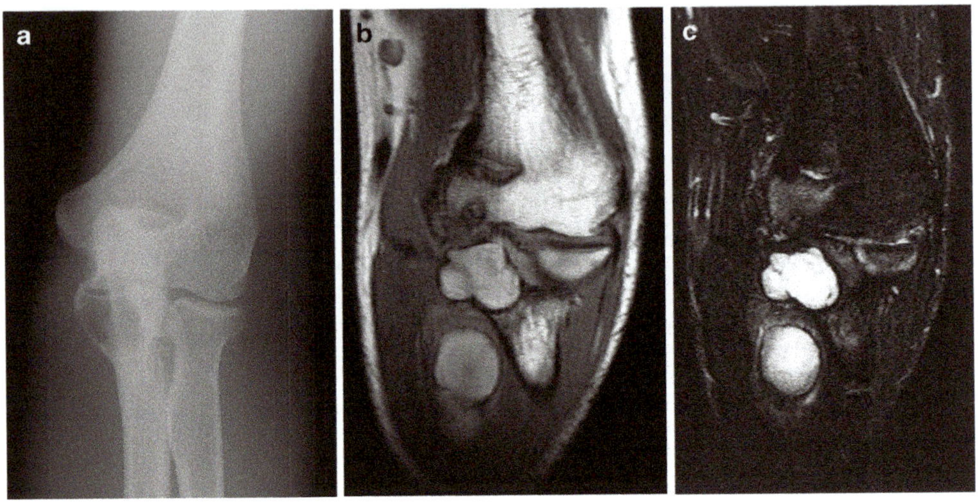

Fig. 10.72

History

A 28-year-old man with "easy bruising" and elbow pain.

Imaging Findings

The AP radiograph (a) of the elbow shows a lucent lesion in the ulna, near the coronoid process. There is no internal mineralization or cortical breakthrough. There is also soft tissue swelling of the proximal forearm. On the MRI, the lesion in the ulna is hyperintense on the T1-weighted MR image (b) and remains bright on the STIR image (c). There is a soft tissue component with identical MR characteristics in the medial soft tissues which is contiguous with the osseous lesion (not shown).

Differential Diagnosis (Best 3)

Subchondral cyst (based on radiograph)
Intraosseous lipoma
Hemophiliac pseudotumor

Discussion

The appearance of the lucent lesion in the ulna is fairly nonspecific and could include many lesions in this age group: subchondral cyst, giant cell tumor, aneursymal bone cyst, fibrous dysplasia, and solitary bone cyst. However, the MR characteristics are fairly unique. Most of the lesions listed above would be hypointense on T1-weighted imaging. This lesion is hyperintense on T1 indicating that it contains fat, hemorrhage, proteinaceous fluid, or melanin (rarely). The lesion is bright on the STIR image; thus, it does not contain fat. Lesions containing proteinaceous material or hemorrhage should be high on the differential and, with the clinical history of "easy bruising," a hemophiliac pseudotumor should be suspected.

Diagnosis

Hemophiliac pseudotumor

Key Points

- Common subtypes: hemophilia A (factor VIII) and hemophilia B (factor IX).
- Autosomal recessive—expressed in men and carried by women.
- Hemarthrosis is characteristic (70–95%) and occurs in: knee>elbow>ankle>hip>shoulder.
- Hemarthrosis leads to hypertrophied synovium with hyperemia.
- Hyperemia in skeletally immature patients leads to epiphyseal overgrowth, physeal fusion, and skeletal shortening.
- Radiographic findings: widened intercondylar notch, osteopenia, erosive changes, degenerative joint disease, and pseudotumors.
- Pseudotumors of hemophilia can occur as (1) slow growing expanding hemorrhagic masses in the soft tissues which erode into the adjacent bone and are more common in proximal bones like the femur and pelvis, (2) rapidly developing lesions in the bone due to intraosseous hemorrhage and are more common in distal small cancellous bones.
- Treatment can involve embolization, surgical curettage/bone grafting, and irradiation.

Suggested Reading

Yu W, Lin Q, Guermazi A, Yu X, et al. Comparison of radiography, CT and MR imaging in detection of arthropathies in patients with haemophilia. Hemophilia. 2009;15:1090–6.
Rodriguez-Merchan EC. The haemophilic pseudotumor. Haemophilia. 2002;8:12–6.

Case 73

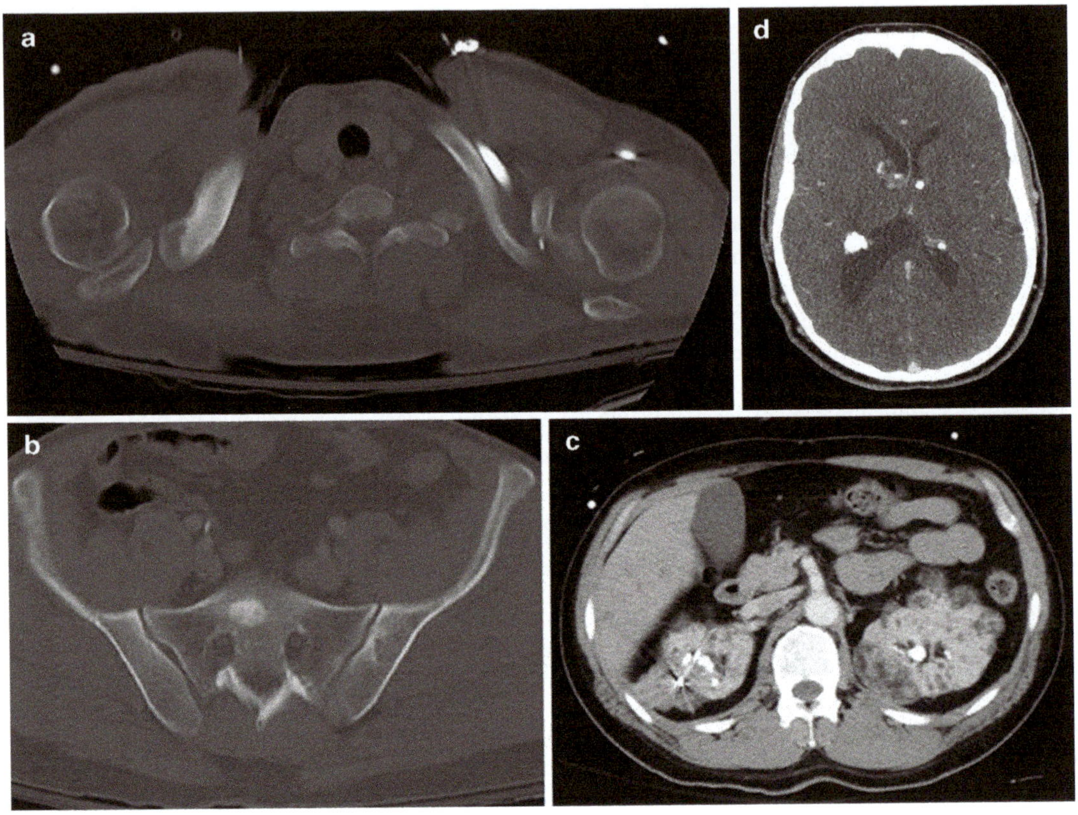

Fig. 10.73

History

A 56-year-old man with chronic illness.

Imaging Findings

Axial CT images (a and b) show sclerotic lesions in the right clavicle and sacrum. The axial abdominal CT image (c) shows numerous heterogeneous renal masses, many of which contain fat. An embolization clip is seen in the right kidney. The axial CT image (d) of the head shows dense subependymal calcifications adjacent to both ventricles, with mild right sided hydrocephalus.

Differential Diagnosis (Best 3)

Bone islands
Sclerotic metastases
Tuberous sclerosis

Discussion

The sclerotic lesions in the clavicle and sacrum are nonspecific and the most common diagnosis would include bone islands or sclerotic metastases. However, given the other systemic findings (renal angiomyolipomas and subependymal nodules), tuberous sclerosis would be the best diagnosis.

Diagnosis

Tuberous Sclerosis (Bourneville's disease)

Key Points

- Autosomal dominant disease with no racial or gender bias.
- Defects in the tumor suppression genes *TSC2* and *TWC1* lead to proliferations of hamartomas.
- Classic triad: (1) epileptic seizures, (2) mental retardation, and (3) skin lesions.
- Numerous systemic findings with the most common being: adenoma sebaceum, shagreen patches, facial angiofibromas, cortical tubers, subependymal nodule (can calcify), subependymal giant cell astrocytomas, cardiac rhabdomyomas, renal angiomyolipomas, dental enamel pits, and periungual fibromas.
- 50% of patients with tuberous sclerosis have some sort of renal lesion (angiomyolipomas, cysts, and aneurysms) and 50% of patients with renal angiomyolipomas have tuberous sclerosis.
- Bone findings include (1) bone cysts and (2) dense sclerotic deposits. Often have sclerotic deposits in the spine and pelvis. These lesions do not expand the bone and rarely present before puberty. Identifying other manifestations of tuberous sclerosis will help distinguish this entity from sclerotic metastases.
- Tuberous sclerosis, neurofibromatosis, and polyostotic fibrous dysplasia are all neuroectodermal and mesodermal dysplasias with all three germ layers potentially involved.

Suggested Reading

Baskin HJ. The pathogenesis and imaging of the tuberous sclerosis complex. Pediatr Radiol. 2008;38:936–52.

Case 74

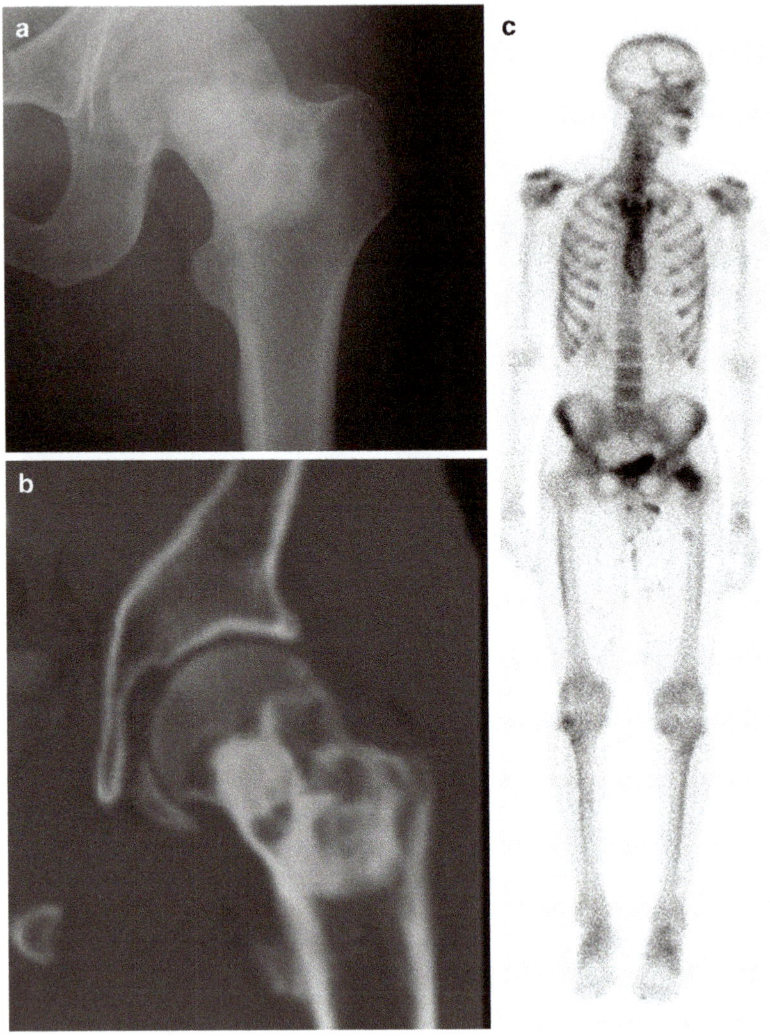

Fig. 10.74

History

A 42-year-old man with left hip pain.

Imaging Findings

AP radiograph (a) shows a moderately well-circumscribed, geographic, dense mixed lucent and sclerotic lesion in the left femoral neck. CT image (b) shows irregular and globular sclerosis, including a focally thick sclerotic rim, and slight bone expansion. Bone scan (c) shows diffusely increased activity in the lesion, without additional lesions.

Differential Diagnosis (Best 3)

Fibrous dysplasia
Liposclerosing myxofibrous tumor (LSMFT)
Treated metastasis or brown tumor (hyperparathyroidism)

Discussion

LSFMT is a mixed lucent and sclerotic lesion that often occurs in the proximal femur and often contains globular and/or irregular mineralization, with a well-defined, often extensively sclerotic rim. Radiographic distinction from fibrous dysplasia, another mixed lucent and sclerotic lesion that is common in the proximal femur, may be difficult. LSMFT tends to have higher signal intensity than fibrous dysplasia (except cystic FD) on fluid-sensitive MRI sequences, due to its myxoid component, and it may contain minute speckles of fat on MRI. When LSFMT is less dense, intraosseous lipoma with involutional change may have a similar appearance. History and presence of additional imaging imaging findings can help to exclude treated metastasis or a brown tumor.

Diagnosis

Liposclerosing myxofibrous tumor (LSMFT)

Key Points

- Benign fibroosseous lesion with heterogeneous and variable composition.
- Majority of lesions occur in the intertrochanteric proximal femur (85% in proximal femur and 91% of those are intertrochanteric).
- Can present as an incidental finding or with pain or pathologic fracture.
- Typically occur in middle-aged adult.
- Globular and/or irregular matrix mineralization (72%) that can extend to margin; sclerotic rim of variable thickness (100%); and bone expansion (28%).
- Does not contain much, if any fat, on imaging—small speckles may be visible on MRI.
- Potential for sarcomatous degeneration (10–16% in two small series).

Suggested Reading

Kransdorf MJ, Murphey MD, Sweet DE. Liposclerosing Myxofibrous Tumor: A Radiologic–Pathologic-Distinct Fibro-osseous Lesion of Bone with a Marked Predilection for the Intertrochanteric Region of the Femur. Radiology. 1999;212:693–8.
Corsi A, De Maio F, Ippolito E, et al. Monostotic fibrous dysplasia of the proximal femur and liposclerosing myxofibrous tumor: which one is which? J Bone Miner Res. 2006;21(12):1955–8.

Case 75

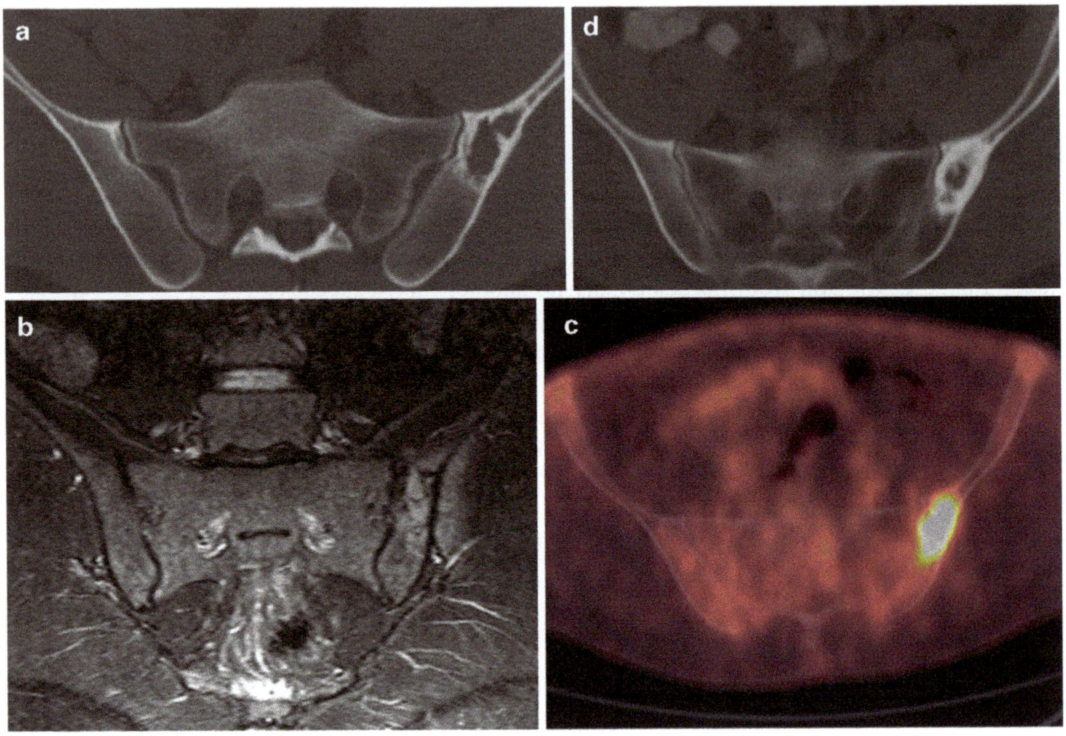

Fig. 10.75 (**d**) Eighteen months after treatment

History

A 42-year-old man with lower extremity numbness and paresthesias.

Imaging Findings

On the pelvic CT image (a), there is a lobulated, geographic, lucent lesion in the left iliac bone, adjacent to the SI joint, with a thin sclerotic rim and a small amount of nonaggressive periosteal new bone formation. On the STIRMR image (b), the lesion is homogeneous in signal and slightly hyperintense to muscle, with faint surrounding muscle and bone edema. PET/CT scan (c) shows increased activity in the bone lesion, which resolved after treatment. Follow-up CT after treatment (d) shows increased sclerosis of the lesion.

Differential Diagnosis

POEMS syndrome with sclerotic mycloma
Giant cell tumor
Fibrous dysplasia

Discussion

While multiple myeloma typically does not have a sclerotic rim, the rare sclerotic form of myeloma can present this way. Fibrous dysplasia can also occur in this location, but should not have periosteal new bone or surrounding edema, unless fractured. Giant cell tumor can elicit surrounding edema, but most giant cell tumors lack a sclerotic rim and GCT is unusual in the iliac bone (3% of GCTs). In this case, serum protein electrophoresis (SPEP) revealed IgG gammopathy and electromyography (EMG) showed polyneuropathy. The initial PET showed increased activity in the lesion, which disappeared after radiation treatment.

Diagnosis

POEMS syndrome with sclerotic myeloma

Key Points

- Sclerotic myeloma is very rare and can occur independently or as part of POEMS syndrome (polneuropathy, organomegaly, endocrinopathy, monoclonocal gammopathy, and skin changes).
- Etiology of POEMS is unknown, but may relate to chronic overproduction of proinflammatory factors and other cytokines, such as vascular endothelial growth factor.
- All patients with POEMS have peripheral neuropathy and a monoclonal plasma cell disorder.
- 85% have elevated serum monoclonal protein, usually lambda light chain.
- 97% of POEMs case will have a "sclerotic" lesion; solitary in 45%, multiple lesions in 55%.
- The sclerotic lesion does not have to be large or uniformly sclerotic: it can be a very small sclerotic focus, can have a mixed-lytic sclerotic pattern, or can have just a thin sclerotic rim.
- Often occurs in the pelvis, spine, ribs, and proximal extremities.
- Random bone marrow aspiration/biopsy often nondiagnostic.
- POEMS has a younger onset (median age 51 years) and longer survival than standard myeloma; it is treated with radiation for local disease. If multiple lesions, treated with chemotherapy.
- Serum or plasma VEGF levels usually elevated; can be followed for response to therapy.
- Features characteristic of classic multiple myeloma are not found in POEMS: anemia, hypercalcemia, renal failure, bone pain, pathologic fractures, and abundant bone marrow plasma cells.

Suggested Reading

Dispenzieri A. POEMS syndrome: 2011 update on diagnosis, risk-stratification, and management. Am J Hematol. 2011;86(7):591–601.
Hall F, Gore S. Osteosclerotic myeloma variants. Skeletal Radiol. 1988;17:101–5.
Kyle RA, Rajkumar SV. Criteria for diagnosis, staging, risk stratification and response assessment of multiple myeloma. Leukemia. 2009;23(1):3–9.

Index of Cases

Case 1 Non-ossifying fibroma
Case 2 Parosteal osteosarcoma
Case 3 Chondroblastoma
Case 4 Intraosseous lipoma
Case 5 Myositis ossificans
Case 6 Osteoid osteoma
Case 7 Giant cell tumor
Case 8 Enchondroma
Case 9 Multiple myeloma
Case 10 Osteosarcoma (conventional)
Case 11 Chondrosarcoma (malignant degeneration of cartilage cap)
Case 12 Primary Non-Hodgkin lymphoma (B cell) of bone
Case 13 Osteopoikilosis
Case 14 Stress fracture
Case 15 Aneurysmal bone cyst
Case 16 Paget disease
Case 17 Dentigerous cyst
Case 18 Distal biceps tendon repair pseudolesion
Case 19 Polyostotic fibrous dysplasia
Case 20 Enchondroma with endosteal scalloping
Case 21 Myelofibrosis
Case 22 Bone island
Case 23 Giant Cell Tumor
Case 24 Hyperparathyroidism (brown tumor)
Case 25 Calcific tendonitis (resorptive phase)
Case 26 Osteochondroma with reactive bursitis/hematoma
Case 27 Simple bone cyst
Case 28 Hemophiliac pseudotumor
Case 29 Hematopoietic marrow (red marrow)
Case 30 Osteopathia striata
Case 31 Lytic metastasis (lung cancer)
Case 32 Paget disease with sarcomatous transformation
Case 33 Telangiectatic osteosarcoma
Case 34 Chordoma
Case 35 Intraosseous lipoma
Case 36 Intraosseous hemangioma
Case 37 Hereditary multiple exostoses (HME)
Case 38 Osteoma
Case 39 Pscudoaneurysm (popliteal artery)
Case 40 Clear cell chondrosarcoma
Case 41 Osteoid Osteoma (intra-articular)
Case 42 Osteonecrosis (avascular necrosis)
Case 43 Supracondylar process
Case 44 Healed non-ossifying fibroma

Index

J.S. Wu and M.G. Hochman, *Bone Tumors: A Practical Guide to Imaging*,
DOI 10.1007/978-1-4419-0808-7,

www.ingramcontent.com/pod-product-compliance
Ingram Content Group UK Ltd.
Pitfield, Milton Keynes, MK11 3LW, UK
UKHW050228160926
475610UK00003B/79
* 9 7 8 1 4 4 1 9 0 8 0 7 0 *